T0259585

Primary Care of the Medically Underserved

Editors

VINCENT MORELLI
ROGER J. ZOOROB
JOEL J. HEIDELBAUGH

PRIMARY CARE:
CLINICS IN OFFICE PRACTICE

www.primarycare.theclinics.com

Consulting Editor
JOEL J. HEIDELBAUGH

March 2017 • Volume 44 • Number 1

ELSEVIER

1600 John F. Kennedy Boulevard • Suite 1800 • Philadelphia, Pennsylvania, 19103-2899

http://www.theclinics.com

PRIMARY CARE: CLINICS IN OFFICE PRACTICE Volume 44, Number 1
March 2017 ISSN 0095-4543, ISBN-13: 978-0-323-50984-8

Editor: Jessica McCool
Developmental Editor: Colleen Dietzler

© **2017 Elsevier Inc. All rights reserved.**

This periodical and the individual contributions contained in it are protected under copyright by Elsevier, and the following terms and conditions apply to their use:

Photocopying
Single photocopies of single articles may be made for personal use as allowed by national copyright laws. Permission of the Publisher and payment of a fee is required for all other photocopying, including multiple or systematic copying, copying for advertising or promotional purposes, resale, and all forms of document delivery. Special rates are available for educational institutions that wish to make photocopies for non-profit educational classroom use. For information on how to seek permission visit www.elsevier.com/permissions or call: (+44) 1865 843830 (UK)/(+1) 215 239 3804 (USA).

Derivative Works
Subscribers may reproduce tables of contents or prepare lists of articles including abstracts for internal circulation within their institutions. Permission of the Publisher is required for resale or distribution outside the institution. Permission of the Publisher is required for all other derivative works, including compilations and translations (please consult www.elsevier.com/permissions).

Electronic Storage or Usage
Permission of the Publisher is required to store or use electronically any material contained in this periodical, including any article or part of an article (please consult www.elsevier.com/permissions). Except as outlined above, no part of this publication may be reproduced, stored in a retrieval system or transmitted in any form or by any means, electronic, mechanical, photocopying, recording or otherwise, without prior written permission of the Publisher.

Notice
No responsibility is assumed by the Publisher for any injury and/or damage to persons or property as a matter of products liability, negligence or otherwise, or from any use or operation of any methods, products, instructions or ideas contained in the material herein. Because of rapid advances in the medical sciences, in particular, independent verification of diagnoses and drug dosages should be made.

Although all advertising material is expected to conform to ethical (medical) standards, inclusion in this publication does not constitute a guarantee or endorsement of the quality or value of such product or of the claims made of it by its manufacturer.

Primary Care: Clinics in Office Practice (ISSN: 0095–4543) is published quarterly by Elsevier Inc., 360 Park Avenue South, New York, NY 10010-1710. Months of issue are March, June, September, and December. Periodicals postage paid at New York, NY and additional mailing offices. Subscription prices are $232.00 per year (US individuals), $451.00 (US institutions), $100.00 (US students), $283.00 (Canadian individuals), $511.00 (Canadian institutions), $175.00 (Canadian students), $355.00 (international individuals), $511.00 (international institutions), and $175.00 (international students). Foreign air speed delivery is included in all *Clinics* subscription prices. All prices are subject to change without notice. POSTMASTER: Send address changes to *Primary Care: Clinics in Office Practice*, Elsevier Periodicals Customer Service, 11830 Westline Industrial Drive, St. Louis, MO 63146. Customer Service Health Sciences Division, Subscription Customer Service, 3251 Riverport Lane, Maryland Heights, MO 63043. **Customer Service: 1-800-654-2452 (U.S. and Canada); 314-447-8871 (outside U.S. and Canada). Fax: 314-447-8029. E-mail: journalscustomerservice-usa@elsevier.com (for print support); journalsonlinesupport-usa@elsevier.com (for online support).**

Reprints. For copies of 100 or more, of articles in this publication, please contact the Commercial Reprints Department, Elsevier Inc., 360 Park Avenue South, New York, NY 10010-1710. Tel. 212-633-3874; Fax: 212-633-3820; E-mail: reprints@elsevier.com.

Primary Care: Clinics in Office Practice is covered in *MEDLINE/PubMed (Index Medicus)* and *EMBASE/ Excerpta Medica, Current Contents/Clinical Medicine,* and *ISI/BIOMED.*

Contributors

CONSULTING EDITOR

JOEL J. HEIDELBAUGH, MD, FAAFP, FACG
Clinical Associate Professor, Departments of Family Medicine and Urology, Clerkship Director, Department of Family Medicine, University of Michigan Medical School, Ann Arbor, Michigan; Ypsilanti Health Center, Ypsilanti, Michigan

EDITORS

VINCENT MORELLI, MD
Department of Family and Community Medicine, Meharry Medical College, Nashville, Tennessee

ROGER J. ZOOROB, MD, MPH
Professor and Chair, Department of Family and Community Medicine, Baylor College of Medicine, Houston, Texas

JOEL J. HEIDELBAUGH, MD, FAAFP, FACG
Clinical Associate Professor, Departments of Family Medicine and Urology, Clerkship Director, Department of Family Medicine, University of Michigan Medical School, Ann Arbor, Michigan; Ypsilanti Health Center, Ypsilanti, Michigan

AUTHORS

TERESA L. BECK, MD, FAAFP
Assistant Professor, Program Director, Emory Family Medicine Residency Program, Department of Family and Preventive Medicine, Emory School of Medicine, Atlanta, Georgia

JONATHAN A. BECKER, MD
Associate Professor, Department of Family and Geriatric Medicine, University of Louisville, Louisville, Kentucky

DANIEL L. BEDNEY, MD
Resident, Department of Family and Community Medicine, Meharry Medical College, Nashville, Tennessee

JULIANA BERENYI, DO
University of Rochester Family Medicine Resident, Rochester, New York

RAMON CANCINO, MD, MSc
Chief Medical Officer, Mattapan Community Health Center, Assistant Professor of Family Medicine and Community Health Sciences, Boston University School of Medicine, Boston, Massachusetts

ARIE (ERIC) DADUSH, MD
Resident, Department of Family and Community Medicine, Meharry Medical College, Nashville, Tennessee

LAUREN DeCAPORALE-RYAN, PhD
Assistant Professor, Departments of Psychiatry, Medicine, and Surgery, University of Rochester Medical Center, Rochester, New York

KONSTANTINOS E. DELIGIANNIDIS, MD, MPH, FAAFP
Director, House Calls Education Program, Northwell Health Solutions, New Hyde Park, New York

NEERAV DESAI, MD
Assistant Professor, Division of Adolescent Medicine & Young Adult Health, Monroe Carell Jr. Children's Hospital at Vanderbilt, Vanderbilt University Medical Center, Nashville, Tennessee

MATHEW DEVINE, DO
Associate Medical Director, Highland Family Medicine; Assistant Professor, Department of Family Medicine, Associate Medical Director, Accountable Health Partners, Rochester, New York

OMOTAYO FAWIBE, MD
Occupational Medicine Resident, Department of Family and Community Medicine, Meharry Medical College, Nashville, Tennessee

LUZ M. FERNANDEZ, MD
Assistant Professor, Department of Family and Geriatric Medicine, University of Louisville, Louisville, Kentucky

SHERYL B. FLEISCH, MD
Assistant Professor of Psychiatry and Medical Director, Homeless Health Services at Vanderbilt, Vanderbilt Street Psychiatry, Vanderbilt University School of Medicine, Nashville, Tennessee

SANDRA J. GONZALEZ, MSSW, LCSW
Instructor, Department of Family and Community Medicine, Baylor College of Medicine, Houston, Texas

SAMUEL NEIL GRIEF, MD, FCFP
Associate Professor, Department of Family Medicine, University of Illinois at Chicago, Chicago, Illinois

MICHAEL HAYDEN, MD
Department of Internal Medicine, School of Medicine, Meharry Medical College, Nashville, Tennessee

QUEEN HENRY-OKAFOR, PhD, FNP-BC
Family Nurse Practitioner Program, Assistant Professor, Vanderbilt University School of Nursing, Nashville, Tennessee

PAUL HUTCHINSON, PhD
Associate Professor, Global Community Health Sciences, Tulane University School of Public Health and Tropical Medicine, New Orleans, Louisiana

MEDHAT KALLINY, MD, PhD
Assistant Professor, Department of Family and Community Medicine, Meharry Medical College, Nashville, Tennessee

ALICIA ANN KOWALCHUK, DO
Assistant Professor, Department of Family and Community Medicine, Baylor College of Medicine, Houston, Texas

THIEN-KIM LE, MD
Department of Family and Preventive Medicine, PGY2 Resident, Emory School of Medicine, Atlanta, Georgia

ROBERT S. LEVINE, MD
Department of Family and Community Medicine, Professor, Baylor College of Medicine, Houston, Texas

MAGDALENE LIM, PsyD
Psychology Fellow, Departments of Psychiatry and Medicine, University of Rochester Medical Center, Rochester, New York

JUDITH GREEN McKENZIE, MD, MPH
Division of Occupational Medicine, Associate Professor, Department of Emergency Medicine, Hospital of the University of Pennsylvania, Philadelphia, Pennsylvania

MARIA C. MEJIA de GRUBB, MD, MPH
Department of Family and Community Medicine, Assistant Professor, Baylor College of Medicine, Houston, Texas

JOHN PAUL MILLER, MD
Program Director, Bakersfield Memorial Family Medicine Residency Program; Assistant Clinical Professor, Department of Family Medicine, University of California Irvine School of Medicine, Bakersfield, California

VINCENT MORELLI, MD
Department of Family and Community Medicine, Meharry Medical College, Nashville, Tennessee

CHARLES P. MOUTON, MD, MS
Department of Family and Community Medicine, School of Medicine, Meharry Medical College, Nashville, Tennessee

ROBERTSON NASH, PhD, ACNP, BC
Assistant in Medicine, Vanderbilt Comprehensive Care Clinic, Vanderbilt Health at One Hundred Oaks, Nashville, Tennessee

OLUWADAMILOLA O. OLAKU, MD, MPH
Office of Cancer Complementary and Alternative Medicine, National Cancer Institute, Bethesda, Maryland; Kelly Services, Rockville, Maryland

BRIAN C. REED, MD
Department of Family and Community Medicine, Associate Professor, Baylor College of Medicine, Houston, Texas

MARY ELIZABETH ROMANO, MD, MPH
Assistant Professor, Division of Adolescent Medicine & Young Adult Health, Monroe Carell Jr. Children's Hospital at Vanderbilt, Vanderbilt University Medical Center, Nashville, Tennessee

MEGHA K. SHAH, MD, MSc
Department of Family and Preventive Medicine, Assistant Professor, Emory School of Medicine, Atlanta, Georgia

MOHAMAD A. SIDANI, MD, MS
Department of Family and Community Medicine, Professor, Baylor College of Medicine, Houston, Texas

JANET H. SOUTHERLAND, DDS, PhD, MPH
Department of Oral and Maxillofacial Surgery, School of Dentistry, Meharry Medical College, Nashville, Tennessee

JEFFREY STEINBAUER, MD
Department of Family and Community Medicine, Professor, Baylor College of Medicine, Houston, Texas

EMMANUEL A. TAYLOR, MSc, DrPH
Center to Reduce Cancer Health Disparities, National Cancer Institute, Rockville, Maryland

CAROL ZIEGLER, DNP, APRN, NP-C, RD
Assistant Professor, Vanderbilt University School of Nursing, Family Nurse Practitioner and Instructor, Department of Family and Community Medicine, Meharry Medical College, Nashville, Tennessee

ROGER J. ZOOROB, MD, MPH
Professor and Chair, Department of Family and Community Medicine, Baylor College of Medicine, Houston, Texas

Contents

Foreword: Political Agendas Aside   xv

Joel J. Heidelbaugh

Preface   xvii

Vincent Morelli and Roger J. Zoorob

An Introduction to Primary Care in Underserved Populations: Definitions, Scope, and Challenges   1

Vincent Morelli

> This article addresses the scope of the problem primary care physicians face when caring for the underserved, both nationally and internationally. It touches on the statistics used to define medically underserved communities, the pervasiveness of poverty, and how primary care physician shortages may soon reach a crisis point. The definitions of socioeconomic status, allostatic load, and structural violence are also reviewed.

Medically Underserved Areas

Primary Care Issues in Rural Populations   11

Konstantinos E. Deligiannidis

> Rural populations have different demographics and health issues compared to their metropolitan counterparts, including higher mortalities from ischemic heart disease, chronic obstructive pulmonary disease, unintentional injuries, motor vehicle accidents, and suicide. Rural primary care physicians (PCPs) have a unique position in counseling, preventing, and treating common issues that are specific to rural populations, such as motor vehicle accidents, unintentional injuries, pesticide poisoning, occupational respiratory illnesses, and mental illness. They are also in a unique position to address prevention and social determinants of health. Rural PCPs can use multiple strategies to improve access to medical care.

Primary Care Issues in Inner-City America and Internationally   21

Ramon Cancino

> Inner-city patient populations are high-risk for poor outcomes, including increased risk of mortality. Barriers to delivering high-quality primary care to inner-city patients include lack of access, poor distribution of primary care providers (PCPs), competing demands, and financial restraints. Health care issues prevalent in this population include obesity, diabetes, cancer screening, asthma, infectious diseases, and obstetric and prenatal care. Population health management and quality improvement (QI) activities must target disparities in care. Partnering with patients and focusing on social determinants of health and medical care are key areas in which to focus to improve overall health outcomes in this population.

Medically Underserved Populations

Medical Care for Undocumented Immigrants: National and International Issues   e1

Teresa L. Beck, Thien-Kim Le, Queen Henry-Okafor, and Megha K. Shah

The number of undocumented immigrants (UIs) varies worldwide, and most reside in the United States. With more than 12 million UIs in the United States, addressing the health care needs of this population presents unique challenges and opportunities. Most UIs are uninsured and rely on the safety-net health system for their care. Because of young age, this population is often considered to be healthier than the overall US population, but they have specific health conditions and risks. Adequate coverage is lacking; however, there are examples of how to better address the health care needs of UIs.

This article can be accessed online at http://www.primarycare.theclinics.com/.

Pediatric and Adolescent Issues in Underserved Populations   33

Neerav Desai and Mary Elizabeth Romano

Children and adolescents in underserved populations have health care risks that are different from those of the adult population. Providers need to be aware of these needs and the available resources. Providers should work with school and community organizations to provide timely and appropriate preventive health care and screen for medical and mental health problems that occur more commonly in these high-risk patient populations.

Women's Select Health Issues in Underserved Populations   47

Luz M. Fernandez and Jonathan A. Becker

The purpose of this article is to review women's health issues that affect underserved populations. Certain groups have a lack of health care resources or inability to access resources. Individuals encounter barriers to accessing health care due to socioeconomic status, transportation, intimate partner issues, and distrust of the health care system. These factors lead to health care disparities and a lack of appropriate care or quality care as it pertains to breast cancer screening, cervical cancer screening, and obtaining contraceptive care. Identifying available resources in response to community-based needs assessment is among the tools available to combat these inequalities.

Geriatric Care Issues: An American and an International Perspective   e15

Mohamad A. Sidani, Brian C. Reed, and Jeffrey Steinbauer

As the global population ages, there is an opportunity to benefit from the increased longevity of a healthy older adult population. Healthy older individuals often contribute financially to younger generations by offering financial assistance, paying more in taxes than benefits received, and providing unpaid childcare and voluntary work. Governments must address the challenges of income insecurity, access to health care, social isolation, and neglect that currently face elderly adults in many countries.

A reduction in disparities in these areas can lead to better health outcomes and allow societies to benefit from longer, healthier lives of their citizens.

This article can be accessed online at http://www.primarycare.theclinics. com/.

Medical Care of the Homeless: An American and International Issue   **57**

Sheryl B. Fleisch and Robertson Nash

Homeless persons die significantly younger than their housed counterparts. In many cases, relatively straightforward primary care issues escalate into life-threatening, expensive emergencies. Poor health outcomes driven by negative interactions between comorbid symptoms meet the definition of a health syndemic in this population. Successful primary care of patients struggling with homelessness may result in long-term lifesaving measures along with decreased expenditure to hospital systems. This primary prevention requires patience, creativity, and acknowledgment that the source of many confounders may lay outside the control of these patients.

Specific Medical Issues Faced by the Underserved

Cardiovascular Health Disparities in Underserved Populations   **e37**

Charles P. Mouton, Michael Hayden, and Janet H. Southerland

African Americans are at increased risk for hypertension, hyperlipidemia, obesity, and diabetes, which contribute to the burden of cardiovascular disease (CVD). The disparities of CVD in underserved populations require targeted attention from primary care clinicians to eliminate. Primary care can provide this targeted care for their patients by assessing cardiovascular risk, addressing blood pressure control, and selecting appropriate intervention strategies. Using community resources is also effective for addressing CVD disparities in the underserved population.

This article can be accessed online at http://www.primarycare.theclinics. com/.

Occupational Health and Sleep Issues in Underserved Populations   **e73**

Medhat Kalliny and Judith Green McKenzie

Sleep disorders and occupational hazards, injuries, and illnesses impact an individual's overall health. In the United States, substantial racial, ethnic, and socioeconomic disparities exist in sleep and occupational health. Primary care physicians working in underserved communities should be aware of this disparity and target these higher-risk populations for focused evaluation and intervention.

This article can be accessed online at http://www.primarycare.theclinics. com/.

Infectious Disease Issues in Underserved Populations   **67**

Samuel Neil Grief and John Paul Miller

Infectious disease has a major impact on the health outcomes of underserved populations and is reported at significantly higher rates among these populations compared with the general population. Overcoming barriers and obstacles to health care access is key to addressing the disparity regarding the prevalence of infectious disease. Enhancing cultural competency and educating practitioners about underserved populations' basic health needs; optimizing health insurance for the underserved; increasing community resources; and improving access to comprehensive, continuous, compassionate, and coordinated health care are strategies for diminishing the burden of infectious disease in underserved populations.

Cancer in the Medically Underserved Population   87

Oluwadamilola O. Olaku and Emmanuel A. Taylor

Cancer is characterized by uncontrolled growth and spread of abnormal cells. It is the second most common cause of death in the United States, and a significant proportion can be prevented. Underrepresented and underserved populations are less likely to receive routine medical procedures and experience a lower quality of health services. Despite the increase in cancer screening, there are disparities in the incidence and mortality of various cancers. These disparities are not fully explained by the correlations between minority race and lower socioeconomic status or minority race and insurance status. Considerations for global cancer control in low-resource settings are presented.

Psychological Issues in Medically Underserved Patients   99

Mathew Devine, Lauren DeCaporale-Ryan, Magdalene Lim, and Juliana Berenyi

The US population has a subset of those that are underserved who are in need of primary care and also suffer from mental health disorders. In this article, categories of underserved populations are described. Each section defines the population being presented, identifies the mental health problems each is likely to encounter, explores the barriers that prevent access to care, and identifies potential methods to minimize such barriers. The ways in which psychiatric issues vary in underserved settings compared with the general population are differentiated. Recommendations are offered for primary care physicians to support improved recognition and management of psychosocial stressors and psychiatric illness among the underserved.

Substance Use Issues Among the Underserved: United States and International Perspectives   113

Alicia Ann Kowalchuk, Sandra J. Gonzalez, and Roger J. Zoorob

Substance use affects people of all ages, cultures, and socioeconomic levels. Most underserved populations have lower rates of substance use than the general population in a given society, excluding tobacco use. The impact of substance use is more severe, however, in the underserved, with higher rates of incarceration, job loss, morbidity, and mortality. Innovative solutions are being developed to address these differences. Working together, underserved patients with substance use problems can be helped on their journeys toward health and wholeness.

Diet and Obesity Issues in the Underserved   127

Maria C. Mejia de Grubb, Robert S. Levine, and Roger J. Zoorob

The goal of this article is to inform new directions for addressing inequalities associated with obesity by reviewing current issues about diet and obesity among socioeconomically vulnerable and underserved populations. It highlights recent interventions in selected high-risk populations, as well as gaps in the knowledge base. It identifies future directions in policy and programmatic interventions to expand the role of primary care providers, with an emphasis on those aimed at preventing obesity and promoting healthy weight.

Exercise and Sports Medicine Issues in Underserved Populations   141

Vincent Morelli, Daniel L. Bedney, and Arie (Eric) Dadush

Primary care providers can make a strong argument for exercise promotion in underserved communities. The benefits are vitally important in adolescent physical, cognitive, and psychological development as well as in adult disease prevention and treatment. In counseling such patients, we should take into account a patient's readiness for change and the barriers to exercise.

Environmental Justice and Underserved Communities   155

Vincent Morelli, Carol Ziegler, and Omotayo Fawibe

Underserved communities suffer from environmental inequities. Gases lead to hypoxia and respiratory compromise, ozone to increased respiratory illnesses and decreased mental acuity, and mercury to prenatal cognitive disabilities and antisocial behaviors. Lead toxicity is associated with developmental delays. Cadmium is linked with cancer. The smaller sizes of air pollution particulate matter are pathogenic and are associated with cardiovascular and pulmonary disease and nervous system disorders. Bisphenol A is being studied for possible links to cancer and pregnancy risks. Physicians should be aware of these dangers, especially in underserved communities and populations. Investigating possible environmental risks and education are key.

Climate Change and Underserved Communities   171

Carol Ziegler, Vincent Morelli, and Omotayo Fawibe

Climate change is the greatest global health threat of the twenty-first century, yet it is not widely understood as a health hazard by primary care providers in the United States. Aside from increasing displacement of populations and acute trauma resulting from increasing frequency of natural disasters, the impact of climate change on temperature stress, vector-borne illnesses, cardiovascular and respiratory illnesses, and mental health is significant, with disproportionate impact on underserved and marginalized populations. Primary care providers must be aware of the impact of climate change on the health of their patients and advocate for adaptation and mitigation policies for the populations they serve.

A Look Towards the Future

International Comparisons in Underserved Health: Issues, Policies, Needs and Projections   **185**

Paul Hutchinson and Vincent Morelli

> Health care globally has made great strides; for example, there are lower rates of infant and maternal mortality. Increased incomes have led to lower rates of diseases accompanying poverty and hunger. There has been a shift away from the infectious diseases so deadly in developing nations toward first-world conditions. This article presents health care statistics across age groups and geographic areas to help the primary care physician understand these changes. There is a special focus on underserved populations. New technologies in health and health care spending internationally are addressed, emphasizing universal health care. The article concludes with recommendations for the future.

PRIMARY CARE:
CLINICS IN OFFICE PRACTICE

FORTHCOMING ISSUES

June 2017
Integrative Medicine
Deborah S. Clements and Melinda Ring,
Editors

September 2017
Geriatrics
Demetra Antimisiaris, *Editor*

December 2017
Gastroenterology
Rick Kellerman and Laura Mayans,
Editors

RECENT ISSUES

December 2016
Hematologic Diseases
Maureen Okam Achebe and Aric Parnes,
Editors

September 2016
Allergy Primer for Primary Care
Michael A. Malone, *Editor*

June 2016
Psychiatric Care in Primary Care Practice
Janet Albers, *Editor*

ISSUE OF RELATED INTEREST

Nursing Clinics, September 2015 (Vol. 50, Issue 3)
Rural and Other Medically Underserved Populations
JoAnn S. Oliver and Sandra Millon Underwood, *Editors*
http://www.nursing.theclinics.com/

THE CLINICS ARE AVAILABLE ONLINE!
Access your subscription at:
www.theclinics.com

Foreword
Political Agendas Aside

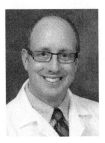

Joel J. Heidelbaugh, MD, FAAFP, FACG
Consulting Editor

Many students in medical, nursing, and physician-assistant training programs seek out opportunities to provide health care for underserved populations both in the United States and abroad. Most medical training institutions have connections to free clinics, homeless clinics, and other venues to provide such experiences, while many are located in urban areas and care for multicultural populations. While the fervor for providing such care continues to grow, why do we continue to have such a shortage of health care providers caring for underserved populations? Do we not understand the unique needs of these populations? Do we lack the adequate time and resources to help them? Is the wealthiest country in the world not able to make a difference?

So how do we define an "underserved population"? The reality is that every day in our practices, we likely care for patients that may fit into this category. And, unfortunately, we may not always consider the disadvantages and challenges inherent in communication and care for these patients, as illiteracy and comprehension rates are greater than the average public. While the main provision of the Affordable Care Act is to provide access and coverage to a primary care provider, the challenge remains in creating adequate and timely access, not to mention the ability to provide the care that these underserved populations need and may not even be aware of.

This issue of *Primary Care: Clinics in Office Practice* provides an exceptionally broad and practical overview on how to approach health care in underserved populations. It begins with a strategy on defining the scope and inherent challenges, applying these concepts to rural and inner city populations. As the politicians continue to argue over what to do with undocumented immigrants, health care providers need a cogent plan on how to best care for their medical and psychosocial needs. Underserved populations encompass men, women, and children across the lifespan, and through the elder years into geriatric populations. As the number of homeless persons continues to grow, both resources and provider knowledge need to keep pace with how to best care for these people.

Prim Care Clin Office Pract 44 (2017) xv–xvi
http://dx.doi.org/10.1016/j.pop.2016.12.002
0095-4543/17/© 2016 Published by Elsevier Inc.

Underserved populations across the world are disadvantaged with respect to receiving appropriate care for cancer, chronic diseases such as cardiovascular disease, infectious diseases, psychological disorders, and substance abuse. Optimistically, there are viable and cost-effective strategies to improve outcomes in underserved populations relative to these conditions. With provider education, these patients can improve nutrition, augment exercise, modify environmental and lifestyle factors, and decrease substance abuse rates with our guidance.

I am indebted to Drs Vincent Morelli and Roger Zoorob for creating the unique concept for this issue of *Primary Care: Clinics in Office Practice*, and for inviting me to participate as a guest editor. I would also like to thank our authors and experts, who contributed very robust and well-referenced articles on topics relevant to the care of underserved populations. While *Primary Care: Clinics in Office Practice* is viewed predominantly as a medical journal, it is my hope that this issue has a much broader reach to public policymakers and health care advocates, so that we can better understand the dire need for attention toward these populations and shape health care coverage toward greater equality. Leaving political agendas aside, we all have the ethical obligation to place a greater emphasis on understanding and caring for underserved populations across the globe.

Joel J. Heidelbaugh, MD, FAAFP, FACG
Departments of Family Medicine and Urology
University of Michigan Medical School
Ann Arbor, MI 48109, USA

Ypsilanti Health Center
200 Arnet Suite 200
Ypsilanti, MI 48198, USA

E-mail address:
jheidel@umich.edu

Preface

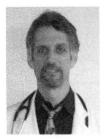 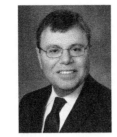

Vincent Morelli, MD   Roger J. Zoorob, MD, MPH
Editors

As primary care physicians on the frontlines of the world's health care delivery system, most of us are tasked daily with providing care for the underserved—the homeless, the aged, the undocumented, the uninsured, and so forth. These populations not only experience significant barriers to care but also face unique medical risks and exposures. Our medical training, though excellent in many aspects, fails to adequately spotlight these populations and discuss their unique medical needs. We hope that this publication will help overcome this deficiency and offer primary care physicians a new perspective when caring for these segments of our population.

Also, as we have researched and written for this issue, we have realized how important our social policies are in affecting the health of our citizens. We hope that policymakers will take the time to consider the information contained in this issue when setting future health care policies.

Finally, we are honored to serve as guest editors for this issue of *Primary Care: Clinics in Office Practice*, and we feel privileged to have worked with such a distinguished group of collaborators. Many thanks to our contributing authors, who have worked diligently to make their articles scholarly and clinically relevant. We also thank the Departments of Family and Community Medicine at Meharry Medical College and Baylor College of Medicine for providing us with the support needed to complete this

Prim Care Clin Office Pract 44 (2017) xvii–xviii
http://dx.doi.org/10.1016/j.pop.2016.12.001
0095-4543/17/© 2016 Published by Elsevier Inc.

primarycare.theclinics.com

project. Finally, thanks to our editors at Elsevier, without whose help this project would never have been accomplished.

Vincent Morelli, MD
Department of Family and Community Medicine
Meharry Medical College
1005 Dr D.B. Todd Boulevard
Nashville, TN 37208, USA

Roger J. Zoorob, MD, MPH
Family and Community Medicine
Baylor College of Medicine
3701 Kirby Drive, Suite 600
Houston, TX 77098, USA

E-mail addresses:
morellivincent@yahoo.com (V. Morelli)
roger.zoorob@bcm.edu (R.J. Zoorob)

An Introduction to Primary Care in Underserved Populations
Definitions, Scope, and Challenges

Vincent Morelli, MD

KEYWORDS

- MUA • MUP • HPSA • Underserved area • Underserved population • Allostatic load
- Socioeconomic status

KEY POINTS

- Medically underserved areas (MUAs) and medically underserved populations (MUPs) are determined by the Health Resources and Services Administration (HRSA) by measuring 4 variables: (1) ratio of primary care physicians (PCPs) per 1000 population, (2) infant mortality rate, (3) percentage of the population below the poverty level, and (4) percentage of the population age 65 or over.
- In a given area or population, each of these variables is measured and then converted to a weighted value using conversion tables.
- In 2015, more than 16% of the US population lived in poverty, up from 14.3% in 2009; approximately 14% of seniors and 18% of children are impoverished.
- Low socioeconomic status (SES) has been linked to poorer metabolic profiles (eg, body mass index [BMI], fasting glucose, glycosylated hemoglobin, and lipid profiles), higher blood pressure, lower heart rate variability, higher levels of inflammatory markers, more risky behaviors (eg, smoking, drinking, and drug use), and higher overall higher allostatic load (AL).

INTRODUCTION

MUAs and MUPs are determined by the HRSA by measuring 4 variables: (1) ratio of PCPs per 1000 population, (2) infant mortality rate, (3) percentage of the population below the poverty level, and (4) percentage of the population age 65 or over.

In a given area or population, each of these variables is measured and then converted to a weighted value using conversion tables (see HRSA MUA/Ps: Index of

The author of this work reports no direct financial interest in the subject matter or any material discussed in this article.

Department of Family Medicine and Community Medicine, Meharry Medical College, Nashville, TN 37208, USA

E-mail address: vmorelli@mmc.edu

Medical Underservice Data Tables at: http://www.hrsa.gov/shortage/mua/imutables. html). The 4 weighted values are then totaled to obtain an "underserved score." Areas or populations that score below 62 are designated as medically underserved, with lower scores indicating greater need. Areas and populations scoring above 62 (from 62 to 100) are designated as adequately served. Federally Qualified Health Centers, which include Community Health Centers and Rural Health Clinics, often provide care in underserved areas/populations and are eligible for federal support.

Despite concerns over the limitations of the HRSA definition of "underserved,"[1,2] for the purposes of this publication, the HRSA definition is used, as stated previously. This article focuses on areas/populations with a disproportionate number of elderly, high infant mortality rates, low access to primary care, and high poverty rates.

SCOPE OF THE PROBLEM: A CLOSER LOOK AT THE VARIABLES MEASURED IN DESIGNATING MEDICALLY UNDERSERVED AREAS AND MEDICALLY UNDERSERVED POPULATIONS
Poverty

In 2015, more than 16% of the US population lived in poverty, up from 14.3% in 2009. Approximately 14% of seniors and 18% of children are impoverished.[3] In 2013, United Nations International Children's Emergency Fund (UNICEF) found the United States to have the second highest child poverty rates of the 35 developed countries studied.[4] Currently in the United States, poverty is defined as earnings of less than $11,700 for an individual or less than $24,250 for a family of 4.

The most recent international data[5] document that, in 2012, 12.7% of the world's population lived at or below $2 a day (purchasing power parity), meaning that close to a billion people were impoverished. This is a vast improvement from the 37% impoverished in 1990, when almost 2 billion people lived in World Bank–defined poverty. This astounding improvement is largely accounted for by China's remarkable economic turnaround. Still, global poverty remains a significant issue with significant public health issues.

The Elderly

United States census data documented an elderly population of 43.1 million in 2012 and predicts that it will double to 83.7 million by 2050.[6] Internationally, population aging, resulting from decreasing mortality and declining fertility, is also taking place. The number of people over age 60 increased from 9.2% in 1990 to 11.7% in 2013 and will reach 21.1% by 2050. By that year, the number of older people will have doubled – from 841 million in 2013 to more than 2 billion.[7]

Infant Mortality

Defined as deaths of infants under 1 year of age per 1000 live births, this ratio is often used as an indicator of the level of health in a country. Worldwide, the infant mortality rate is approximately 42/1000 to 50/1000 live births.[8] The overall US infant mortality rate is 5.3/1000 live births,[9] with higher rates occurring in underserved areas. This article focuses on select underserved populations both in the Untied States and internationally, with infant mortality rates on the higher end of the spectrum.

Primary Care Physician Shortages

Currently, there are 778,000 practicing physicians in the United States. Approximately one-half of them are engaged in primary care, but approximately one-half are over the age of 50; almost one-third are projected to retire in the next 10 years.[10] Compounding the problem is that currently, just 25% of medical school graduates go into and remain in primary care.[11] The reasons for this are no secret: lower primary care salaries, busier work load, perceived lifestyle, high medical school debt, excessive administrative requirements, and relative lack of prestige.

In 2006, in response to the projected shortage of PCPs, medical schools agreed to increase enrollment by 30%. Congress, however, in its 1997 Balanced Budget Act, froze residency training funds (Congress/Medicare funds 80% of residency training slots), leaving the country with an increased number of medical school graduates and a looming shortage of residency training slots. It is projected that by 2017 there will not be enough residency slots for US medical school graduates,[10] resulting in little impact on PCP shortages — an unfathomable error in policy and an egregious disservice to expectant medical students and underserved populations.

For this article, it is important to define what is meant by a primary care shortage. For federal grant funding purposes, the HRSA designates a Health Professional Shortage Area (HPSA) as one with a PCP-to-population ratio of less than 1 PCP per 3500 residents. HRSA notes, however, that this ratio, used since the 1970s, is used for federal granting purposes only and that the primary care needs of a community vary depending on age, poverty levels, percentage of underserved, and so forth. HRSA also notes that their estimates do not take into account the availability of ancillary care providers, such as nurse practitioners (NPs) or physician assistants (PAs). Although the 1:3500 ratio has been a long-standing norm used to identify high-need areas in the United States, HRSA notes that there is no universally accepted critical shortage ratio. With this in mind, when designating underserved areas and populations for this publication, it is probably best to use the combined MUA and MUP index, as stated previously, rather than rely solely on a specific physician-to-population ratio.

Internationally the World Health Organization (WHO) differs in degree with the HRSA figures that designate HPSAs and advocates at least 1 PCP per 1000 people to sufficiently care for populations in developed countries.[12] Again, the 1/1000 ratio is likely a gross underestimation of need for disproportionately elderly populations with complicated medical conditions or in impoverished areas, where patients have more critical presentations and a greater burden of disease.

The WHO designates countries with a total physician/patient ratio of less than 1.13/1000 as having a critical physician shortage; 44% of WHO Member States report falling in this category, most in Africa, Southeast Asia, or Central America. Currently, the United States has approximately 2.5 total doctors per 1000 people but has 10 states with fewer than 1 PCP per 1000 residents.[13]

Note: in absolute numbers, the 2013 HRSA Health Workforce report[14] predicts that despite an 8% increase in the number of PCPs by 2020, there will still be a shortage of 20,000 such physicians — with the caveat that NPs and PAs will fill much of this gap. With a projected 30% increase in NPs and 60% increase in PAs, the Workforce report predicts the shortage of primary care providers nationwide will be cut down to just 6000.[14] Currently, the WHO also estimates a shortage of 4.3 million physicians, nurses and other health workers worldwide.[12]

UNINSURED THUS UNDERSERVED

Data from 2015 document approximately 37 to 43 million uninsured Americans,[15] down from 48 to 50 million uninsured prior to the implementation of the Patient Protection and Affordable Care Act.[16]

KEY CONCEPTS FOR PRIMARY CARE PHYSICIANS WORKING IN UNDERSERVED AREAS

It is important to review concepts of SES, AL, and structural violence. SES, usually defined by lower educational achievement, substandard income attainment, and/or low occupational status, is an important contributor to health. Low SES has been linked to poorer metabolic profiles (eg, BMI, fasting glucose, glycosylated hemoglobin, and lipid profiles),[17–19] higher blood pressure, lower heart rate variability,[20] higher levels of inflammatory markers,[21,22] more risky behaviors (eg, smoking, drinking, and drug use), and higher overall higher AL (discussed later).[23,24]

The concept of AL was born out of the realization that social, environmental, and economic stressors can significantly and simultaneously affect the functioning of multiple interconnected biologic systems (eg, endocrine, immune, digestive, neurologic, and cardiovascular) and that an objective measurement of SES effect would be useful.[25]

The basic idea of AL is that stress-induced changes (eg, secreted hormones and blood pressure increases) that are adaptive in the short run can cause changes leading to disease over the longer term. McEwen[26] found that one of the most potent of stressors (contributors to AL) was competitive interaction between animals of the same species and that this stress contributed to the formation of dominance hierarchies, where lower-ranking animals have been found to have impaired cognitive function and higher burdens of disease.

The quantification of AL has evolved and improved over time. Early methods, such as measured by Evans,[27] quantified 6 factors that documented the effect of stress on the body: resting systolic blood pressure, resting diastolic blood pressure, BMI, overnight urinary cortisol, overnight urinary epinephrine, and overnight urinary norepinephrine. Later and more comprehensive methods, such as those used by Zilioli and colleagues,[28,29] measured up to 24 biomarkers across 7 physiologic domains (ie, cardiovascular, lipid metabolism, glucose metabolism, inflammation, sympathetic nervous system response, parasympathetic nervous system response, and hypothalamic pituitary axis) to assess AL. As with SES, multiple studies[30–32] have documented that higher ALs are associated with negative health outcomes — many of which are discussed in the articles that follow.

It is important for PCPs to realize that both lower SES and higher AL experienced in childhood carry their untoward effects into adulthood,[29,33–35] where AL has been documented to increase negative adult health outcomes and increase all-cause mortality.[36] AL has been proved a stronger predictor of morbidity and mortality than SES or any single health parameter.[37,38] This is because AL accounts for stressors that accumulate with prolonged exposure; thus, what may be small changes in individual parameters will, over time, be accounted for in a more comprehensive fashion by measurement of the cumulative AL, all of which is to say that AL is a significant predictor of dysregulation and untoward health effects and that PCPs working in underserved environments need to be aware of the concept and its potential health effects.[30,31,39]

That being said, PCPs should be encouraged by the knowledge that interventions geared toward the reductions in AL may significantly decrease morbidity and mortality.[38] Because decreased AL has been documented in those with religious ties,[40] stronger social connections,[41] and a greater sense of meaning/purpose,[28,42] holistic interventions taking such factors into consideration are important in health promotion in underserved communities.

Closely related to AL, is the concept of "structural violence." Structural violence is any suffering caused by the structure and institutions of a society that put individuals (especially marginalized individuals) in harm's way. PCPs should be cognizant of the outcomes of structural violence — unequal access to wages, resources, political power, education, health care, or legal standing and so forth — that can contribute to poor health. Some investigators argue that not only can structural violence lead to physical violence[43] but also structural violence alone can produce suffering and death as often as direct violence, although the damage is more insidious, more widespread, and more difficult to repair.[44]

As discussed in the articles that follow, structural violence, SES, and AL play a contributory role in several maladies, including sleep disorders,[45–48] substance abuse,[49,50] psychological disorders,[51–54] appetite dysregulation and obesity,[55,56] and cardiovascular disease.[57,58]

Although much structural violence and AL may be caused or alleviated by governmental policy, it is important for PCPs to be aware of the effects of low SES and high AL if they are to ameliorate untoward individual health effects and provide optimal service when working in underserved areas or with underserved populations.

In the articles that follow, underserved areas are examined, both rural and urban, and issues are highlighted that PCPs working in these environments should be aware of. Disease entities and social and psychological issues that PCPs should be prepared for are spotlighted, to help them focus their attention and best allocate their resources.

In addition to examining underserved areas, underserved peoples are looked at. Health issues that occur disproportionately in underserved populations are discussed — again with the intent to make physicians working with these populations aware of their unique medical challenges. The populations addressed are immigrants, the elderly, underserved children, the homeless, and underserved women.

The last main section of this issue takes an in-depth look at disease categories that overly affect underserved individuals. Infectious diseases, occupational and sleep issues, cardiovascular risks, psychological conditions, substance use problems, cancer risks, diet and obesity disparities, environmental inequities, and exercise questions and sedentary lifestyle in these populations are explored. These articles highlight the "neglected diseases of the underserved" so that PCPs working in these areas will be more aware of their likelihood. For example, the infectious disease article discusses Chagas disease, an underappreciated cause of heart failure in underserved populations in the United States (see Samuel Neil Grief and John Paul Miller's article, "Infectious Disease Issues in Underserved Populations," in this issue). It discusses cysticercosis presenting as headaches or seizures; toxocariasis, the helminth infection caused by ingestion of soil infected with cat or dog feces, with its links to diminished lung and cognitive function; toxoplasmosis, with possible links not only to HIV but also to psychiatric and mood disorders; and trichomoniasis, which has a 10-times higher incidence than among Mexican-American or non-Hispanic white women. Such infectious diseases of the underserved are fully discussed and their unrecognized links to cardiovascular, respiratory, and psychiatric maladies and so forth (conditions ordinarily thought of as noncommunicable diseases) are explored.[59]

The final article discusses the changing morbidity and mortality trends in underserved communities worldwide (see Vincent Morelli and Paul Hutchinson's article, "International Comparisons in Underserved Health - Issues, Policies, Needs and Projections," in this issue). Policy change recommendations are made to address these shifting patterns of disease. In an ever-shrinking world of increasing international travel, both diseases and social ills will continue to cross geographic boundaries and disproportionately affect the most vulnerable underserved peoples. International cooperation and coordination of policy focused on primary care of the underserved is important to avert future public health crises and continue to build a socially aware and enfranchising world.

REFERENCES

1. Kviz FJ, Flaskerud JH. An evaluation of the index of medical underservice. Results from a rural consumer survey. Med Care 1984;22:877–89.
2. Goldsmith LJ, Ricketts TC. Proposed changes to designations of medically underserved populations and health professional shortage areas: effects on rural areas. J Rural Health 1999;15:44–54.
3. Short, Kathleen, "The research supplemental poverty measure: 2012" U.S. Census Bureau, P60–247, Current Population Reports, 2013. Available at: www.census.gov/prod/2013pubs/p60-247.pdf. Accessed December 1, 2015.
4. Adamson P. Child well-being in rich countries: A comparative overview. Innocenti Report Card 11. Florence (Italy): UNICEF Office of Research; 2013. p. 7. Available at: http://www.unicef-irc.org/publications/pdf/rc11_eng.pdf. Accessed December 1, 2015.
5. The World Bank: Poverty overview. Available at: http://www.worldbank.org/en/topic/poverty/overview. Accessed December 1, 2015.
6. Ortman JM, Velkoff VA, Hogan H. United States Census Bureau. An aging nation: The older population in the United States. Population estimates and projections, 2014. Available at: www.census.gov/prod/2014pubs/p25-1140.pdf. Accessed December 1, 2015.
7. United Nations, Department of Economic and Social Affairs, Population Division, 2013. World Population Ageing, page xii. Available at: http://www.un.org/en/development/desa/population/publications/pdf/ageing/WorldPopulationAgeing2013.pdf. Accessed December 1, 2015.
8. Wikipedia: the free encyclopedia. List of countries by infant mortality rate. Available at: https://en.wikipedia.org/wiki/List_of_countries_by_infant_mortality_rate. Accessed December 3, 2015.
9. United Nations, Department of Economic and Social Affairs, Population Division, page 7. World population prospects, the 2015 revision. Available at: esa.un.org/unpd/wpp/publications/files/key_findings_wpp_2015.pdf. Accessed December 1, 2015.
10. Frisch S. The primary care physician shortage. BMJ 2013;347:f6559.
11. Chen C, Petterson S, Phillips RL, et al. Toward graduate medical education (GME) accountability: Measuring the outcomes of GME institutions. Acad Med 2013;88:1267–80.
12. World Health Organization. Models and tools for health workforce planning and projections. Geneva (Switzerland): Human Resources for Health Observer; 2010. Issue No. 3. Available at: http://apps.who.int/iris/bitstream/10665/44263/1/9789241599016_eng.pdf. Accessed December 1, 2015.
13. United Health Foundation. America's Health Rankings. Primary care physicians: United States. Available at: http://www.americashealthrankings.org/all/pcp. Accessed December 1, 2015.
14. U.S. Department of Health and Human Services. HRSA Health Workforce. Projecting the supply and demand for primary care practitioners through 2020, November 2013. Available at: http://bhpr.hrsa.gov/healthworkforce/supplydemand/usworkforce/primarycare/primarycarebrief.pdf. Accessed December 1, 2015.
15. Karman KG, Eibner C. Changes in health insurance enrollment since 2013: evidence from the RAND health reform opinion study. Santa Monica (CA): The Rand Corporation ; 2014. Available at: http://www.rand.org/pubs/research_reports/RR656.html. Accessed December 1, 2015.

16. Levy J, editor. U.S., Uninsured rate dips to 11.9% in first quarter. Washington, DC: Gallup; 2015. Available at: http://www.gallup.com/poll/182348/uninsured-rate-dips-first-quarter.aspx. Accessed December 1, 2015.
17. Loucks EB, Magnusson KT, Cook S, et al. Socioeconomic position and the metabolic syndrome in early, middle, and late life: Evidence from NHANES 1999–2002. Ann Epidemiol 2007;17:782–90.
18. McLaren L. Socioeconomic status and obesity. Epidemiol Rev 2007;29:29–48.
19. Senese LC, Almeida ND, Fath AK, et al. Associations between childhood socioeconomic position and adulthood obesity. Epidemiol Rev 2009;31:21–51.
20. Sloan RP, Huang MH, Sidney S, et al. Socioeconomic status and health: Is parasympathetic nervous system activity an intervening mechanism? Int J Epidemiol 2005;34:309–15.
21. Loucks EB, Pilote L, Lynch JW, et al. Life course socioeconomic position is associated with inflammatory markers: The Framingham Offspring Study. Soc Sci Med 2010;71:187–95.
22. Gruenewald TL, Cohen S, Matthews KA, et al. Association of socioeconomic status with inflammation markers in black and white men and women in the Coronary Artery Risk Development in Young Adults (CARDIA) study. Soc Sci Med 2009;69:451–9.
23. Crimmins EM, Kim JK, Seeman TE. Poverty and biological risk: The earlier "aging" of the poor. J Gerontol A Biol Sci Med Sci 2009;64:286–92.
24. Seeman TE, Singer BH, Rowe JW, et al. Price of adaptation – allostatic load and its health consequences: MacArthur studies of successful aging. Arch Intern Med 1999;159:1176.
25. Gerdes L, Tegeler CH, Lee SW. A groundwork for allostatic neuro-education. Front Psychol 2015;6:1224.
26. McEwen BS. Protective and damaging effects of stress mediators. N Engl J Med 1998;338:171–9.
27. Evans GW. A multimethodological analysis of cumulative risk and allostatic load among rural children. Dev Psychol 2003;39:924–33.
28. Zilioli S, Slatcher RB, Ong AD, et al. Purpose in life predicts allostatic load ten years later. J Psychosom Res 2015;79:451–7.
29. Gruenewald TL, Karlamangla AS, Hu P, et al. History of socioeconomic disadvantage and allostatic load in later life. Soc Sci Med 2012;74:75–83.
30. McEwen BS. Protection and damage from acute and chronic stress: Allostasis and allostatic overload and relevance to the pathophysiology of psychiatric disorders. Ann N Y Acad Sci 2004;1032:1–7.
31. McEwen BS. Physiology and neurobiology of stress and adaptation: central role of the brain. Physiol Rev 2007;87:873–904.
32. Diez Roux AV. Conceptual approaches to the study of health disparities. Annu Rev Public Health 2012;33:41–58.
33. Tamayo T, Herder C, Rathmann W. Impact of early psychosocial factors (childhood socioeconomic factors and adversities) on future risk of type 2 diabetes, metabolic disturbances and obesity: A systematic review. BMC Public Health 2010;10:525.
34. Widom CS, Horan J, Brzustowicz L. Childhood maltreatment predicts allostatic load in adulthood. Child Abuse Negl 2015;47:59–69.
35. Tomasdottir MO, Sigurdsson JA, Petursson H, et al. Self reported childhood difficulties, adult multimorbidity and allostatic load. A cross-sectional analysis of the Norwegian HUNT Study. PLoS One 2015;10(6):e0130591.

36. Seeman TE, McEwen BS, Rowe JW, et al. Allostatic load as a marker of cumulative biological risk: MacArthur studies of successful aging. Proc Natl Acad Sci U S A 2001;98:4770–5.
37. Karlamangla AS, Singer BH, McEwen BS, et al. Allostatic load as a predictor of functional decline. MacArthur studies of successful aging. J Clin Epidemiol 2002;55(7):696–710.
38. Karlamangla AS, Singer BH, Seeman TE. Reduction in allostatic load in older adults is associated with lower all-cause mortality risk: MacArthur studies of successful aging. Psychosom Med 2006;68:500–7.
39. McEwen BS. Stress, adaptation, and disease: Allostasis and allostatic load. Ann N Y Acad Sci 1998;840:33–44.
40. Maselko J, Kubzansky L, Kawachi I, et al. Religious service attendance and allostatic load among high-functioning elderly. Psychosom Med 2007;69:464–72.
41. Seeman TE, Singer BH, Ryff CD, et al. Social relationships, gender, and allostatic load across two age cohorts. Psychosom Med 2002;64:395–406.
42. Lindfors P, Lundberg O, Lundberg U. Allostatic load and clinical risk as related to sense of coherence in middle-aged women. Psychosom Med 2006;68:801–7.
43. Copp JE, Kuhl DC, Giordano PC, et al. Intimate partner violence in neighborhood context: the roles of structural disadvantage, subjective disorder, and emotional distress. Soc Sci Res 2015;53:59–72.
44. Winter DA, Leighton DC. Structural violence. In: Christie DJ, Wagner RV, Winter DA, editors. Peace, conflict, and violence: peace psychology for the 21st century. Englewood Cliffs (NJ): Prentice-Hall; 2001. p. 99–201.
45. McEwen BS, Karatsoreos IN. Sleep deprivation and circadian disruption: Stress, allostasis, and allostatic load. Sleep Med Clin 2015;10:1–10.
46. Juster RP, McEwen BS. Sleep and chronic stress: new directions for allostatic load research. Sleep Med 2015;16:7–8.
47. Clark AJ, Dich N, Lange T, et al. Impaired sleep and allostatic load: Cross-sectional results from the Danish Copenhagen Aging and Midlife Biobank. Sleep Med 2014;15:1571–8.
48. Chen X, Redline S, Shields AE, et al. Associations of allostatic load with sleep apnea, insomnia, short sleep duration, and other sleep disturbances: Findings from the National Health and Nutrition Examination Survey 2005 to 2008. Ann Epidemiol 2014;24:612–9.
49. Chen E, Miller GE, Brody GH, et al. Neighborhood poverty, college attendance, and diverging profiles of substance use and allostatic load in rural African American youth. Clin Psychol Sci 2015;3:675–85.
50. Doan SN, Dich N, Evans GW. Childhood cumulative risk and later allostatic load: Mediating role of substance use. Health Psychol 2014;33:1402–9.
51. Juster RP, McEwen BS, Lupien SJ. Allostatic load biomarkers of chronic stress and impact on health and cognition. Neurosci Biobehav Rev 2010;35:2–16.
52. Pettorruso M, De Risio L, Di Nicola M, et al. Allostasis as a conceptual framework linking bipolar disorder and addiction. Front Psychiatry 2014;5:173.
53. Hintsa T, Elovainio M, Jokela M, et al. Is there an independent association between burnout and increased allostatic load? Testing the contribution of psychological distress and depression. J Health Psychol 2016;21(8):1576–86.
54. Misiak B, Frydecka D, Zawadzki M, et al. Refining and integrating schizophrenia pathophysiology - relevance of the allostatic load concept. Neurosci Biobehav Rev 2014;45:183–201.
55. Sinha R, Jastreboff AM. Stress as a common risk factor for obesity and addiction. Biol Psychiatry 2013;73(9):827–35.

56. Katz DA, Sprang G, Cooke C. The cost of chronic stress in childhood: Understanding and applying the concept of allostatic load. Psychodyn Psychiatry 2012;40:469–80.
57. Ippoliti F, Canitano N, Businaro R. Stress and obesity as risk factors in cardiovascular diseases: A neuroimmune perspective. J Neuroimmune Pharmacol 2013;8: 212–26.
58. Sabbah W, Watt RG, Sheiham A, et al. Effects of allostatic load on the social gradient in ischaemic heart disease and periodontal disease: Evidence from the Third National Health and Nutrition Examination Survey. J Epidemiol Community Health 2008;62:415–20.
59. Hotez PJ. Neglected parasitic infections and poverty in the United States. Plos Negl Trop Dis 2014;8:e3012.

Primary Care Issues in Rural Populations

Konstantinos E. Deligiannidis, MD, MPH, FAAFP

KEYWORDS

- Rural • Determinants of health • Prevention • Treatment • Adherence • Access
- Training • Retention

KEY POINTS

- Rural populations have different demographics and health issues compared with metropolitan populations, with higher rates of mortality.
- Rural primary care physicians (PCPs) must be familiar with treating and counseling for conditions faced more commonly in their patient population, such as occupational respiratory illness.
- Rural PCPs can address treatment, prevention, and social determinants of health.
- Multiple strategies can be used by rural PCPs to address access, such as the use of mid-level health care professionals, electronic visits, and other technology.

INTRODUCTION

The Institute of Medicine defines primary care as "the provision of integrated, accessible health care services by clinicians who are accountable for addressing a large majority of personal health care needs, developing a sustained partnership with patients, and practicing in the context of family and community."[1] Primary care physicians (PCPs) have the benefit of caring for patients from a longitudinal perspective and developing rapport and relationships with patients and their families, often across generations. Physicians receive a great benefit from assisting patients with multiple medical and psychosocial issues, both acute and chronic. However, along with these benefits that primary care gives to the physician, the specialty also presents challenges in addressing the health of patients, families, and communities. Moreover, these challenges are particularly prominent in rural communities. This article discusses some of the issues that rural PCPs face, such as health problems that are more common in rural populations, disease prevention and adherence issues, access to health care services, and educational issues.

Disclosure: The author has nothing to disclose.
Northwell Health Solutions, House Calls Program, 1983 Marcus Ave. Suite C102, New Hyde Park, NY 11042, USA
E-mail address: kdeligiann@northwell.edu

HEALTH PROBLEMS FACED IN RURAL POPULATIONS

Rural populations have a different population demographic and face a different set of medical issues, which bring about challenges for family physicians. Statistics compiled in the Rural-Urban Chartbook in 2014 revealed that there are differences between metropolitan and nonmetropolitan (including both micropolitan and rural) areas. For instance, as populations move from metropolitan areas to nonmetropolitan areas, the age distribution tends to get older, and the percentage of population in the rural counties that is 65 years old or older is higher in nonmetropolitan counties compared with metropolitan counties. This pattern is seen in all regions of the United States.[2] Furthermore, the highest levels of poverty in the South and West regions of the United States are in rural counties (whereas the highest levels in the Midwest and the Northeast were in large metropolitan counties).[2]

Substance Use

Tobacco use also affects nonmetropolitan counties more than metropolitan counties. The highest percentage of men and women who smoke are in nonmetropolitan and rural counties. Furthermore, the highest percentage of adolescents who smoke is in the rural and nonmetropolitan counties. Again, this is true for all regions of the United States, except the West, where adolescent smoking was the second highest percentage.[2]

Self-reported alcohol consumption varies across the regions of the United States, with the highest percentage of individuals who report alcohol consumption living in the nonmetropolitan/rural areas in the West, whereas in the South it is the smallest percentage (compared with metropolitan counties).[2]

Moreover, substance use treatment admission rates are higher in nonmetropolitan areas for stimulants, although treatment admission rates are lower for opiates in rural areas. The challenge with this statistic is that the rate of opiate use disorder may not correlate with the treatment admission rates. Although there is evidence that the availability of prescription opiates has increased, and more so in rural areas,[3] care must be taken in interpreting these statistics, because 94% of people who are prescribed opiates do not develop opiate use disorder.[4,5]

Obesity and Physical Inactivity

The highest percentages of the population that are obese are in the nonmetropolitan/rural counties in all regions of the United States.[2] Perhaps surprisingly, the highest percentages of the population who are physically inactive are in the nonmetropolitan/rural populations of the Midwest and the South. The large metropolitan counties in the Northeast are an exception.[2]

Mental Health

Nationally, mental illness in men and women is more prevalent in nonmetropolitan and rural counties, with a higher percentage of women with mental illness compared with men. Similar rates also occurred for serious mental illness, which is defined as mental/behavioral/emotional disorder that results in serious functional impairment.[2]

Other Medical Issues

Other health issues seen in primary care are also more prominent in rural communities. Adolescent birth rates are highest in nonmetropolitan/rural areas nationally, especially in the South and the West.[2] Limitation of activity because of chronic health conditions is highest nationally in rural counties.[2] In addition, the percentage of the population with edentulism (the condition of being toothless) is highest in nonmetropolitan/rural counties, regardless of income level.[2] This may be because the supply of dentists in rural areas decreases as urbanization increases, with approximately one-third as many dentists in rural counties as in large metropolitan counties.[2]

MORTALITY

Nationally, infant mortalities are higher in rural counties, but this varies by region. All-cause death rates are greater in children and young adults (1–24 years old) in nonmetropolitan/rural counties compared with their metropolitan counterparts nationally (with some variation among regions for male gender).[2] Nationally, all-cause mortalities for working-age adults (25–64 years old) and elderly ($\geq$65 years old) are higher in nonmetropolitan/rural counties than metropolitan counties.[2]

Mortality Causes

The death rate from ischemic heart disease rates for men and women is highest in rural counties, as is the chronic obstructive pulmonary disease (COPD)–related death rate.[2] Similarly, death rates from unintentional injuries and motor vehicle accidents (for both genders 1–42 years old) is highest in nonmetropolitan/rural areas, with the number of male deaths approximately double the number of female deaths.[2] Furthermore, suicide rates were highest in nonmetropolitan/rural areas in each of the 4 regions of the United States.[2]

SPECIFIC RURAL ISSUES, WITH THEIR PREVENTION AND COUNTERMEASURES

PCPs have a unique position in counseling, preventing, and treating common issues that are specific to rural populations, such as motor vehicle accidents, unintentional injuries, pesticide poisoning, and occupational respiratory illnesses.

Motor Vehicle Accidents and Unintentional Injuries

Although "one-third of all motor vehicle accidents occur in rural areas, two-thirds of motor vehicle deaths occur on rural roads."[6] Furthermore, "rural residents are also nearly twice as likely as urban residents to die from unintentional injuries other than motor vehicle accidents."[6] Unintentional injuries may occur from farm equipment; working with livestock; and falls from ladders, grain binds, and other heights. PCP in rural areas should therefore help with addressing this by counseling on safe driving and on preventing occupational hazards that are specific to their location. In addition, physicians should have a fundamental knowledge of trauma care (eg, laceration repair, care of fractures) and be readily able to communicate with emergency medical services (EMS). Communication with EMS regarding medical records and medical history has been identified as a need to address, especially with electronic medical records and electronic communication.[7]

Organophosphate Poisoning

Organophosphate poisoning usually occurs as a form of intentional exposure (eg, suicide attempt), and rarely as accidental exposure. Note that adults and children are affected differently. Exposure, and subsequent poisoning, can occur via absorption through the skin, inhalation, or ingestion. Although exposures are declining because of the phasing out by the Environmental Protection Agency of the common household and agricultural organophosphate insecticides,[8] it still is important for PCPs to be aware of the signs, symptoms, and treatment of organophosphate poisoning. Symptoms in adults include muscarinic effects (eg, diaphoresis, diarrhea, urinary incontinence, miosis, bradycardia, bronchospasm, emesis, excess lacrimation, salivation), nicotinic effects (eg, fasciculations, cramping, weakness), and central nervous system effects (eg, anxiety, emotional lability, confusion, ataxia, tremors, and seizures). In children, seizure and coma are the most common presentations. Physical examination findings include decreased (or increased) respirations, bradycardia, tachycardia, hypotension or hypertension, and paralysis, as well as impaired memory, confusion, irritability, lethargy, and psychosis. Removal from exposure is paramount. PCPs or EMS personnel need to control the airways and administer oxygen, and possibly even need to intubate the patient, although atropine administration may eliminate the need for intubation. Central lines should be established, pulse oximetry and electrocardiography should be monitored, and arrhythmias should be treated accordingly.

Tick-borne Illnesses

Several tick-borne illnesses are found in rural areas, and are variable in different regions of the United States. The Northeast and upper Midwest of the United States are likely to encounter anaplasmosis, babesiosis, Powassan disease, tularemia, and Lyme disease (either from *Borrelia burgdorferi*, *Borrelia mayonii*, or *Borrelia miyamotoi*).[9] The Pacific coast can also experience anaplasmosis, Lyme, tick-borne relapsing fever (TBRF), tularemia, and 364D rickettsiosis.[9] Rocky Mountain states may see Colorado tick fever, TBRF, and tularemia. Southern tick-associated rash illness (STARI) can be seen in southeastern and eastern states; TBRF can be seen in the western half of the United States. Ehrlichiosis is seen in south-central and southeastern states.[9]

PCPs should be aware of the most common symptoms of tick-related illnesses, such as fever and chills, headache, fatigue, and muscle aches. Also, rashes may occur, such as erythema migrans (in Lyme, STARI), small pink nonpruritic macules to petechiae (in Rocky Mountain spotted fever), or skin ulcers (in tularemia). Most of these tick-borne illnesses can be treated with antibiotics, and prompt start of antibiotics when indicated may help reduce the severity of symptoms.

Occupational Respiratory Illnesses

Other issues that can occur specific to rural areas include farmer's hypersensitivity pneumonitis (FHP, or farmer's lung), organic dust toxicity syndrome (ODTS, or silo unloader's syndrome), silo filler's disease, and asthma. These conditions have different causes. For instance, FHP is related to the inhalation of mold spores. Thus, it is important for physicians to counsel patients to reduce the exposure to spores (eg, by avoiding working in confined dusty areas; by increasing ventilation to remove spores; by using mold inhibitors; and by harvesting, baling, and storing grains in a manner to reduce mold growth). Similar recommendations can be made for ODTS, which occurs from organic dust. Silo filler's disease occurs from the inhalation of nitrogen dioxide, so it is important for PCPs to counsel patients on reducing the risk of developing this, such as never entering the silo 2 to 3 days after filling, using portable gas monitors to monitor levels in the silo, and wearing an N95-rated dust mask if entering the silo after the 3-week postfilling period.[10] In addition, counseling with regard to these issues also helps with reducing the risk for asthma exacerbation. Further information is available online.[10,11]

Stress/Anxiety

Although droughts, floods, pests, natural disasters, financial instability, and isolation occur at every location, people living or working in rural environments may be especially vulnerable. Practicing rural PCPs should be aware of mental health issues and be able to offer counseling and support. Furthermore, the US Preventive Services Task force issued a grade B recommendation that "screening for depression in the general adult population should be implemented with adequate systems in place to ensure accurate diagnosis, effective treatment, and appropriate follow-up."[12] Although screening is important, PCPs should also be able to provide treatment or referral to mental health professionals. However, given the disparity between rural and urban areas with regard to access to mental health providers, PCPs may need to use other strategies to address this issue (discussed later).

Other Common Medical Conditions

In a recent National Health Report, the 10 leading causes of death in the United States were cardiovascular disease, cancer, chronic pulmonary disease, stroke, unintentional injuries, Alzheimer, diabetes, pneumonia and influenza, kidney disease, and suicide.[13] Some have been shown to have a major difference in rates of occurrence between rural and metropolitan areas (as discussed earlier). However, there are others (pneumonia and influenza), for which there are no readily available statistics that differentiate incidences between rural and urban communities, and so it is difficult to extrapolate whether there are major differences between the two areas.

PREVENTION IN RURAL AREAS

As mentioned earlier, there are many health issues that are more prominent in rural areas compared with urban areas. The top 20 Rural Healthy People 2020 national objectives that are recognized as priorities by rural stakeholders are the following: access to quality health services, nutrition and weight status, diabetes, mental health, substance abuse, heart disease and stroke, physical activity and health, older adults, maternal and child health, tobacco use, cancer, education and community-based programs, oral health, quality of life and well-being, immunizations and infectious diseases, public health infrastructure, family planning and sexual health, injury and violence prevention, social determinants of health, and health communication and health IT.[14] Although it is important to treat illnesses, it is also important to help prevent some illnesses by addressing social determinants of health.

For instance, in order to prevent heart disease, stroke, COPD, and lung cancer, smoking cessation and prevention are important. Public policy measures (eg, cigarette tax, age limits to purchase), motivational interviewing (for behavior change), nicotine replacement therapy, and other types of pharmacotherapy (bupropion, varenicline) all play a role. Furthermore, physical inactivity and obesity are important to prevent by counseling behavior change. Motivational interviewing is helpful but must also be met with resources in the area. Rural PCPs must be able to use creativity in helping patients be physically active and improve on dietary changes. For instance, walking/running clubs are used in some rural areas of the United States, as well as cooking classes coordinated by medical professionals and community members.

ADHERENCE

Adherence to lifestyle modification is challenging, no matter the behavior change. Likewise, adherence to medical advice and guidelines is also challenging. For instance, in patients who are breast cancer survivors, physical activity is associated with a decreased all-cause mortality, breast cancer mortality, and recurrence.[15,16] However, only 19% of rural breast cancer survivors meet physical activity guidelines.[17] Recommendations for clinicians that have been suggested include targeting self-efficacy and prescribing physical activity regimens that are tailored to the patient and the patient's abilities.[17]

Another study [18] showed that in a Latino population with diabetes in rural California, food insecurity was independently associated with not receiving foot examinations, dilated eye examinations, medication underuse, and not having control of a composite measure of diabetes control. The recommendation for "clinicians and health systems is to aggressively address social issues such as food insecurity in addition to improving standard diabetes medical management."[18] This recommendation includes "screening of patients at high risk for food insecurity and aggressively referring patients to nutrition services. and rethinking target A1c goals for patients with food insecurity."[18] As is evident with the previous 2 medical issues, social determinants of health are key influences of health, and rural PCPs need to be creative in addressing social issues to improve the health of the population.

ADDRESSING ACCESS IN RURAL AREAS
Improving Access to Medical Care

Just as there are differences between rural and metropolitan areas in rates of medical conditions, there are also differences in the supply of physicians. The supply of almost every subspecialty is less in nonmetropolitan areas compared with metropolitan areas. Large metropolitan counties have approximately 380.5 physicians per 100,000 population, whereas rural counties have approximately 118.3 per 100,000 population.[2] As mentioned earlier, the highest priority for Rural Healthy People 2020 is access to quality health services.[14] Improving access is addressed later.

Personnel

There are several steps that communities and policy makers have taken to address access to primary care in rural communities. First is the use of midlevel or advanced practice clinicians, such as nurse practitioners and physician assistants who can see patients, usually as part of a team. Another important aspect to the clinical team approach to patient care is the use of nurses, including visiting nurses or town nurses, to visit patients between visits with their clinicians. Other clinical team approaches involve pharmacists with a pharmacist collaborative practice agreement, by which pharmacists are authorized to provide medication management under protocol. However, the scope of authorization varies throughout the United States.

Visit types

Another approach that rural PCPs use to address access is the use of home visits and group visits. Some patients struggle with transportation, or are disabled, so that leaving their homes requires a taxing effort, making it difficult for them to get to their health care facilities. To address this access problem, rural PCPs can go to the homes of patients. The benefit to this approach is that PCPs are able to learn more about their patients and about their lives, environment, and context, further enabling them to take better care of their patients. Group visits can be held for patients who have a common condition (eg, diabetes, obesity, asthma). In this scenario, education and even clinician visits can be used to address multiple patients at the same time, thereby increasing access by seeing more patients in the time in which a clinician would typically see an individual. This approach improves access and also provides a social network for patients to teach each other how they manage their chronic conditions and help each other in their illnesses.

Technology

With the rapid development of technology, other methods have been added to the clinician's toolkit in caring for the rural population. One strategy is the use of e-visits. E-visits, whether they are part of the electronic medical record or a separate secure messaging program, involve patients entering their relevant clinical information into the message, which the PCP receives. The provider makes an assessment and communicates the clinical decision to the patient electronically. A possible scenario is one in which a female patient with no significant past medical history has dysuria, urinary frequency, and urgency, similar to her urinary tract infections in the past. She sends a message to her PCP who then may decide to call in an antibiotic for her.

Another technological advancement is the role of telemedicine, which is being used in areas where subspecialist access is limited. For example, PCPs may connect patients with dermatologists or psychiatrists via telemedicine platforms to assist them in diagnosis and treatment of conditions for which their subspecialist involvement is needed. Furthermore, the use of Project ECHO (Extension for Community Healthcare Outcomes; http://echo.unm.edu) networks may assist rural PCPs in the diagnosis and management of conditions such as hepatitis C, human immunodeficiency virus, and even chronic pain so that the issue can be treated by rural PCPs.

In addition, there has been a shift in the health care marketplace with the development of urgent care clinics. Urgent care clinics (some affiliated with drug-store chains, some independent, and some affiliated with hospital systems) have had the effect of increasing access to health care and avoidance of the emergency departments for nonemergency health care needs. However, these centers can also lead to fragmented care if used frequently.

Improving Training and Retention of Rural Primary Care Physicians

Rural areas experience physician shortages, as mentioned earlier, but this is not new, and has been a concern for decades.[19] This shortage has been the focus of many programs to increase the supply of both medical students and residents interested in practicing in rural areas, as well retaining them after graduation. This goal poses a challenge, not just because of the patient demographics in the rural communities but also because of the challenges of "lower reimbursements for services, clinician lifestyle considerations, spousal career needs, and, for those physicians with children, school quality."[20]

In order to help with recruitment and retention of physicians to rural areas, the federal government has used 3 approaches: Area Health Education Centers (AHECs), National Health Service Corps (NHSC), and Federally Qualified Health Centers (FQHCs). AHECs provide connections with academic institutions to allow training experiences in the ambulatory setting, not just for medical students but for all health professions students. The NHSC provides scholarships and loan repayment programs to physicians from allopathic and osteopathic schools practicing in underserved areas (not just rural but also urban). In addition, FQHCs are health centers that provide comprehensive primary care to patients with limited access to health care, not just in rural areas but in urban areas as well. Furthermore, some states offer loan repayment programs and scholarship programs for those interested in, and committed to, rural practice.

According to the American Academy of Family Physicians, "two of the strongest predictors that a physician will choose rural practice are specialty and background: family physicians are more likely than those with less general training to go into rural practice, and physicians with rural backgrounds are more likely to locate in rural areas than those with urban backgrounds."[21] Other factors that correlate with an increased likelihood that a physician will choose rural practice include training at a medical school with a mission to train rural physicians, osteopathic training, training that includes rural components, and participation in the NHSC. However, those who are prepared not just to practice medicine but also to live in a rural area are more likely to stay in the rural area long term.[22]

SUMMARY

Rural PCPs know their patients and their communities well, being key members of their communities. They also are positioned to be involved what the Institute of Healthcare Improvement calls the Triple Aim: optimizing health system performance with improving the patient experience of care (including quality and satisfaction), improving the health of populations, and reducing the per capita cost of health care.[23] Although rural populations have higher rates of medical conditions than their metropolitan counterparts, and have less access to quality health care, rural PCPs can use technology and health care professionals in a team-based approach to improve the health of their community. However, it is critical to note that policy makers are also key to improving rural health, because policies can produce changes to determinants of health. In this current climate of using quality metrics for pay for performance, many metrics have limited evidence and may not lead to better health outcomes. Therefore, policy makers need to transform the current system of metrics to include metrics that are patient centered, evidence based, and address social determinants of health.[24]

REFERENCES

1. Donaldson MS, Yordy KD, Lohr KN, et al, editors. Primary care: America's health in a new era. Washington, DC: Committee on the Future of Primary Care Services, Division of Health Care Services, Institute of Medicine. National Academy Press; 1996.
2. Meit M, Knudson A, Gilbert T, et al. The 2014 update of the rural-urban Chartbook. Bethesda (MD): Rural Health Reform Policy Research Center, University of North Dakota Center for Rural Health and the NORC Walsh Center for Rural Health Analysis; 2014. Available at: https://ruralhealth.und.edu/projects/health-reform-policy-research-center/pdf/2014-rural-urban-chartbook-update.pdf.
3. Keyes KM, Cerda M, Brady JE, et al. Understanding the rural-urban differences in nonmedical prescription opioid use and abuse in the United States. Am J Public Health 2014;104(2):e52–9.
4. Substance Abuse and Mental Health Services Administration, Results from the 2011 National Survey on Drug Use and Health: Summary of National Findings, NSDUH Series H-44, HHS Publication No. (SMA) 12-4713. Rockville (MD): Substance Abuse and Mental Health Services Administration; 2012. Available at: http://www.samhsa.gov/data/NSDUH/2k11Results/NSDUHresults2011.pdf.
5. Jones CM, Paulozzi LJ, Mack KA. Sources of prescription opioid pain relievers by frequency of past-year nonmedical use United States 2008-2011. JAMA Intern Med 2014;174(5):802–3.
6. Goins RT, Williams KA, Carter MW, et al. Perceived barriers to health care access among rural older adults: a qualitative study. J Rural Health 2005;21(3):206–13. Available at: http://ruralhealth.stanford.edu/health-pros/factsheets/disparities-barriers.html.
7. National Conference of State Legislatures. Emergency medical services in rural areas: how can states ensure their effectiveness? Rural Health Brief. Denver (CO): National Conference of State Legislatures; 2000.

8. Sudakin DL, Power LE. Organophosphate exposures in the United States: a longitudinal analysis of incidents reported to poison centers. J Toxicol Environ Health A 2007;70(2):141–7.
9. Centers for Disease Control and Prevention. Available at: http://www.cdc.gov/ticks/diseases/index.html. Accessed March 8, 2016.
10. Murphy DJ. Farm respiratory hazards. University Park (PA): Pennsylvania State University College of Agricultural Sciences Publication; 2013. Available at: http://extension.psu.edu/business/ag-safety/health/e26.
11. Occupational Safety and Health Administration. Safety and Health Topics. United States Department of Labor. Available at: https://www.osha.gov/dsg/topics/agriculturaloperations/hazards_controls.html. Accessed March 8, 2016.
12. Final update summary: Depression in adults: screening. U.S. Preventive Services Task Force. 2016. Available at: http://www.uspreventiveservicestaskforce.org/Page/Document/UpdateSummaryFinal/depression-in-adults-screening1. Accessed March 8, 2016.
13. Johnson NB, Hayes LD, Brown K. National Health Report: leading causes of morbidity and mortality and associated behavioral risk and protective factors – United States, 2005-2013. MMWR Suppl 2014;63(04):3–27.
14. Bolin JN, Bellamy G, Ferdinand AO, et al, editors. Rural healthy people 2020, vol. 1. College Station (TX): Texas A&M Health Science Center School of Public Health, Southwest Rural Health Research Center; 2015. p. i–xii.
15. Friendenreich CM, Gregory J, Kopciuk KA, et al. Prospective cohort study of lifetime physical activity and breast cancer survival. Int J Cancer 2009;124:1954–62.
16. Holick CN, Newcomb PA, Trentham-Dietz A, et al. Physical activity and survival after diagnosis of invasive breast cancer. Cancer Epidemiol Biomarkers Prev 2008;17:379–86.
17. Olson EA, Mullen SP, Rogers LQ, et al. Meeting physical activity guidelines in rural breast cancer survivors. Am J Health Behav 2014;38(6):890–9.
18. Moreno G, Morales LS, Isiordia M, et al. Latinos with diabetes and food insecurity in an agricultural community. Med Care 2015;53(5):423–9.
19. Mareck DG. Federal and state initiatives to recruit physicians to rural areas. Virtual Mentor 2011;13(5):304–9.
20. Rosenblatt RA, Chen FM, Lishner DM, et al. Final report 125: the future of family medicine and implications for rural primary care physician supply. Seattle (WA): WWAMI Rural Health Research Center, University of Washington; 2010.
21. Martin JC, Avant RF, Bowman MA, et al. The future of family medicine: a collaborative project of the family medicine community. Ann Fam Med 2004;2(Suppl 1): S3–32.
22. Rural practice, keeping physicians in (Position Paper). AAFP 2002, 2014 COD. Available at: http://www.aafp.org/about/policies/all/rural-practice-paper.html. Accessed March 8, 2016.
23. Berwick DM, Nolan TW, Whittington J. The triple aim: Care, health, and cost. Health Aff (Millwood) 2008;27(3):759–69.
24. Saver BG, Martin SA, Adler RN, et al. Care that matters: Quality measurement and health care. PLoS Med 2015;12(11):e1001902.

Primary Care Issues in Inner-City America and Internationally

Ramon Cancino, MD, MSc

KEYWORDS

• Inner city • Population • Disparities • Primary care • Cancer

KEY POINTS

- Inner-city patient populations are at high risk for poor outcomes, including increased risk of mortality.
- Barriers to delivering high-quality primary care to inner-city patients include lack of access, poor distribution of primary care providers, competing demands, and financial restraints.
- Health care issues prevalent in this population include obesity, diabetes, cancer screening, asthma, infectious diseases, and obstetric and prenatal care.
- Population health management and quality improvement activities must target disparities in care.
- Partnering with patients and focusing on social determinants of health and medical care are key areas in which to focus to improve overall health outcomes in this population.

The gap between rich and poor continues to widen. According to the Bureau of Labor Statistics, the minimum amount of income the top 10% of full-time wage and salary workers earned was nearly four times as much as what the lowest 10% earned in 1979; this ratio increased to five times by 2014.[1]

Inner-city populations are affected by this gap. The Urban Health Penalty is the observation that "inner city residents suffer the same chronic conditions as people everywhere, but that their situations are made worse by poverty, poor housing conditions, unemployment and other socioeconomic problems."[2] Delivering high-quality primary care to inner-city patients is important and challenging.

PRIMARY CARE IN INNER CITIES

The definition of "primary care" varies, but its principles remain consistent. The World Health Organization (WHO) defines primary care as first-contact, accessible,

Disclosure Statement: The author has nothing to disclose.
Department of Family Medicine, Boston University School of Medicine, 1 BMC Place, Boston, MA 02118, USA
E-mail address: ramon.cancino@gmail.com

Prim Care Clin Office Pract 44 (2017) 21–32
http://dx.doi.org/10.1016/j.pop.2016.09.004
0095-4543/17/© 2016 Elsevier Inc. All rights reserved.

continued, comprehensive, and coordinated care.[3] Other descriptions build on this description adding emphasis on partnership,[4] disease prevention, advocacy,[5] and involvement of family and community, along with the patient.[6]

Inner-cities are usually older densely occupied, deteriorating, and populated by poor, often minority, groups. The Initiative for a Competitive Inner City defines inner-city as a geographic area that has a poverty rate of 20% or higher or a poverty rate of 1.5 times higher than the metropolitan statistical area and an unemployment rate of 1.5 the metropolitan statistical area and/or a median household income of 50% or less than the metropolitan statistical area.[7]

In the United States, about 25% of inner-city inhabitants are middle class, whereas roughly 60% are working class or working poor.[8] Poverty rates for African American and Hispanic populations living in inner-cities can be four to five times that of suburban rates. Disparities exist within cities. One study found 17.5% of inner-city residents were poor compared with 9.1% in other urban areas.[9]

Challenges to delivering primary care to the inner-city include the following:

1. Racism: 16% of whites, 35% of blacks, and 30% of Latinos believe racism in health care is a major problem.[10]
2. Low literacy: 12% to 28% of those ages 16 to 24 are out of school and chronically out of work.[8] Low health literacy contributes to misunderstanding of physician instructions, adherence, and becoming lost to follow-up.[11–13]
3. Competing demands: Personal challenges and economic factors, such as taking time off work, finding child care, and transportation, make accessing care challenging, even when available.[14]
4. Lack of physician resources: Inner-city physicians note financial barriers affect ability to provide medications, equipment, training, and patient education.[15]
5. Poor access:
   a. One in four inner-city residents did not have health insurance as of 2012.[16]
   b. Uninsured adults and those with Medicaid are less likely to get care as soon as wanted compared with adults with private insurance.[17]
   c. Pediatric patients with only Medicaid or Children's Health Insurance Program are less likely to get care as soon as wanted compared with children with any private insurance.[17]
   d. Provider-shortages compound the problem of access.[14] There are only 84 PCPs per 100,000 patients in urban areas.[18] Therefore, there exists a poor distribution of PCPs, which disproportionately affects inner-city areas.[19] In fact, inner-city communities require nearly 13,500 more physicians.[18]
   e. Distance to and long waits contribute to patients' avoidance of care.[14]

The most common health needs facing the inner-cities are explored next. A PCP should be aware of these health issues.

OBESITY

Obesity, defined as body mass index of greater than or equal to 30.0 in adults and as gender-specific weight-for-length greater than or equal to 95th percentile in children, is linked to increased risk for diabetes,[20] cardiovascular disease,[21] cancer,[22] and mortality.[23] Among adults, obesity prevalence increased from 13% to 32% between the 1960s and 2004.

There is an association between urban sprawl and obesity.[24] The inner-city prevalence of overweight and obesity is 21.7% and 22.5%, respectively.[25] Inner-city minority and low-socioeconomic-status groups are disproportionately affected at all ages.

Eleven percent to 16% of inner-city children and adolescents are overweight, and 34% are at risk of overweight.[26,27]

In the inner cities, fresh produce is unavailable or expensive. Inhabitants have less access to safe settings for exercise, increased reliance on television for entertainment of adults and children, easy access to fast-food vendors, and economic pressures limiting time for family meals at home. Children in inner-city schools rely on high fat–high carbohydrate foodstuffs in lunch programs at the same time that school budget cuts often reduce or eliminate physical education programs.[28–30]

DIABETES

The Centers for Disease Control and Prevention estimates 29.1 million people in the United States have diabetes. Of these people, 8.1 million are undiagnosed.[31] A total of 24% of patients admitted to an inner-city hospital were found to have undiagnosed diabetes, so the prevalence of diabetes and of people with diabetic complications may be higher in the inner city.[32] One study demonstrated 33.6% of inner-city patients had diabetic retinopathy.[33]

PCPs should address barriers to adherence among inner-city patients with diabetes. Inner-city inhabitants have poor access to healthy food and safe exercise areas. As many as one in six inner-city inhabitants have a drinking problem.[34] Alcohol intake is associated with poor adherence to recommendations for self-care behaviors among inner-city patients with diabetes.[35] The WHO estimates adherence to long-term therapies is as low as 50% in the developing world, and far lower in less developed countries.[36] Overall, diabetes medication adherence ranges from 25% to 40%.[37,38] Poor adherence to insulin therapy is the leading cause of recurrent diabetic ketoacidosis in inner-city patients.[39]

ASTHMA

The overall US prevalence of asthma is 7.0% in adults and 8.3% in children.[40] The prevalence is 10.9% for those adults and children living below 100% of federal poverty level.[40] The asthma prevalence rate in poor inner-city communities in the United States is twice the national prevalence rate.[41] Those living in inner-city environments experience higher asthma-related morbidity and mortality.[42,43] Furthermore, hospitalization rates for asthma are highest in inner-city neighborhoods. One cause of the increased hospitalizations is the lack of (high cost) inhaled anti-inflammatory medication.[44]

PCPs should address housing and environmental triggers in the asthma patient population. The inner-city housing environment plays a major role in the growing asthma burden in these areas. Environmental concerns include mold, rodent, cockroach, pet, and dust mite allergens.[45] Further contributing to asthma morbidity are the higher concentrations of air pollutant particulate matter and nitrogen dioxide, and secondhand smoke found in inner-city homes.[45,46]

CANCER SCREENING

Cancer screening is a complicated process, lending itself to risk of failure. Patients with low socioeconomic status have a disproportionally higher burden of gastrointestinal diseases (eg, colorectal cancer) that are commonly prevented, diagnosed, or treated with endoscopy.[47–49] Inner-city patients avoid attending appointments for invasive screening procedures. One study reported a nonattendance rate of 21% at an inner-city teaching hospital in London.[50] Another study at a large safety-net health care system found a 42% no-show rate.[51] Screening for other cancers, such as breast and cervical cancers, is also low in the inner-city.[52]

Previous studies have concluded language barriers,[53] socioeconomic status,[54] attitudes,[55] cost,[56] fear,[56] lack of knowledge,[57] and lack of insurance[58] contribute to lower screening rates. The PCP, therefore, plays an important role in communicating the importance of cancer screening and should develop systems to ensure proper patient education and follow-up of referrals and appointments.

HUMAN IMMUNODEFICIENCY VIRUS

There is an estimated 1.2 million persons aged 13 and older with human immunodeficiency virus (HIV) in the United States.[59] With a prevalence of 2.4%, low-income inner-city residents are at greater risk for HIV than those living above the poverty line.[60,61]

Drug use in the inner-city contributes to this problem. Crack cocaine users, and women who have sex in exchange for money or drugs, are at high risk for HIV infection. Drug use also promotes the indirect transmission of HIV via such sexual exchanges.[62] Advances in HIV treatment have had a positive impact on most risk groups in an HIV clinical setting,[63] and care and life expectancy have improved dramatically,[64] but these improvements have not been shared equally. Persons of low income strata have not benefitted from improvements.[65]

Infection rates are particularly high in the inner cities especially among African Americans,[66] persons below the poverty line,[67] and injection drug users.[68] Therefore, PCPs should standardize HIV screening, which can also decrease stigma. Furthermore, providers should develop therapeutic relationships with HIV-positive patients. In inner-city populations, challenges include access, retention in care, and adherence to treatment regimens.[65]

VIOLENCE

Violence is one of the leading causes of death in all parts of the world for ages 15 to 44.[69] Many large cities have a high prevalence of gang homicides and victims of gang homicides are often younger. Between 27% and 42% of victims are 15 to 19 years.[70] Between 50% and 96% of inner-city youth have been exposed to community violence, which is higher than other environments.[71,72]

Intimate partner violence (IPV), including rape and assault, affects 1.5 million women and 834,700 men in the United States annually.[73] Nearly 50% report experiencing IPV, with more than 18% reporting IPV during the previous year.[74] Inner-city single-mother households have increased risk of prolonged poverty, child abuse, and violence.[8]

PCPs to inner-city patients should speak to their patients about home and neighborhood safety, because the PCP may be the patient's only access to reliable advice.

MENTAL ILLNESS

In the United States 7.6% of persons 12 years of age and older self-reported depression in any 2-week period 2009 to 2012.[75] The same report showed that those living below the poverty level were nearly 2.5 times more likely to have depression than those at or above the level of poverty.

The inner-city environment plays a role. Community violence exposure increases risk of posttraumatic stress, aggression, and other mental health problems.[76,77] Other inner-city conditions that increase the prevalence of mental health conditions include being lower income and social class, especially among urban, predominantly ethnic minority youth.[78–80] In inner-cities, an association between depression, substance abuse, IPV, and HIV infection rates has been documented.[81]

The PCP should make screening for depression and substance abuse part of standard practice of the clinical examination. Doing so can help to decrease stigma around such diagnoses.

OTHER HEALTH ISSUES

Although overall smoking prevalence rates have declined over the past three decades,[82] prevalence rates for inner-city African Americans remain high (33%–54%). Prevalence in one inner-city is 60% in health care settings and 52% in housing developments.[83,84]

Homes painted between 1884 and 1978 can have high lead levels. There is no safe level of lead exposure and elevated levels result in lower scores in intelligence scales,[85] poor schooling outcomes,[86] and increased risk for antisocial and delinquent behavior.[87] Lead levels have been found to be higher in inner-city areas disproportionately affecting the children and minority populations.[88–90]

Obstetric outcomes are important markers of population health. Low birth weight (<2500 g) increases outcome of fetal and neonatal death, respiratory distress syndrome, blindness, deafness, and hydrocephaly. One inner-city population had a six-fold increase in the risk of low birthweight in association with financial problems.[91] Inner-city sub-Saharan Africa found a 10.2% incidence of low birth weight children.[92]

SOCIAL DETERMINANTS OF HEALTH MUST BE ADDRESSED BY PRIMARY CARE PROVIDERS

PCPs should be aware that clinical disease is not the only factor that can impact health. Issues that should be addressed include social determinants of health, which include stress, social exclusion, unemployment, social support, food, and transport.[93] Initiatives, such as that described in the report *Promoting Health Equity: A Resource to Help Communities Address Social Determinants of Health*, have given guidance to community health centers and organizations to address social determinants of health to improve outcomes.[94]

QUALITY IMPROVEMENT AND POPULATION HEALTH MANAGEMENT CAN HELP IMPROVE PATIENT OUTCOMES

The 2010 National Healthcare Disparities Report emphasizes the need for "improvements in quality and progress reducing disparities with respect to certain populations, including residents of inner-city areas." Awareness of disparities in inner-city health outcomes allows the PCP to focus care delivery. This is especially important with increasing momentum to tie financial reimbursement to quality of care delivered to patient populations.

Quality of care metrics can include diabetes control and cancer screening. Inner-city practices tie QI activities to quality metrics. Many inner-city practices form QI committees and teams to develop projects to improve quality of care. One method that is often used in QI activities is the Institute for Healthcare Improvement's Model for Improvement. Examples of projects include using measures as indicators of improvement in community health centers to show significant improvement in prevention and screening measures for chronic diseases, such as diabetes and asthma[95–97]; and focusing on communication, teamwork, process, and workflow to improve delivery of patient services.[98] Social determinants of health impact health care quality in the inner-city but is not often enough linked to QI activities.[99]

Inner-city PCPs can use quality metrics to target populations at risk for health care disparities and allocate resources to improve health. Targeted breast health navigators have been shown to improve outcomes in inner-city women.[100,101] Case management improved glycemic control, blood pressure, and cholesterol in a population of inner-city patients with diabetes.[102]

PARTNERSHIPS

An inner-city PCP should understand how partnerships with federal, state, and community-based organizations can facilitate delivery of services to patients. The National Center for Medical Legal Partnership has partnered with multiple entities to decrease housing violations, which are often tied to poor outcomes in inner-city pediatric asthma patients.[103] The South Bronx Asthma Partnership used asthma education and empowerment to work with patients and families in partnership with health care providers and community programs.[104] Navigation programs in inner-city hospitals have enhanced cancer treatment and education.[101,105] The WHO cites collaboration between primary care, community services, and specialty care as key to delivering care to these patients.[106]

As the name suggests, the PCP can be a patient's first contact with the health care system, but delivering high-quality primary care to inner-city patients is fraught with challenges. Poor access, mistrust, miscommunication, low health literacy, and competing priorities can result in poor outcomes for pediatric and adult inhabitants. These outcomes include increased risk of mortality, malignancy, and hospital utilization. Nevertheless, these sorts of outcomes highlight the important role PCPs play in using all tools available to identify, contact, and treat patients in this high-risk population. These outcomes also suggest the PCP's importance in providing comprehensive preventive care and in partnering with communities to educate patients of all ages on health-related topics. As care delivery models evolve, the PCP is entrusted to ensure that voice is given to inner-city populations such that these models decrease rather than magnify the disparities of care delivered to this population.

REFERENCES

1. A look at pay at the top, the bottom, and in between: Spotlight on statistics: U.S. Bureau of Labor Statistics. Available at: http://www.bls.gov/spotlight/2015/a-look-at-pay-at-the-top-the-bottom-and-in-between/home.htm. Accessed January 24, 2016.
2. Inner-city health care. American College of Physicians. Ann Intern Med 1997; 126(6):485–90.
3. Main terminology. 2016. Available at: http://www.euro.who.int/en/health-topics/Health-systems/primary-health-care/main-terminology. Accessed January 24, 2016.
4. Donaldson M, Yordy K, Vanselow N. Defining primary care: an interim report. Washington, DC: National Academies Press; 1994. Available at: http://www.nap.edu/catalog/9153. Accessed January 24, 2016.
5. American Academy of Family Physicians. Primary Care. AAFP's definition of primary care related terms and appropriate usage recommendations. Available at: http://www.aafp.org/about/policies/all/primary-care.html#use. Accessed February 15, 2016.
6. Starfield B, Shi L, Macinko J. Contribution of primary care to health systems and health. Milbank Q 2005;83(3):457–502.
7. In America's War on Poverty, Inner Cities Remain the Front Line | @icicorg. Available at: http://www.icic.org/connection/blog-entry/blog-in-americas-war-on-poverty-inner-cities-remain-the-front-line. Accessed March 12, 2016.

8. Patterson O. The real problem with America's inner cities. The New York Times 2015. Available at: http://www.nytimes.com/2015/05/10/opinion/sunday/the-real-problem-with-americas-inner-cities.html. Accessed March 13, 2016.
9. Weinberg D. Poverty estimates for places in the United States. Washington, DC: Center for Economic Studies, U.S. Census Bureau; 2005. Available at: https://ideas.repec.org/p/cen/wpaper/05-12.html. Accessed March 12, 2016.
10. Lillie-Blanton M, Brodie M, Rowland D, et al. Public perceptions race, ethnicity, and the health care system: public perceptions and experiences. Med Care Res Rev 2000;57(Suppl 1):218–35.
11. Beitler JJ, Chen AY, Jacobson K, et al. Health literacy and health care in an inner-city, total laryngectomy population. Am J Otolaryngol 2010;31(1):29–31.
12. Schillinger D, Piette J, Grumbach K, et al. Closing the loop: physician communication with diabetic patients who have low health literacy. Arch Intern Med 2003;163(1):83–90.
13. Paasche-Orlow MK, Riekert KA, Bilderback A, et al. Tailored education may reduce health literacy disparities in asthma self-management. Am J Respir Crit Care Med 2005;172(8):980–6.
14. Heaman MI, Sword W, Elliott L, et al. Barriers and facilitators related to use of prenatal care by inner-city women: perceptions of health care providers. BMC Pregnancy Childbirth 2015;15:2.
15. Lara M, Allen F, Lange L. Physician perceptions of barriers to care for inner-city Latino children with asthma. J Health Care Poor Underserved 1999;10(1):27–44.
16. Targeting inner cities will increase the Nation's Insured | @icicorg. Available at: http://www.icic.org/connection/blog-entry/blog-targeting-inner-cities-will-increase-the-nations-insured. Accessed March 27, 2016.
17. 2014 National Healthcare Quality & Disparities Report. 2015. Available at: http://www.ahrq.gov/research/findings/nhqrdr/nhqdr14/index.html. Accessed February 15, 2016.
18. Graham Center Policy One-Pagers: Unequal distribution of the U.S. primary care workforce - American Family Physician. Available at: http://www.aafp.org/afp/2013/0601/od1.html. Accessed March 13, 2016.
19. Reynolds PP. A legislative history of federal assistance for health professions training in primary care medicine and dentistry in the United States, 1963-2008. Acad Med 2008;83(11):1004–14.
20. Egede LE, Zheng D. Modifiable cardiovascular risk factors in adults with diabetes: prevalence and missed opportunities for physician counseling. Arch Intern Med 2002;162(4):427–33.
21. Wang G, Zheng ZJ, Heath G, et al. Economic burden of cardiovascular disease associated with excess body weight in U.S. adults. Am J Prev Med 2002;23(1):1–6.
22. Bhaskaran K, Douglas I, Forbes H, et al. Body-mass index and risk of 22 specific cancers: a population-based cohort study of 5·24 million UK adults. Lancet 2014;384(9945):755–65.
23. Calle EE, Thun MJ, Petrelli JM, et al. Body-mass index and mortality in a prospective cohort of U.S. adults. N Engl J Med 1999;341(15):1097–105.
24. Lopez R. Urban sprawl and risk for being overweight or obese. Am J Public Health 2004;94(9):1574–9. Available at: http://www.ncbi.nlm.nih.gov/pmc/articles/PMC1448496/. Accessed January 25, 2016.
25. Isasi C, Whiffen A, Campbell E, et al. High prevalence of obesity among inner-city adolescent boy in the Bronx, New York: forgetting out boys. Prev Chronic

Dis 2011;8(1):A23. Available at: http://www.cdc.gov/pcd/issues/2011/jan/10_
0009.htm. Accessed January 25, 2016.

26. Wang Y, Beydoun MA. The obesity epidemic in the United States—gender, age, socioeconomic, racial/ethnic, and geographic characteristics: a systematic review and meta-regression analysis. Epidemiol Rev 2007;29(1):6–28.

27. Pan L, May AL, Wethington H, et al. Incidence of obesity among young US children living in low-income families, 2008–2011. Pediatrics 2013;132(6):1006–13.

28. Lopez RP, Hynes HP. Obesity, physical activity, and the urban environment: public health research needs. Environ Health 2006;5:25.

29. Leyden KM. Social capital and the built environment: the importance of walkable neighborhoods. Am J Public Health 2003;93(9):1546–51.

30. Candib LM. Obesity and diabetes in vulnerable populations: reflection on proximal and distal causes. Ann Fam Med 2007;5(6):547–56.

31. 2014 Statistics Report | Data & Statistics | Diabetes | CDC. Available at: http://www.cdc.gov/diabetes/data/statistics/2014statisticsreport.html.   Accessed January 25, 2016.

32. Weijers RN, Bekedam DJ, Oosting H. The prevalence of type 2 diabetes and gestational diabetes mellitus in an inner city multi-ethnic population. Eur J Epidemiol 1998;14(7):693–9.

33. Broadbent DM, Scott JA, Vora JP, et al. Prevalence of diabetic eye disease in an inner city population: the Liverpool Diabetic Eye Study. Eye (Lond) 1999;13(Pt 2):160–5.

34. Simon DDG, Eley JW, Greenberg RS, et al. A survey of alcohol use in an inner-city ambulatory care setting. J Gen Intern Med 1991;6(4):295–8.

35. Johnson KH, Bazargan M, Bing EG. Alcohol consumption and compliance among inner-city minority patients with type 2 diabetes mellitus. Arch Fam Med 2000;9(10):964–70.

36. Geest SD, Sabaté E. Adherence to long-term therapies: evidence for action. Eur J Cardiovasc Nurs 2003;2(4):323.

37. Feldman BS, Cohen-Stavi CJ, Leibowitz M, et al. Defining the role of medication adherence in poor glycemic control among a general adult population with diabetes. PLoS One 2014;9(9):e108145.

38. Cramer JA. A systematic review of adherence with medications for diabetes. Diabetes Care 2004;27(5):1218–24.

39. Randall L, Begovic J, Hudson M, et al. Recurrent diabetic ketoacidosis in inner-city minority patients behavioral, socioeconomic, and psychosocial factors. Diabetes Care 2011;34(9):1891–6.

40. CDC - Asthma - Most Recent asthma data. Available at: http://www.cdc.gov/asthma/most_recent_data.htm. Accessed February 6, 2016.

41. Crain EF, Weiss KB, Bijur PE, et al. An estimate of the prevalence of asthma and wheezing among inner-city children. Pediatrics 1994;94(3):356–62.

42. Bryant-Stephens T. Asthma disparities in urban environments. J Allergy Clin Immunol 2009;123(6):1199–206 [quiz: 1207–8].

43. Gold DR, Wright R. Population disparities in asthma. Annu Rev Public Health 2005;26(1):89–113.

44. Gottlieb DJ, Beiser AS, O'Connor GT. Poverty, race, and medication use are correlates of asthma hospitalization rates. A small area analysis in Boston. Chest 1995;108(1):28–35.

45. Matsui EC, Hansel NN, McCormack MC, et al. Asthma in the inner city and the indoor environment. Immunol Allergy Clin North Am 2008;28(3):665–86.

46. Thorne PS, Kulhánková K, Yin M, et al. Endotoxin exposure is a risk factor for asthma: the national survey of endotoxin in United States housing. Am J Respir Crit Care Med 2005;172(11):1371–7.

47. Jemal A, Siegel R, Xu J, et al. Cancer statistics, 2010. CA Cancer J Clin 2010; 60(5):277–300.

48. Kinsey T, Jemal A, Liff J, et al. Secular trends in mortality from common cancers in the United States by educational attainment, 1993–2001. J Natl Cancer Inst 2008;100(14):1003–12.

49. Siegel RL, Jemal A, Thun MJ, et al. Trends in the incidence of colorectal cancer in relation to county-level poverty among blacks and whites. J Natl Med Assoc 2008;100(12):1441–4.

50. Corfield L, Schizas A, Williams A, et al. Non-attendance at the colorectal clinic: a prospective audit. Ann R Coll Surg Engl 2008;90(5):377–80.

51. Kazarian ES, Carreira FS, Toribara NW, et al. Colonoscopy completion in a large safety net health care system. Clin Gastroenterol Hepatol 2008;6(4):438–42.

52. Collins KS, Hall AG, Neuhaus C, et al. US minority health: A chartbook. 1999. Available at: http://www.commonwealthfund.org/~/media/files/publications/chartbook/1999/may/u-s-minority-health-a-chartbook/collins_usminority-pdf.pdf. Accessed March 13, 2016.

53. Green AR, Peters-Lewis A, Percac-Lima S, et al. Barriers to screening colonoscopy for low-income Latino and white patients in an urban community health center. J Gen Intern Med 2008;23(6):834–40.

54. Baquet CR, Horm JW, Gibbs T, et al. Socioeconomic factors and cancer incidence among blacks and whites. J Natl Cancer Inst 1991;83(8):551–7.

55. Chavez LR, Hubbell FA, Mishra SI, et al. The influence of fatalism on self-reported use of Papanicolaou smears. Am J Prev Med 1997;13(6):418–24.

56. Jennings K. Getting a Pap smear: focus group responses of African American and Latina women. Oncol Nurs Forum 1997;24(5):827–35. Available at: http://europepmc.org/abstract/med/9201736. Accessed February 7, 2016.

57. Meissner HI, Potosky AL, Convissor R. How sources of health information relate to knowledge and use of cancer screening exams. J Community Health 1992; 17(3):153–65.

58. Jennings-Dozier K, Lawrence D. Sociodemographic predictors of adherence to annual cervical cancer screening in minority women. Cancer Nurs 2000;23(5): 350–6 [quiz: 357–8].

59. Prevalence of diagnosed and undiagnosed HIV infection—United States, 2008–2012. Available at: http://www.cdc.gov/mmwr/preview/mmwrhtml/mm6424a2.htm?s_cid=mm6424a2_e. Accessed May 3, 2016.

60. Dinenno EA, Oster AM, Sionean C, et al. Piloting a system for behavioral surveillance among heterosexuals at increased risk of HIV in the United States. Open AIDS J 2012;6:169–76.

61. Raj A, Bowleg L. Heterosexual risk for HIV among black men in the United States: A call to action against a neglected crisis in black communities. Am J Mens Health 2012;6(3):178–81.

62. Edlin BR, Irwin KL, Faruque S, et al. Intersecting epidemics: crack cocaine use and HIV infection among inner-city young adults. N Engl J Med 1994;331(21): 1422–7.

63. Moore RD, Keruly JC, Bartlett JG. Improvement in the health of HIV-infected persons in care: reducing disparities. Clin Infect Dis 2012;55(9):1242–51.

64. van Sighem A, Gras L, Reiss P, et al. Life expectancy of recently diagnosed asymptomatic HIV-infected patients approaches that of uninfected individuals. AIDS 2010;24(10):1527–35.

65. Centers for Disease Control and Prevention (CDC). CDC health disparities and inequalities report—United States, 2011. MMWR Morb Mortal Wkly Rep Suppl 2011;60(Suppl):1–124.

66. Hall HI, Hughes D, Dean HD, et al, Centers for Disease Control and Prevention (CDC). HIV infection—United States, 2005 and 2008. MMWR Morb Mortal Wkly Rep Suppl 2011;60(Suppl):87–9.

67. Song R, Hall HI, Harrison KM, et al. Identifying the impact of social determinants of health on disease rates using correlation analysis of area-based summary information. Public Health Rep 2011;126(Suppl 3):70–80.

68. Centers for Disease Control and Prevention (CDC). HIV infection among injection-drug users—34 states, 2004-2007. MMWR Morb Mortal Wkly Rep 2009;58(46):1291–5.

69. Krug EG, Mercy JA, Dahlberg LL, et al. The world report on violence and health. Lancet 2002;360(9339):1083–8.

70. Gang homicides—five U.S. Cities, 2003–2008. Available at: http://www.cdc.gov/mmwr/preview/mmwrhtml/mm6103a2.htm. Accessed May 4, 2016.

71. Zimmerman GM, Messner SF. Individual, family background, and contextual explanations of racial and ethnic disparities in youths' exposure to violence. Am J Public Health 2013;103(3):435–42.

72. Gibson CL, Morris SZ, Beaver KM. Secondary exposure to violence during childhood and adolescence: does neighborhood context matter? Justice Q 2009;26(1):30–57.

73. Tjaden P, Thoennes N. Full report of the prevalence, incidence, and consequences of violence against women: findings from the National Violence Against Women Survey. Washington, DC: U.S. Department of Justice, Office of Justice Programs, National Institute of Justice; 2000. Available at: https://www.google.com/search?q=Tjaden+PG%2C+Thoennes+N.+Full+Report+of+the+Prevalence%2C+Incidence%2C+and+Consequences+of+Violence+Against+Women%3A+Findings+from+the+National+Violence+Against+Women+Survey.+Washington%2C+DC%3A+U.S.+Dept.+of+Justice%2C+Office+of+Justice+Programs%2C+National+Institute+of+Justice%3B+2000.&oq=Tjaden+PG%2C+Thoennes+N.+Full+Report+of+the+Prevalence%2C+Incidence%2C+and+Consequences+of+Violence+Against+Women%3A+Findings+from+the+National+Violence+Against+Women+Survey.+Washington%2C+DC%3A+U.S.+Dept.+of+Justice%2C+Office+of+Justice+Programs%2C+National+Institute+of+Justice%3B+2000.&aqs=chrome..69i57.193j0j4&sourceid=chrome&ie=UTF-8. Accessed May 4, 2016.

74. El-Bassel N, Gilbert L, Witte S, et al. Intimate partner violence and substance abuse among minority women receiving care from an inner-city emergency department. Womens Health Issues 2003;13(1):16–22.

75. Pratt LA, Brody DJ. Depression in the US household population, 2009–2012. NCHS Data Brief 2014;(172):1–8. Available at: http://198.246.124.22/nchs/data/databriefs/db172.pdf. Accessed March 12, 2016.

76. McDonald CC, Richmond TR. The relationship between community violence exposure and mental health symptoms in urban adolescents. J Psychiatr Ment Health Nurs 2008;15(10):833–49.

77. Pastore DR, Fisher M, Friedman SB. Violence and mental health problems among urban high school students. J Adolesc Health 1996;18(5):320–4.

78. Brooks-Gunn J, Duncan GJ. The effects of poverty on children. Future Child 1997;7(2):55–71.
79. McLoyd VC. Socioeconomic disadvantage and child development. Am Psychol 1998;53(2):185–204.
80. McLeod JD, Shanahan MJ. Trajectories of poverty and children's mental health. J Health Soc Behav 1996;37(3):207–20.
81. Oldenburg CE, Perez-Brumer AG, Reisner SL. Poverty matters: contextualizing the syndemic condition of psychological factors and newly diagnosed HIV infection in the United States. AIDS 2014;28(18):2763–9.
82. Giovino GA, Henningfield JE, Tomar SL, et al. Epidemiology of tobacco use and dependence. Epidemiol Rev 1995;17(1):48–65.
83. Ahluwalia JS, McNagny SE, Clark WS. Smoking cessation among inner-city African Americans using the nicotine transdermal patch. J Gen Intern Med 1998; 13(1):1–8.
84. Resnicow K, Futterman R, Weston RE, et al. Smoking prevalence in Harlem, New York. Am J Health Promot 1996;10(5):343–6.
85. Needleman HL, Gunnoe C, Leviton A, et al. Deficits in psychologic and classroom performance of children with elevated dentine lead levels. N Engl J Med 1979;300(13):689–95. Available at: http://www.nejm.org/doi/full/10.1056/NEJM197903293001301. Accessed March 13, 2016.
86. Fergusson DM, Horwood LJ, Lynskey MT. Early dentine lead levels and educational outcomes at 18 years. J Child Psychol Psychiatry 1997;38(4):471–8. Available at: http://onlinelibrary.wiley.com/doi/10.1111/j.1469-7610.1997.tb01532.x/abstract. Accessed March 13, 2016.
87. Needleman HL, Riess JA, Tobin MJ, et al. Bone lead levels and delinquent behavior. JAMA 1996;275(5):363–9. Available at: http://jama.jamanetwork.com/ARTICLE.ASPX?ARTICLEID=395592. Accessed March 13, 2016.
88. Mielke HW, Gonzales CR, Powell ET, et al. Environmental and health disparities in residential communities of New Orleans: the need for soil lead intervention to advance primary prevention. Environ Int 2013;51:73–81.
89. Mielke HW, Blake B, Burroughs S, et al. Urban lead levels in Minneapolis: the case of the Hmong children. Environ Res 1984;34(1):64–76. Available at: http://www.sciencedirect.com/science/article/pii/0013935184900768. Accessed March 13, 2016.
90. Mielke HW, Anderson JC, Berry KJ, et al. Lead concentrations in inner-city soils as a factor in the child lead problem. Am J Public Health 1983;73(12):1366–9.
91. Binsacca DB, Ellis J, Martin DG, et al. Factors associated with low birthweight in an inner-city population: the role of financial problems. Am J Public Health 1987; 77(4):505–6. Available at: http://ajph.aphapublications.org/doi/abs/10.2105/AJPH.77.4.505. Accessed March 13, 2016.
92. Olusanya BO, Ofovwe GE. Predictors of preterm births and low birthweight in an inner-city hospital in sub-Saharan Africa. Matern Child Health J 2010;14(6): 978–86.
93. Marmot M. Social determinants of health inequalities. Lancet 2005;365(9464): 1099–104.
94. Brennan Ramirez L, Baker E, Metzler M. Promoting health equity: a resource to help communities address social determinants of health. Atlanta (GA): U.S.: Department of Health and Human Services; Centers for Disease Control and Prevention; 2008. Available at: http://www.cabdirect.org/abstracts/20103345471.html. Accessed March 13, 2016.

95. Landon BE, Hicks LS, O'Malley AJ, et al. Improving the management of chronic disease at community health centers. N Engl J Med 2007;356(9):921–34.

96. Woods ER, Bhaumik U, Sommer SJ, et al. Community Asthma Initiative: evaluation of a quality improvement program for comprehensive asthma care. Pediatrics 2012;129(3):465–72.

97. Sequist TD, Adams A, Zhang F, et al. Effect of quality improvement on racial disparities in diabetes care. Arch Intern Med 2006;166(6):675–81.

98. Taylor CR, Hepworth JT, Buerhaus PI, et al. Effect of crew resource management on diabetes care and patient outcomes in an inner-city primary care clinic. Qual Saf Health Care 2007;16(4):244–7.

99. Fiscella K, Franks P, Gold MR, et al. Inequality in quality: addressing socioeconomic, racial, and ethnic disparities in health care. JAMA 2000;283(19):2579–84. Available at: http://jama.jamanetwork.com/article.aspx?articleid=192714. Accessed March 12, 2016.

100. Battaglia TA, Roloff K, Posner MA, et al. Improving follow-up to abnormal breast cancer screening in an urban population. Cancer 2007;109(S2):359–67.

101. Phillips C, Rothstein J, Beaver K, et al. Patient navigation to increase mammography screening among inner city women. J Gen Intern Med 2011;26(2):123–9.

102. Shea S, Weinstock RS, Starren J, et al. A randomized trial comparing telemedicine case management with usual care in older, ethnically diverse, medically underserved patients with diabetes mellitus. J Am Med Inform Assoc 2006; 13(1):40–51.

103. Public/private partnership to address housing and health care for children with asthma. Health Affairs. Available at: http://healthaffairs.org/blog/2015/07/22/publicprivate-partnership-to-address-housing-and-health-care-for-children-with-asthma/. Accessed March 13, 2016.

104. NACI: South Bronx Asthma Partnership works to empower health care providers and parents of asthma patients. Available at: http://www.nhlbi.nih.gov/health-pro/resources/lung/naci/naci-in-action/south-bronx.htm. Accessed March 13, 2016.

105. Robinson-White S, Conroy B, Slavish KH, et al. Patient navigation in breast cancer: a systematic review. Cancer Nurs 2010;33(2):127–40.

106. World Health Organization, World Organisation of National Colleges, Academies and Academic Associations of General Practitioners/Family Physicians, editors. Integrating mental health into primary care: a global perspective. Geneva (Switzerland): World Health Organization, Wonca; 2008.

Pediatric and Adolescent Issues in Underserved Populations

Neerav Desai, MD*, Mary Elizabeth Romano, MD, MPH

KEYWORDS

- LGBT youth • Foster/kinship care • Juvenile justice system • Refugee health
- Native American health

KEY POINTS

- Children and adolescents in underserved populations have unique health care needs.
- Resources are available for pediatric/adolescent providers to facilitate delivery of care to high-risk children/adolescents.
- Being aware of the health care issues in this underserved pediatric/adolescent population can ensure that preventive health care needs are met as well as screening for physical and mental health needs that require additional intervention.

INTRODUCTION

Children and adolescents in underserved populations experience health care disparities that are unique. These disparities include access to care, continuity of care, and confidentiality issues. This article reviews which groups are underserved, why they are underserved, and how pediatric providers can best care for them. The following pediatric populations are discussed:

- Inner city
- Rural
- American Indians and Alaskan Natives (AIAN)
- International refugees
- Lesbian/gay/bisexual/transgender/questioning/intersex (LGBT)
- Foster care/kinship care
- Juvenile detention
- Homeless

Disclosure: The authors have nothing to disclose.
Division of Adolescent Medicine & Young Adult Health, Monroe Carell Jr. Children's Hospital at Vanderbilt, Vanderbilt University Medical Center, One Hundred Oaks, 719 Thompson Lane, Suite 36300, Nashville, TN 37204, USA
* Corresponding author.
E-mail address: neerav.desai@vanderbilt.edu

Inner City Youth

Inner city areas are defined as the central section of an urbanized area in which poorer residents live, older housing structures exist, and there is the highest population density. In the United States, most inner city populations are nonwhite. Children in these areas are at higher risk for moderate to severe asthma, trauma and violence, lead poisoning, malnutrition (including obesity), psychiatric, and substance use disorders.[1] Higher rates of sexually transmitted infections (STIs) and pregnancies are also well documented in urban and inner city areas.[2]

Pediatric providers can use strategies to engage inner city youth to improve health care outcomes. They should promote the pediatric medical home model of care. This model ensures that acute visits, ongoing chronic care, sports physicals, and possibly behavioral health are managed in 1 location by the same providers who are closely familiar with each child's history. It engenders trust and cuts down on unnecessary tests and procedures usually done in retail-based or urgent care settings.[3] Another strategy is the development of school-based health centers. They augment access to care and with proper communication can fit into the medical home model of care.[4] School-based health centers have repeatedly been shown to reduce unnecessary pediatric emergency department visits and have improved quality of asthma care.[5]

Rural Pediatric Populations

Rural areas are defined as those not within a designated urban area.[6] Health care, schools, groceries, and other necessities are harder to access in these areas, presenting challenges to long-term health outcomes. Poverty rates and children and adolescents living in poverty are higher in rural areas and parental education levels are lower.[7]

Two vulnerable pediatric populations in rural areas are those that have special health care needs and those who need subspecialty care. Children with special health care needs are defined as having 1 or more of the following: limitations in performance ability, use of multiple prescription drugs, and requirement of specialized therapies or services.[7] In rural areas, they are less likely to be seen by a trained pediatric provider compared with their urban peers.[7] The data also show significant delays in access to therapists and dentists compared with their urban counterparts. Children in rural areas who need subspecialty care have the most difficulty accessing pediatrics-trained cardiologists, neurologists, gastroenterologists, and psychiatrists. Many of these families have the added burden of cost and time because they are forced to drive long distances to access specialists.

Health care systems must adapt to the disparity faced by rural children by incorporating new technology and promoting the medical home model. The increasing use of telemedicine in rural pediatrics has shown promise, especially in accessing subspecialty care.[8] The most pressing question related to implementation of telemedicine centers is the lack of standardized insurance reimbursements for these services. Moreover, according to the summary of the Pediatrician Workforce Policy Statement developed by the American Academy of Pediatrics (AAP): "More primary care pediatricians will be needed to care for the increasing number of children who have significant chronic health problems and who will require more medical and surgical care from pediatric physicians throughout their childhood. In addition, there will be an increased demand for general pediatricians" because, according to AAP, there is a "decrease in the number of family physicians providing care for children and the limited number of non-physician clinicians interested in pediatric careers."[9,10]

Native American Youth

AIAN youth are a well-studied underserved segment of the population, representing about 1% of all US children.[11] The key demographic contributors to health care disparity are emphasized in **Table 1**.[12]

The largest contributions to morbidity and mortality in AIAN youth are accidents and injuries. Data show that AIAN youth are involved in much higher rates of violent crimes, injuries, and accidents compared with the general population.[13] AIAN adolescents engage in more risk-taking behavior, including not wearing seatbelts, drinking and driving, and riding with someone who is impaired.[14]

The data focusing on physical health reveals much higher rates of obesity and dental caries, which could be affected by diet, education, and health care access.[15,16] The disparity in infant mortality and Sudden Infant Death Syndrome, and the lack of prenatal care compared with the general population, are also alarming. The AIAN community has 5 times the rate of fetal alcohol syndrome (FAS) compared with geographically similar nonnatives.[17] The burden of FAS is distributed across the entire childhood spectrum and affects adult caregivers as well.

Several mental health disparities exist between AIAN youth and their nonnative geographic peers. In one study in Appalachia, substance use was prevalent in 9% of Indian children compared with 3.8% of white children.[18] Perhaps the greatest disparity is seen in the suicide rates among AIAN youth, which are from 3 to 6 times greater than in their nonnative peers.[19,20]

Pediatric providers face a combination of these disparities and some barriers in working with AIAN children. One large barrier to engagement is the inherent distrust the Native American community has for government-backed initiatives, as mentioned in the Broken Promises Letter of Transmittal.[21] Another is a lack of funding for Indian Health Services, which in 2004 was allocated $1914 per patient per year (compared with $3803 per year spent on federal prisoners).[22] The best providers can integrate into the environment and understand which health care priorities and goals are most important to the community. In addition, culturally appropriate community and school-based education has been shown to be best adapted, as shown in health curriculums that prioritize Native American values.[23] In addition, and perhaps most importantly for pediatric providers, the role of the extended family and joint health care decision making is a key part of many Native American cultures.[24]

International Refugee Health in Pediatrics

The United States pediatric refugee population is a diverse group that varies greatly by region and city. Although the numbers vary, roughly 18,000 to 20,000 pediatric refugees are resettled to the United States every year.[25] Refugees and asylum seekers are distinct from immigrants because they have been forced to leave their countries of origin because of persecution or fear of persecution.[26] It may take up to 18 months

Table 1
Adult demographics for American Indians and Alaskan Natives that affect child health

	AIAN Adults (%)	General Population Adults (%)
Individuals below poverty	27	15.6
High school diploma	71	80
Bachelor's degree	11.5	24.4
Unemployment	14–35 (regional variation)	7

for refugee applications to be considered and approved, which results in a lag time of vulnerability.[27]

Refugee children are particularly vulnerable to inequalities in health care caused by several factors, including language and communication barriers, underinsured parents, and a complex maze of support services.[28] Pediatric providers should be aware that the most vulnerable time is between 8 and 24 months after resettlement, because of the lapse in family benefits, including stipends, vocational training, and health insurance, that occurs around 8 months after migration. Refugee families are generally undertrained in accessing school resources, health care facilities, insurance providers, and vocational prospects by the time their benefits expire.[28]

Some pediatric health care issues that have a higher prevalence in refugee patients are shown in **Box 1**.[29] Refugee children are at particularly high risk for violence in their places of origin and in refugee camps before resettlement, which predisposes them to physical and mental health issues. Providers should screen for these issues over multiple visits using culturally appropriate methods and suitable communication methods. **Box 2** provides resources for clinicians. Pediatric providers usually complete an initial domestic health assessment that is specific to each state and in conjunction with the refugee resettlement agency. Frontloading services and interventions for refugee children are recommended because of problems of access and availability.

Health Care for Lesbian, Gay, Bisexual, and Transgender Adolescents

According to Youth Risk Behavior Surveillance System (YRBS) 2011, 4.5% of 9th to 12th graders identify as LGBT and 4.5% report questioning their sexual/gender identity.[1] Health care disparities in the LGBT population are well documented.[30]

Box 1
Initial and ongoing screening for pediatric refugee health

Initial and ongoing health care issues in refugee children

Malnutrition

Micronutrient deficiencies

Immunization schedules

Parasitic diseases

Tuberculosis

STIs

Female genital cutting and mutilation

Dental problems

Lead screening

Emerging infectious diseases (Ebola, Zika)

Depression

Anxiety

Posttraumatic stress disorder

Rheumatic heart disease

Adapted from Seery T, Boswell H, Lara A. Caring for refugee children. Pediatr Rev 2015;36:323–38.

Box 2
Valuable resources for clinicians caring for refugee families

Ethnomed (Integrating cultural medicine into practice)
  http://ethnomed.org

Cultural Orientation Resource Center
  http://www.culturalorientation.net

BRYCS (Building Refugee Youth and Children's Services)
  http://www.brycs.org/publications/index.cfm

US Centers for Disease Control and Prevention (CDC) Refugee Health Profiles
  www.cdc.gov/immigrantrefugeehealth

Adapted from Seery T, Boswell H, Lara A. Caring for refugee children. Pediatr Rev 2015;36:323–38.

Healthy People 2010 included a companion document that outlined the need for more information about the health status of the LGBT population in order to document and address the factors that contribute to health disparities.[31] Healthy People 2020 used these data to create health goals specific to the disparities of the LGBT population.[32] These disparities include:

- LGBT youth are 2 to 3 times more likely to attempt suicide
- LGBT youth are more likely to be homeless
- Men having sex with men are at higher risk of human immunodeficiency virus (HIV) and other STIs
- Transgender individuals have a high prevalence of HIV/STIs, victimization, mental health issues, and suicide and are less likely to have health insurance than heterosexual or LGBT individuals
- LGBT populations have the highest rates of tobacco, alcohol, and other substance use[31]

Providers should identify LGBT adolescents and young adults and screen for risk and protective factors. LGBT youth must also contend with discrimination, limited social support, and limited contact with other LGBT adults. Providers should train all staff about LGBT health to create a safe clinical environment and should ensure confidentiality and proactively share these policies with patients and families, including when a breach of confidentiality is indicated. Laws vary by state and can be accessed at http://www.guttmacher.org/sections/adolescents.php.

LGBTI youth may be reluctant to use insurance for fear of disclosure to parents through explanation of benefits information. As a result, public clinics may be a preferred option and see a larger proportion of LGBT youth and young adults.

The HEADSSS (home, education/employment/eating, activities, drugs, sexuality, suicide/depression, safety) mnemonic is a useful interview tool to ensure that a thorough risk assessment is done, and this is outlined in **Table 2**.[33]

Pregnancy risk is an issue for all sexually active female patients. Teen pregnancy rates are higher in lesbian and bisexual youth than in heterosexual teens.[30] All sexually active adolescent girls should be counseled on contraceptive options and all sexually active adolescents should be educated on the use of emergency contraception.

STI screening should be done based on behaviors, not sexual orientation and gender identity. Specific STI screening and treatment guidelines are delineated by the US Centers for Disease Control and Prevention (CDC).[34] Providers should be aware and proactive about transgender youths' comfort and preferences for

Table 2	
HEADSSS psychosocial assessment tool	
H	Home: where do you live; with whom do you live; relationships at home; violence at home
E	Education: what grade are you in; school performance; changes in school performance; favorite subjects; future plans/goals; problems at school with bullying, suspension
	Employment: hours; effect on school performance
	Eating: history of dieting; concerns about weight/body; exercise habits
A	Activities: activities with friends; activities with families; extracurricular activities/sports; hobbies; television/media use
D	Drugs: tobacco, alcohol, or substance use; frequency of use; social use vs using alone; CRAFFT questionnaire if concerns for abuse
S	Sexuality: romantic relationships; interested in boys/girls/both; sexual activity (ask about types of sexual activity; have you ever used birth control; have you ever been pregnant; have you have had an STI or STI testing; is family aware of sexual activity or sexual/gender identity; safe sex practices)
S	Suicide/depression: are you more sad, irritable, or anxious than usual; do you have a lack of interest in activities or difficulty with sleep or energy; are you more isolated; any thoughts of killing yourself, hurting yourself or other; have you ever tried to kill yourself or hurt yourself?
S	Safety: seatbelt use; helmet/protective equipment use; texting and driving; ridden with someone who was impaired; exposure to violence at home, at school; history of physical or sexual abuse; bullying at school; cyber bullying; access to guns

Abbreviation: CRAFFT, car, relax, alone, forget, friends, trouble.
Adapted from Goldenring J RD. Getting into adolescent heads: An essential update. Contemp Pediatr 2004;21:64.

genitourinary examinations. Many clinics provide accessible, reliable, and accurate information through Web sites and pamphlets about sexual education for all youth, including LGBT youth.

According to the Substance Abuse and Mental Health Services Administration, substance abuse disorders among LGBT youth are almost double those of their heterosexual peers.[35] Substance use is linked to high-risk sexual behaviors, motor vehicle accidents, and suicide attempts, further putting LGBT youth at risk for morbidity and mortality. Referrals for treatment should be pursued aggressively.[34]

LGBT youth are also at risk for physical violence and bullying as documented by a 2013 report showing that:

- Among LGBT youth, 43% reported being victims of physical dating violence versus 29% of heterosexual youth
- Among LGBT youth, 59% reported emotional abuse versus 46% of heterosexual youth
- Transgender and female youth report the highest rates of victimization[36]

LGBT youth have higher rates of suicide attempts compared with their heterosexual peers.[31] The risk is further increased in LGBT youth who are homeless, in foster care, or in juvenile detention centers. Providers should screen LGBT youth for depression and suicidality, assessing social support and bullying issues and asking directly about suicidal ideation. They should also ask about acceptance by family. LGBT youth who experience parental rejection are more likely to experience negative health outcomes and have issues with depression, suicidality, and substance use.[31] Providers can work with patients and families to promote acceptance strategies and increase positive support.

Health Care in the Juvenile Justice System

Adolescents in the juvenile justice system are at risk, as shown in the 2010 Survey of Youth in Residential Placement:

- Among youth offenders in custody, 69% have some type of health care need
- Dental, vision, or hearing needs were reported by 37%
- More than one-quarter of those interviewed needed care for illness, injury, or some other health care need that was not listed[37]
- Adolescents with fetal alcohol spectrum disorder (FASD) are over-represented in the juvenile justice populations: 35% of adolescents 12 years of age or older with FASD have been incarcerated at some point[38]

Health issues in this population range from common problems that have been neglected, to consequences of exposure, to violence or poor living conditions and high-risk behaviors.

Health care services received while in detention may be affected by length of stay. On admission, all juveniles should be screened for medical or mental health problems requiring immediate attention. For those that are in custody for 7 days or longer, more comprehensive adolescent health services should be provided. Adolescents in juvenile detention typically receive fragmented medical care because of inconsistent living situations, being in custody or a detention facility, and frequent running away from their home environments.[39]

Immediate health issues that should be assessed and addressed appropriately include:

- Infectious diseases, such as tuberculosis, scabies, lice
- Substance use disorders that may result in withdrawal with abrupt cessation
- Psychiatric emergencies, such as suicidal or homicidal ideation
- Chronic medical problems that require continuation of daily medications

Comprehensive evaluation should include a medical assessment that addresses vision, hearing, and dental needs. These needs are more frequently reported as unmet compared with other health care issues.[37] Adolescents in juvenile detention should be assessed for a history of traumatic injuries. These youth report higher rates of interpersonal violence and have been found to have higher rates of traumatic brain injury.[40]

They also have higher rates of risky sexual activity and pregnancy than the general adolescent population.[37] A pelvic examination may be indicated in adolescent girls with genitourinary symptoms. Pregnancy testing should be done in all postmenarchal girls. When possible, contraception should be offered to all adolescent girls. Routine vaccines, including hepatitis A and B, meningitis, and human papilloma virus should also be completed. Adolescent vaccine recommendations as per the CDC are available at http://www.cdc.gov/vaccines/hcp/acip-recs.

All adolescents should have comprehensive mental health screening by a trained mental health professional because substance use and suicide attempts are reported at higher rates in juvenile detention.[39] This screening should be done on admission and as part of ongoing care, and includes:

- Initial assessment within 24 hours of admission
- Comprehensive assessment as soon as possible

- Accessing previous records from families, schools, mental health providers
- Rescreening as part of transition/release from custody
- Regular screenings during periods of confinement[39]

An evidence-based screening tool should be used. One such tool specifically developed for adolescents and young adults in juvenile detention is the Massachusetts Youth Screening Instrument Second Version (MAYSI-2).[41] MAYSI-2 is a 52-item self-reported questionnaire. It requires 10 minutes to complete and is not biased to age, ethnicity, or gender.

Health Care for Adolescents and Children in Foster Care

The number of children and adolescents (aged 0–21 years) living in foster and kinship care has decreased from its peak in 2002.[42] Almost 614,000 children, up to age 21 years, spent some time in foster care in 2013. In 2002 that number was approximately 814,000.[42] Kinship care is a term used to designate those who, by court order, are living with extended family and not their biological parents. More than 70% of children and adolescents in foster care have a documented history of abuse and greater than 80% have had significant exposure to violence. Health care issues in this group are often the result of inconsistent access to health care, previously chaotic home environments, and a history of trauma, which includes the placement into foster care. Health care providers also encounter barriers when providing care to this population, which includes limited access to medical history, poorly identified consent protocols, and limited resources. The AAP has detailed guidelines for the provision of medical care to children and adolescents in the foster care system.[42] Whenever possible, every effort should be made to establish a medical home for children and adolescents in foster care, including:

- Obtaining a copy of signed consents from the foster care agency
- Keeping consent paperwork as part of each child's permanent health record
- Maintaining contact information for each child's caseworker in the health record
- Providing a summary of the visit to the caseworker after each health care visit

The AAP recommends evaluation by a pediatric or adolescent provider within 72 hours of placement into foster care. This evaluation should be done sooner if there are concerns for acute needs or abuse. Three visits within the first 3 months of placement are recommended with more comprehensive evaluations occurring at 30 and 60 days. **Box 3** provides a comprehensive outline of these visits.[42]

Health Care for Homeless Youth and Adolescents

According to a 2013 report, 1 in 30 children in the United States are homeless, equating to approximately 2.5 million children.[43] Homelessness includes anyone who lacks a permanent residence, lives in a place that is not designed for human living (ie, car, park), lives in temporary living arrangements, or is in imminent risk of losing housing. Populations at risk for homelessness include parents who have a history of substance use, job loss, mental illness, previous military service, or a history of domestic violence and physical or sexual abuse.[44] Among adolescents, previous placement in foster care, school expulsion, and identifying as LGBT are all risk factors for homelessness.[44]

Box 3
Health care visits for youth and adolescents in foster/kindship care

Initial health visit (within 72 hours):

- Identify health conditions requiring immediate attention
  - Review health information
  - Review trauma history
  - Review of systems
  - Symptom-targeted examination
- Identify health/behavioral conditions relevant to placement decisions
  - Child abuse screen
    - Growth parameters, vital signs
    - Skin examination
    - External genitourinary examination
  - Developmental surveillance/screen
  - Mental health screen
    - Suicidality, homicidality
    - Exposure to violence
    - Substance use/abuse
    - History of violent behaviors
  - Sexual health screen
    - Pregnancy test
    - STI screening

Comprehensive health visit (within 30 days):

- Review available health information
  - Records from previous providers, caregivers if available
  - Immunization review
  - Complete physical examination
- Identify acute and chronic health conditions
  - Child abuse screen
  - Trauma screen
  - Mental health screen for mood/conduct disorders, suicidality, behavioral issues
- Health maintenance
  - School performance
  - Adolescent risk review (sexual history, substance use history)
- Develop an individualized treatment plan
  - Dental referral
  - Hearing and vision screening/referral
  - STI screening, contraceptive counseling
  - Mental health referral
  - Psychoeducational testing
  - Laboratory screening: complete blood count, lipid panel, lead level
  - Communicate with caseworker, schedule follow-up appointments

Comprehensive health visit (within 90 days):

- Identify acute and chronic health conditions
  - Growth parameters
  - Physical examination
- Assess ongoing stressors
  - Mental health screening
  - Interaction/relationship between child and foster parents
  - Assess for abuse/neglect
- Health maintenance
  - Update immunizations
  - Reassess school performance
  - Adolescent risk review

- Update treatment plan
  - Follow up on referrals and recommendations
  - Reviewed individualized education plan
  - Communicate with caseworker, schedule follow-up appointments

Adapted from Szilagyi MA, Rosen DS, Rubin D, et al. Health care issues for children and adolescents in foster care and kinship care. Pediatrics 2015;136:e1142–66.

Children who are homeless face significant health challenges, including complicated access to care, interrupted education, and trauma. Children and adolescents who are homeless may have chosen to leave home, but many are escaping abusive or neglectful homes or rejection because of sexual orientation or gender identity. Minors have the added barrier of lacking an adult caregiver, issues with consent, and lack of access to health insurance. An exact number of uninsured homeless youth is not available. Many homeless youth are eligible for state-funded insurance programs and eligibility has increased with the Affordable Care Act. A difficult application process and disconnectedness from family can make it difficult for youth to access these services.[45] Health care providers should work with community resources to facilitate access to and enrollment in health insurance programs.

A list of common health conditions with higher prevalence in homeless youth is provided in **Box 4**.[44] Providers should screen for housing insecurity and inquire about options for storing and securing medications. Providers should offer information about insurance enrollment and, if possible, provide an avenue for access. They can use the medical home model to alleviate the fragmentation of care. Practitioners should also be mindful of communication, transportation, and cost when developing a treatment plan. Providers can obtain state-specific statistics about the homeless population in their area in the State Report Card on Homelessness at www.homelesschildrenamerica.org. Pediatric providers can advocate for homeless youth by partnering with schools, community outreaches, and caseworkers to ensure continuity and coordination of care. State-specific laws are available from the National Association for the Education of Homeless Children and Youth at http://naehcy.org/sites/default/files/pdf/State%20by%20state%20overview.pdf.

Box 4
Common conditions in homeless youth

Infectious diseases (recurrent respiratory infections, infectious diarrhea)

Malnutrition (obesity and failure to thrive)

Dermatologic disease

Asthma

Poor dentition, dental caries

Mental health disorders

Substance use/abuse

Poor academic performance

SUMMARY

A variety of children and adolescents are underserved in the United States. What stands out are the common challenges each population faces, including access to care, poverty, marginalization, vulnerability, and issues of confidentiality. This article emphasizes the essential role that pediatric and adolescent providers play in the health care of these individuals by being informed and creating a welcoming and culturally appropriate environment.

REFERENCES

1. CDC Youth Risk Behavior Survey. 2011. Available at: www.cdc.gov/features/yrbs. Accessed February 26, 2016.
2. Kann L, Olsen EO, McManus T, et al. Sexual identity, sex of sexual contacts, and health-risk behaviors among students in grades 9-12–youth risk behavior surveillance, selected sites, United States, 2001-2009. MMWR Surveill Summ 2011; 60(7):1–133.
3. Committee on Practice and Ambulatory Medicine. AAP principles concerning retail-based clinics. Pediatrics 2014;133(3):e794–7.
4. Council on School Health. School-based health centers and pediatric practice. Pediatrics 2012;129(2):387–93.
5. Brindis CD, Klein J, Schlitt J, et al. School-based health centers: accessibility and accountability. J Adolesc Health 2003;32(6 Suppl):98–107.
6. What is rural? Available at: https://ric.nal.usda.gov/what-rural. Accessed February 26, 2016.
7. Skinner AC, Slifkin RT. Rural/urban differences in barriers to and burden of care for children with special health care needs. J Rural Health 2007;23(2):150–7.
8. Ray KN, Demirci JR, Bogen DL, et al. Optimizing telehealth strategies for subspecialty care: recommendations from rural pediatricians. Telemed J E Health 2015; 21(8):622–9.
9. Basco WT, Rimsza ME, Committee on Pediatric Workforce, et al. Pediatrician workforce policy statement. Pediatrics 2013;132(2):390–7.
10. Committee on Pediatric Workforce. Enhancing pediatric workforce diversity and providing culturally effective pediatric care: implications for practice, education, and policy making. Pediatrics 2013;132(4):e1105–16.
11. Flores G, Res CP. Technical report: racial and ethnic disparities in the health and health care of children. Pediatrics 2010;125(4):E979–1020.
12. US Census Bureau. We the people: American Indians and Alaska Natives in the United States.
13. Manson SM, Beals J, Klein SA, et al. Social epidemiology of trauma among two American Indian reservation populations. Am J Public Health 2005;95(5):851–9.
14. Blum RW, Harmon B, Harris L, et al. American Indian–Alaska Native youth health. JAMA 1992;267(12):1637–44.
15. Jackson MY. Height, weight, and body mass index of American Indian schoolchildren, 1990-1991. J Am Diet Assoc 1993;93(10):1136–40.
16. Jones C. Indian Health Service oral health survey of American Natives. Preface. J Public Health Dent 2000;60(Suppl 1):236–7.
17. May PA, Gossage JP. Estimating the prevalence of fetal alcohol syndrome. A summary. Alcohol Res Health 2001;25(3):159–67.
18. Costello EJ, Farmer EMZ, Angold A, et al. Psychiatric disorders among American Indian and white youth in Appalachia: The Great Smoky Mountains study. Am J Public Health 1997;87(5):827–32.

19. Harrop AR, Brant RF, Ghali WA, et al. Injury mortality rates in native and non-native children: a population-based study. Public Health Rep 2007;122(3):339–46.

20. Wallace LJD, Patel R, Dellinger A. Injury mortality among American Indian and Alaska native children and youth - United States, 1989-1998. JAMA 2003; 290(12):1570–1.

21. US Commission on civil rights. Broken promises evaluating the Native American health care system. 2004. Available at: http://www.usccr.gov/pubs/nahealth/nabroken.pdf. Accessed February 26, 2016.

22. US Commission on Civil Rights. A quiet crisis: federal funding and unmet needs in Indian country. 2004. Available at: http://www.usccr.gov/pubs/na0703/na0204.pdf. Accessed February 26, 2016.

23. Stokes SM. Curriculum for Native American students: using Native American values. Read Teach 1997;50(7):576–84.

24. LaFromboise TD, Trimble JE, Mohatt GV. Counseling intervention and American Indian tradition: an integrative approach. In: Atkinson DR, Morian G, Sue DW, editors. Counseling American minorities. Madison (WI): Brown & Benchmark Publishers; 1993. p. 119–91.

25. Office of the United Nations High Commissioner for Refugees. Figures at a glance. Available at: http://www.unchr.org/pages/49c3646c11.html. Accessed February 26, 2016.

26. US Department of Homeland Security. Definition of terms. Available at: http://www.dhs.gov/definition-terms#17. Accessed February 26, 2016.

27. US Refugee Admissions Program FAQs. 2013. http://www.state.gov/j/prm/releases/factsheets/2013/210135.htm. Accessed February 26, 2016.

28. Mirza M, Luna R, Mathews B, et al. Barriers to healthcare access among refugees with disabilities and chronic health conditions resettled in the US Midwest. J Immigr Minor Health 2014;16(4):733–42.

29. Seery T, Boswell H, Lara A. Caring for refugee children. Pediatr Rev 2015;36(8): 323–38 [quiz: 339–40].

30. CDC Report. Available at: https://www.cdc.gov/lgbthealth/. Accessed February 26, 2016.

31. Gay and Lesbian Medical Association and LGBT health experts. Healthy People 2010 companion document for lesbian, gay, bisexual, and transgender (LGBT) health. Available at: http://www.glma.org/_data/n_0001/resources/live/Healthy CompanionDoc3.pdf. Accessed February 25, 2016.

32. Healthy People 2020. Available at: http://www.healthypeople.gov/2020/topics-objectives/topic/lesbian-gay-bisexual-and-transgender-health. Accessed February 25, 2016.

33. Goldenring J, Rosen D. Getting into adolescent heads: an essential update. Contemp Pediatr 2004;21(64):76–95.

34. CDC STD Treatment guidelines. 2015. Available at: http://www.cdc.gov/std/tg2015/screening-recommendations.htm. Accessed February 26, 2016.

35. Poirier JM, Francis KB, Fisher SK, et al. Practice brief 1: providing services and supports for youth who are lesbian, gay, bisexual, transgender, questioning, intersex, or two-spirit. 2008.

36. Dank M, Lachman P, Zweig JM, et al. Dating violence experiences of lesbian, gay, bisexual, and transgender youth. J Youth Adolesc 2014;43(5):846–57.

37. Office of Juvenile Justice and Delinquency Prevention. Youth's needs and services: findings from the survey of youth in residential placement. 2010. Available at: https://syrp.org/images/Youth_Needs_and_Services.pdf. Accessed February 26, 2016.

38. Office of Juvenile Justice and Delinquency Prevention. 2012. Available at: http://www.ojjdp.gov/newsletter/238981/sf_2.html. Accessed February 26, 2016.
39. Golzari M, Hunt SJ, Anoshiravani A. The health status of youth in juvenile detention facilities. J Adolesc Health 2006;38(6):776–82.
40. Committee on Adolescence. Health care for youth in the juvenile justice system. Pediatrics 2011;128(6):1219–35.
41. Penn JV, Thomas C. Practice parameter for the assessment and treatment of youth in juvenile detention and correctional facilities. J Am Acad Child Adolesc Psychiatry 2005;44(10):1085–98.
42. Council on Foster Care, Adoption, Kinship Care, Committee on Adolescence, Council on Early Childhood. Health care issues for children and adolescents in foster care and kinship care. Pediatrics 2015;136(4):e1131–40.
43. The National Center on Family Homelessness. America's youngest outcasts 2014: state report card on child homelessness. Available at: www.FamilyHomelessness.org. Accessed February 26, 2016.
44. Council on Community Pediatrics. Providing care for children and adolescents facing homelessness and housing insecurity. Pediatrics 2013;131(6):1206–10.
45. English A, Scott J, Park M. Implementing the Affordable Care Act: how much will it help vulnerable adolescents and young adults? Available at: http://nahic.ucsf.edu/wp-content/uploads/2014/01/VulnerablePopulations_IB_Final.pdf. Accessed February 26, 2016.

Women's Select Health Issues in Underserved Populations

Luz M. Fernandez, MD, Jonathan A. Becker, MD*

KEYWORDS

- Breast cancer • Cervical cancer • Contraception • Health care disparities
- Underserved women

KEY POINTS

- Health care disparities exist among populations with a lack of health care resources or poorer socioeconomic status.
- Barriers to health care include transportation, distrust of the health care system, lack of access to health care, and intimate partner issues.
- There is a lack of availability of cancer screening in poorer nations.
- Creating a needs assessment and using community resources are methods used to combat health care disparities in underserved women.
- Continuity of care and use of allied health professionals improve maternal-fetal outcomes.

INTRODUCTION

Care of the medically underserved presents unique challenges to health care providers. Underserved women lack or have limited access to health care. Combatting health care disparities requires a partnership between the community, its providers, and health care advocates for developing a needs assessment so that resources are used in an effective, efficient, and economically viable manner. Women are especially vulnerable to health care disparities in both industrialized and developing nations. The basis of this is multifactorial with poor socioeconomic status, lack of appropriate cancer screening, lack of reasonable transportation, and unequal gender roles all playing a part. The focus of this article is to outline the health care disparities in underserved women and present solutions to help bridge the health care gap.

The authors have nothing to disclose.
Department of Family and Geriatric Medicine, University of Louisville, Louisville, KY, USA
* Corresponding author. 201 Abraham Flexner Way, Suite 690, Louisville, KY 40202.
E-mail address: jon.becker@louisville.edu

Prim Care Clin Office Pract 44 (2017) 47–55
http://dx.doi.org/10.1016/j.pop.2016.09.008
0095-4543/17/© 2016 Elsevier Inc. All rights reserved.

CANCER SCREENING IN UNDERSERVED WOMEN

Cancer-related health disparities are defined by the National Cancer Institute as "adverse differences in cancer incidence cancer prevalence, cancer mortality, cancer survivorship, and burden of cancer or related health conditions that exist among specific population groups in the United States."[1] The disparity may exist due to age, disability, education, ethnicity, gender, geographic location, income, or race/ethnicity. Women who are uninsured or underinsured have higher incidence of cervical and breast cancers and a more advanced disease than the general population. In the United States, the most vulnerable groups include African Americans/blacks, Asian Americans, Hispanic/Latinos, Native Americans, Alaska Natives, and underserved whites.

CERVICAL CANCER SCREENING
Barriers to Access to Care: Transportation

Women in underserved populations are more vulnerable to cervical cancer than their counterparts due to barriers to access to care.[1,2] Few primary care clinics are situated to serve patients of lower socioeconomic status. Many of these women may not have personal vehicles for transportation, relying instead on friends and/or family or city/local buses for transportation to their clinics.[1] They may arrive late to their office visits due to late buses. Some patients may rely on transportation provided by their insurance companies, which requires calling a specific company with whom the insurance company has a contract at least 3 days in advance of an appointment to arrange transportation.[3] Arriving late to an appointment may result in a lost appointment or the necessity of rescheduling. Repeated missed appointments may result in a patient being dismissed and discharged from the practice.[1–4]

In countries of lower socioeconomic status, reliable and timely transportation may not be available. Many villages in Africa are far from industrialized areas, without dependable transportation. Women may have to travel far distances on foot through treacherous terrain to seek medical care for themselves and their children.[5]

Distrust of the Medical Providers and System

Another barrier to care includes distrust of the medical providers and the medical system in general.[6] Underserved women may have had bad experiences with the health care system and with medical providers who may not be sensitive to their individual needs. They may have experienced refusal to be seen by a medical provider due to either lack of insurance.[6,7] Some may believe that they receive treatment that was less than optimal based on their race, gender, religion, or other factors.[1,2] African American patients may recall the history of experimentation on patients of color. Modern surgical gynecology, founded by J. Marion Sims, has a gruesome foundation in its use of female slaves as his experimental subjects.[8] Still others may recall the Tuskegee Experiment[9] (US Public Health Service 1932–1972). Hispanic/Latino women residing in the United States may not seek health care services so as to not be vulnerable to inquiry about immigration status and face possible deportation.[6]

Fear of Cancer

The data show that precancerous or cancerous lesions of the cervix (and those of the breast as well) are found at more advanced stages in underserved women than in their counterparts.[2,3] The fear of diagnosis of higher-grade lesions perpetuates the avoidance of preventive health care. Many women in this population delay preventive health maintenance and seek care only when they experience symptoms. Because most cervical cancer is asymptomatic until later stages, and the symptoms may be nonspecific, there may be a remarkable delay in care. Underserved women may not understand the importance of routine health maintenance, prevention, and promotion.[2,3]

Confusion over Newer Cervical Cancer Screening Guidelines

Newer guidelines for cervical cancer screening are confusing to patients and providers (**Table 1**).[10] The most recent guidelines issued by the US Preventive Services Task Force (USPSTF) in 2012 move away from yearly Papanicolaou (Pap) smears for women who have never had an abnormal Pap smear in favor of screening with liquid-based cytology and testing for human papillomavirus (HPV), the virus implicated in most cases of cervical dysplasia and cervical cancer (especially strains HPV 16 and HPV 18). Cytology and HPV status (positive for high-risk strains vs negative) guide the screening interval. Women with an abnormal Pap smear should be screened at more frequent intervals. Some underserved women have routine Pap smears only during pregnancy or postpartum period and may not understand the need for cervical cancer screening at other intervals.[10] **Table 1** lists cervical cancer screening guidelines based on age group. These guidelines assume an average-risk woman and do not apply to those with a history of higher-grade precancerous cervical lesions or cervical cancer or who are immunocompromised.

Test Discomfort

Some women delay having a Pap smear because the test is uncomfortable. The discomfort and potential embarrassment of the examination outweigh any perceived benefit of the test.[6,7]

Lack of Availability of Papanicolaou Tests

Many developing countries do not have access to Pap smears for routine cervical cancer screening.[5] Some of these developing nations use an acetic acid solution applied to the cervix of patients to try to indirectly detect the presence of HPV; areas that turn

Table 1			
Summary of US Preventive Services Task Force cervical cancer screening guidelines			
Age	Screening Guideline	Screening Interval	Strength of Recommendation
<21	Not indicated	Not indicated	D
21–29	Cytology	Every 3 y	A
30–65	Cytology alone	Every 3 y	A
30–65	Cytology + HPV DNA testing	Every 5 y if HPV negative	A
>65	Not indicated	Not indicated	D
Women post-hysterectomy with removal of cervix for benign reasons	Not indicated	Not indicated	D

Adapted from Moyer V. Screening for Cervical Cancer: US Preventive Services task force recommendation statement. Ann Intern Med 2012;156:882.

acetowhite are treated as HPV lesions without cytology, HPV DNA testing, or colposcopy with biopsy of suspicious lesions.[7,11,12] Many areas in developing countries do not have physicians to perform these tests. They rely on nurses, allied health care professionals, and/or lay individuals trained in cervical cancer screening and detection and perform the acetic acid crude testing both independently and, when available, under the guidance of a remote physician or other medical provider using telemedicine.[5,11–13]

Special Considerations

Certain cultural practices can make routine female health screenings more challenging. For example, female circumcision, which results in genital mutilation. may make pelvic examinations more difficult because there may be more difficulty inserting a speculum (or it may be impossible to insert a standard speculum) and the experience may be traumatic to the patient.[14,15] The introduction of DNA testing for the detection of higher-risk strains of HPV may help increase cervical cancer screening programs in underserved areas by making DNA swabs more widely available and at a more reasonable cost. DNA swabs could be self-administered by the patients under direction of a trained health care advocate.[16]

Sexual Assault

Sexual violence against women occurs in all countries and spans all socioeconomic statuses. In many countries, sexual assault is used as a form of torture and warfare. Some women are also sold into sexual slavery.[16–18] Women who are at very high risk for cervical dysplasia may not tolerate a pelvic examination. The use of a speculum may trigger flashbacks of sexual assault. Multiple visits with use of desensitization techniques may help patients tolerate the examination over time.[18,19]

SCREENING FOR BREAST CANCER

Breast cancer remains a leading cause of cancer-related death among women worldwide.[20] The highest rates of breast cancer deaths are in areas of lower socioeconomic status with more limited resources.[20–23] These countries may not have universal breast cancer screening programs. To combat this issue, the Breast Health Global Initiative has compiled evidence-based guidelines, which take into account the economic burden of breast cancer screening and treatment.[20–22]

Screening for breast cancer has similar barriers to access for care as cervical cancer screening. Developing countries may not have access to mammography; therefore, breast cancer is generally found at later stages than in countries with a robust breast cancer screening program.[20–22] Poorer countries may use guidelines that lean more heavily on a provider's clinical breast examination and defer mammogram or diagnostic ultrasound for those with abnormal clinical breast examinations. Diagnostic ultrasound may be more available in these countries and may be the test of choice when abnormalities are detected on clinical breast examination.[20–22] DNA testing for mutations that may place women into higher-risk categories for developing breast cancer (such as BRCA mutations) may not be readily available.[21,22] As a result, early breast cancer screening as well as procedures, such as prophylactic mastectomy, prophylactic oophorectomy, and colon cancer screening, may not be available to decrease their risk of developing breast cancer, ovarian cancer, or colon cancer.[20–22]

Some developing countries have not made breast cancer screening a public health priority. This is in part because these countries have a higher incidence of infectious diseases, which take priority in terms of resource allocation. According to the World Health Organization, guidelines for breast cancer screening and treatment are not readily feasible in poor or developing countries.[20,21] **Table 2** describes methods of breast cancer screening based on resource allocation.

Recent guidelines by the USPSTF rate teaching self-breast examinations as a category D (recommend against) recommendation and clinical breast examinations as a category I recommendation (insufficient to assess the additional benefits and harms of clinical breast examination beyond screening mammography in women 40 years or older).

These guidelines are aimed at trying to detect breast cancer at earlier stages because later stages require more intensive treatments and resource allocation. Based on needs assessments, resources for breast cancer screening are allocated to areas in which overall rates are higher.[20–22]

CONTRACEPTIVE CARE IN UNDERSERVED WOMEN

Women of lower socioeconomic status may not have access to contraceptives for many reasons beyond the transportation issues and distrust of the medical system (discussed previously).

Cost

Prior to the passing of the Affordable Care Act in the United States, long-term contraception was cost-prohibitive to many underserved women of lower socioeconomic status.[24,25] Long-acting reversible contraceptive methods, such as intrauterine devices and implantable hormonal contraceptives, are expensive methods that were not affordable to those without contraceptive coverage on their insurance plans.[26] In the United States, undocumented women immigrants do not have access to insurance, including state-sponsored plans, such as Medicaid.[24,25] Clinics not requiring insurance coverage or payment may not offer long-acting reversible contraceptives or lack the necessary supply.[24,25] Methods, such as oral contraceptive pills, hormone-containing vaginal ring, hormone-containing patch, and hormone injections, may also not be readily accessible to these women.[24,25]

Differences in Contraceptive Preferences and Contraceptive Acceptance

Certain contraceptive methods are more popular in some areas than in others. For example, in Latin America and Europe, the intrauterine device is widely accepted and used.[26–28] Select contraceptive methods that provide for a monthly period (such as oral contraceptive pills, hormone pills, and hormone vaginal rings) may be

Table 2
Methods for breast cancer screening based on resource allocation

Method	Resource Poor	Resource Plentiful
Patient education	+	+
Self-breast examinations	+	+
Clinical breast examination (performed by a provider)	+/−	+
Mammography	+/−	+
Diagnostic ultrasound	+	+

Adapted from Anderson BO, Shyyan R, Eniu A, et al. Breast cancer in limited-resource countries: an overview of the Breast Health Global Initiative 2005 Guidelines. Breast J 2006;12:S9.

preferable to some women who believe having regular menses provides reassurance that they are not pregnant.[27] Women may also prefer contraceptive methods they can use without the knowledge of their sexual partners due to social, cultural, and/or religious reasons. In some regions, women may have fear that a contraceptive device would be placed by a health care provider without their explicit informed consent. Moreover, in developing countries, there may be a precedent of experimentation on members of their population.[29–31] For example, the first clinical trials of oral contraceptive pills were performed in Puerto Rico without the explicit informed consent of women participating in the study. Likewise, several developing countries have been sites of forced sterilization. Certain groups in the United States, such as women with mental health disorders or cognitive and other impairments who were institutionalized in the past, were victims of forced sterilization.[29–31]

Perceived side effects of the various contraceptive methods are also a barrier to its use. For example, those who use the contraceptive hormone injections may experience a delay of up to 18 months after their last injection in regaining fertility and becoming pregnant.[26,27] **Table 3** describes potential side effects of contraceptives that may contribute to women's refusal of certain contraceptive methods.

INTIMATE PARTNER VIOLENCE

In the United States, intimate partner violence is prevalent in all socioeconomic groups.[17] Women experiencing physical, verbal, and/or sexual violence may experience fear and shame, which keep them from reporting the abuse to their medical providers.[17,18] Women in the United States who are of limited English proficiency may be unable to report abuses to their medical providers because interpretation of their office visits may be performed through their significant other and not a third party.[17–19] In many situations, even if a third party is present to provide medical interpretation,

Table 3 Potential side effects of contraceptive methods	
Intrauterine device, hormonal	Irregular bleeding/spotting Amenorrhea Weight gain Mood changes
Intrauterine device, copper	Increased menstrual cramping Increased menstrual flow
Hormone implant	Irregular bleeding/spotting Amenorrhea Weight gain Arm pain Mood changes
Hormone injection	Irregular bleeding/spotting Amenorrhea Weight gain Increased risk of osteopenia Delayed fertility on discontinuation Mood changes
Oral contraceptive pills	Weight gain Bloating Mood changes

the significant other may still be present for the entire medical encounter, and the patient may not feel able to recount a history of abuse. In some countries, it is socially acceptable for the male partner to use physical methods of discipline on his female partner.[17–19]

SPECIAL CONSIDERATIONS FOR MATERNAL-FETAL HEALTH

Many developing countries experience a higher rate of death during childbirth than industrialized nations, with the highest incidences in areas of Africa and Asia[32]; 90% of all maternal deaths and 80% of stillbirths are in countries that lack trained health care workers. Contributing factors to these deaths include poverty, poor overall health status, poor health literacy, lack of autonomy for medical decision making, lack of an adequately trained birth attendant, lack of an adequate referral system, inadequate transportation, and poor communication between health centers and communities.[32–34]

The programs that seem most successful in decreasing morbidity and mortality associated with pregnancy, childbirth, and the postpartum period are those that are community based.[32–34] Allied health care workers, such as midwives and volunteers, can educate women on proper care, nutrition, and vaccination (where available) during or after childbirth. Use of local, trained professionals helps increase adherence by eliminating patients' need to travel away from home for health care services.[34–36] It also helps lessen distrust in the medical providers and health care system to receive health information and care from one of their perceived peers. These workers are trained in a variety of skills that range from keeping the baby warm postdelivery and neonatal resuscitation to care of the umbilical cord stump and breastfeeding.[34–36] Studies have shown that the use of local health care advocates (described previously) helps increase breastfeeding rates for the mother and increase immunization rates in both mother and the infant.[32–34] Home visitation has also been shown to decrease antenatal hospital admissions and the rates of cesarean section births.[35–38]

In the United States, methods that have been studied to help in teenage pregnancy have included support via telephone calls, home visits, social support from friends and family, and continuity of care, such as same obstetric provider throughout the whole pregnancy, family doctor to handle prenatal care, postpartum care, and care of the infant; however, these methods have not been shown to have a statistically significant effect on infant mortality in that population.[39] Methods, such as mass media campaigns, community education, and outreach services, still lack data showing effectiveness.[39]

In industrialized, higher-income countries, the leading causes of deaths in infants are congenital anomalies, conditions related to premature birth, and sudden infant death syndrome/sudden or unexpected death in infancy.[37,38] Group antenatal visits are one intervention that may help decrease infant mortality. This is true of in both industrialized and developing countries.[38]

SUMMARY

Underserved women experience health care disparities in the United States and abroad, especially in the areas of cervical or breast cancer screening, and contraception. Additional factors relate to intimate partner violence and prenatal and postpartum care. Understanding these disparities and working with local resources within these communities are among the most promising interventions that will help health care providers and patients partner to reduce these gaps.

REFERENCES

1. Freeman HP, Wingrove BK. Excess cervical cancer mortality: a marker for low access to healthcare in poor communities. Rockville (MD): National Cancer Institute; Center to Reduce Cancer Health Disparities; 2005. NIH Pub. No. 05–5282.
2. Wharam JF, Zhang F, Xu X, et al. National trends and disparities in cervical cancer screening among commercially insured women, 2001–2010. Cancer Epidemiol Biomarkers Prev 2014;23:2366–73.
3. Health care financing administration. National Association of Medicaid Directors' Non-Emergency Transportation Technical Advisory Group. (1998, August). Designing and operating cost effective medicaid non-emergency transportation programs: a guidebook for state medicaid agencies. Available at: http://ntl.bts.gov/lib/12000/12200/12290/medicaid.pdf. Accesed July 17, 2015.
4. Hicks ML, Yap OW, Matthews R, et al. Disparities in cervical cancer screening, treatment and outcomes. Ethn Dis 2006;16:S3.
5. Haar EK, Vonder KK, Schust DJ. Adapting cervical dysplasia screening, treatment and prevention approaches to low resource settings. Int STD Res Rev 2013;1:38–48.
6. Johnson CE, Mues KE, Mayne SL, et al. Cervical cancer screening among immigrants and ethnic minorities:a systematic review using the health belief model. J Low Genit Tract Dis 2008;12:232–41.
7. Goldie SJ, Gaffikin L, Goldhaber-Fiebert J, et al. Cost-effectiveness of cervical-cancer screening in five developing countries. N Engl J Med 2005;353:2158–68.
8. Axelsen DE. Women as victims of medical experimentation: J. Marion Sims' surgery on slave women, 1845-1850. Sage 1985;2:10–3.
9. Green BL, Maisiak R, Wang MQ, et al. Participation in health education, health promotion, and health research by African Americans: effects of the Tuskegee Syphilis Experiment. J Health Educ 1997;28:196–201.
10. Moyer V. Screening for cervical cancer: US preventive services task force recommendation statement. Ann Intern Med 2012;156:880–91.
11. Murillo R, Almonte M, Pereira A, et al. Cervical cancer screening programs in Latin America and the Caribbean. Vaccine 2008;26(Suppl 11):L37–48.
12. Ditzian LR, David-West G, Maza M, et al. Cervical cancer screening in low-and middle-income countries. Mt Sinai J Med 2011;78:319–26.
13. Roger E, Nwosu O. Diagnosing cervical dysplasia using visual inspection of the cervix with acetic acid in a woman in rural Haiti. Int J Environ Res Public Health 2014;11:12304–11.
14. De Silva S. Obstetric sequelae of female circumcision. Eur J Obstet Gynecol Reprod Biol 1989;32:233–40.
15. Toubia N. Female circumcision as a public health issue. N Engl J Med 1994;331:712–6.
16. Dzuba IG, Díaz EY, Allen B, et al. The acceptability of self-collected samples for HPV testing vs. the pap test as alternatives in cervical cancer screening. J Womens Health Gend Based Med 2002;11:265–75.
17. Gandhi S, Rovi S, Vega M, et al. Intimate partner violence and cancer screening among urban minority women. J Am Board Fam Pract 2010;23:343–53.
18. Elliott L, Nerney M, Jones T, et al. Barriers to screening for domestic violence. J Gen Intern Med 2002;17:112–6.
19. McFarlane J, Malecha A, Watson K, et al. Intimate partner sexual assault against women: Frequency, health consequences, and treatment outcomes. Obstet Gynecol 2005;105:99–108.

20. Anderson BO, Shyyan R, Eniu A, et al. Breast cancer in limited-resource countries: an overview of the Breast Health Global Initiative 2005 Guidelines. Breast J 2006;12(Suppl 1):S3–15.
21. Anderson BO, Jakesz R. Breast cancer issues in developing countries: an overview of the Breast Health Global Initiative. World J Surg 2008;32:2578–85.
22. Coughlin SS, Ekwueme DU. Breast cancer as a global health concern. Cancer Epidemiol 2009;33:315–8.
23. Bray F, McCarron P, Parkin DM. The changing global patterns of female breast cancer incidence and mortality. Breast Cancer Res 2004;6:229–39.
24. Peipert JF, Madden T, Allsworth JE, et al. Preventing unintended pregnancies by providing no-cost contraception. Obstet Gynecol 2012;120:1291–7.
25. Burlone S, Edelman AB, Caughey AB, et al. Extending contraceptive coverage under the Affordable Care Act saves public funds. Contraception 2013;87:143–8.
26. Feyisetan B, Casterline JB. Fertility preferences and contraceptive change in developing countries. Int Fam Plan Perspect 2000;26:100–9.
27. Garcia SG, Snow R, Aitken I. Preferences for contraceptive attributes: voices of women in Ciudad Juárez, México. Int Fam Plan Perspect 1997;23:52–8.
28. Narzary PK, Sharma SM. Daughter preference and contraceptive-use in matrilineal tribal societies in Meghalaya, India. J Health Popul Nutr 2013;31:278–89.
29. Bruinius H. Better for all the world: the secret history of forced sterilization and America's quest for racial purity. New York: Vintage Books; 2007.
30. Briggs L. Discourses of forced sterilization in Puerto Rico: the problem with the speaking subaltern. Differences 1998;10:30–3.
31. Hyatt S. A shared history of shame: Sweden's four-decade policy of forced sterilization and the eugenics movement in the United States. Indiana Int Comp Law Rev 1998;8:475–503.
32. Hollowell J, Oakley L, Kurinczuk JJ, et al. The effectiveness of antenatal care programmes to reduce infant mortality and preterm birth in socially disadvantaged and vulnerable women in high-income countries: a systematic review. BMC Pregnancy Childbirth 2011;11:13.
33. Lassi ZS, Das JK, Salam RA, et al. Evidence from community level inputs to improve quality of care for maternal and newborn health: interventions and findings. Reprod Health 2014;11:S2.
34. Osrin D, Prost A. Perinatal interventions and survival in resource-poor settings: which work, which don't, which have the jury out? Arch Dis Child 2010;95:1039–46.
35. Kurinczuk JJ, Hollowell J, Brocklehurst P, et al. Inequalities in infant mortality project briefing paper 1. Infant Mortality: overview and context. Oxford (United Kingdom): National Perinatal Epidemiology Unit; 2009.
36. Callaghan WM, MacDorman MF, Rasmussen SA, et al. The contribution of preterm birth to infant mortality rates in the United States. Pediatrics 2006;118:1566–73.
37. Rosano A, Botto LD, Botting B, et al. Infant mortality and congenital anomalies from 1950 to 1994: an international perspective. J Epidemiol Community Health 2000;54:660–6.
38. Ickovics JR, Kershaw TS, Westdahl C, et al. Group prenatal care and preterm birth weight: results from a matched cohort study at public clinics. Obstet Gynecol 2003;102:1051–7.
39. Little M, Gorman A, Dzendoletas D, et al. Caring for the most vulnerable: a collaborative approach to supporting pregnant homeless youth. Nurs Womens Health 2007;11:458–66.

Medical Care of the Homeless

An American and International Issue

Sheryl B. Fleisch, MD[a], Robertson Nash, PhD, ACNP, BC[b],*

KEYWORDS

- Homelessness • Environment • Smoking • Diabetes mellitus • HIV • Dental
- Sexually transmitted infections • Cardiac disease

KEY POINTS

- Homeless persons die significantly younger than their housed counterparts.
- In many cases, relatively straightforward primary care issues (obesity, hypertension, diabetes mellitus, sexually transmitted infections, urinary tract infections, upper and lower respiratory infections, chronic obstructive pulmonary disease, depression, and poor dental hygiene) escalate into life-threatening, expensive emergencies.
- Poor health outcomes driven by negative interactions between comorbid symptoms meet the definition of a health syndemic in this population.
- Successful primary care of patients struggling with homelessness may result in long-term lifesaving measures along with decreased expenditure to hospital systems.
- This primary prevention requires patience, creativity, and acknowledgment that the source of many confounders may lay outside the control of these patients.

INTRODUCTION

Homeless persons die significantly younger than their housed counterparts.[1] In many cases, relatively straightforward primary care issues (obesity, hypertension, diabetes mellitus, sexually transmitted infections, urinary tract infections, upper and lower respiratory infections, chronic obstructive pulmonary disease [COPD], depression, and poor dental hygiene) escalate into life-threatening, expensive emergencies. The goal of this article is to provide the interested reader with insights gained from serving

Disclosure: The authors of this work report no direct financial interest in the subject matter or any material discussed in this article.
[a] Vanderbilt University School of Medicine, 2215 Garland Avenue, Light Hall, Nashville, TN 37232, USA; [b] Vanderbilt Comprehensive Care Clinic, Vanderbilt Health at One Hundred Oaks, 719 Thompson Lane, Suite 37189, Nashville, TN 37204, USA
* Corresponding author.
E-mail address: Robertson.nash@vanderbilt.edu

Prim Care Clin Office Pract 44 (2017) 57–65
http://dx.doi.org/10.1016/j.pop.2016.09.009
0095-4543/17/© 2016 Elsevier Inc. All rights reserved.

primarycare.theclinics.com

homeless patients, on the street and in shelters. The focus is to highlight factors that exacerbate diseases and complicate care. The authors also hope to provide readers with clinically proven methods to improve the lives of homeless patients.

ENVIRONMENT AS A HEALTH CHALLENGE
Pearl

The outside environment, where homeless people spend most of their time, is a risk factor and driver of poor health outcomes.

For individuals struggling with homelessness, the outside environment is where they will spend most of their time. The outdoors is where they work, sleep, socialize, and live out the functions of daily life. No matter whether hot, cold, raining, or snowing, they must learn how to survive in the environment that surrounds them. It is often this environment that becomes a risk factor and driver of poor outcomes because of exposure-related injuries.

Approximately 700 individuals experiencing homelessness or at risk of homelessness will die from hypothermia yearly in the United States.[2] Signs and symptoms of hypothermia include exhaustion, numbness, cold sensation, shivering, pale, or flushed skin, decreased hand coordination, slurred speech, and confusion.[3] Hypothermia can occur before extreme cold, especially when clothes are wet.

Frostbite, like hypothermia, is a medical emergency. Superficial frostbite often presents with tingling and numbness, whereas deep frostbite that has been present for a long time can present dark and gangrenous. Affected areas could require amputation and need to be checked for infection. It is critical that cities prepare for cold weather, including provision of emergency shelter beds. This includes admission of all homeless persons to shelters no matter their sobriety status or whether they have previously been banned.[4]

Just as cold weather poses significant risks, hot weather does as well. High humidity makes thermoregulation difficult because it is more challenging for sweat to evaporate. Heat cramps, heat exhaustion, and heat stroke are all potential risks, with heat stroke being the most serious. The person will often present with inability to sweat and become hot and dry. He or she may experience chest pain, shortness of breath, headache, abdominal pain, and confusion. This person will require cooling via any means necessary.[5]

Given that homeless persons frequently stay outdoors or within shelters, exposure to insect bites or parasitic infestations is 3 times higher than in the general population.[6] Homeless persons staying in shelters are at particular risk for exposure to scabies, lice, and bedbugs. Lice and scabies are highly contagious and can spread in the confines of close quarters. Spiders, mosquitoes, ticks, fleas, and ants may affect persons staying outdoors, so provision of repellant and proper tenting is important. It is critical to do a thorough history on exposure to insects, particularly those that are communicable, to provide the best medical care to homeless persons.[5]

In addition to weather-related hazards, there are challenges by virtue of simply living on the streets, including being the victim of physical and sexual crimes. From 1999 to 2013, the National Coalition for the Homeless documented 1437 acts of violence against homeless persons, including 375 acts that resulted in death. These acts of violence occurred in 47 states, Puerto Rico, and Washington, DC. Perpetrators were generally male, under 30 years old, and commonly teenagers. It is thought that these numbers are an underrepresentation of hate crimes against homeless persons. Additionally, in a racially diverse sample of homeless mothers, 92% reported experiencing severe physical and/or sexual violence at some point in their lives, with 43% reporting sexual abuse in childhood and 63% reporting intimate partner violence in adulthood.[7]

OCULAR CARE
Pearl

Decreased visual acuity, combined with lack of access to eyeglasses, increases the risk of trauma and sexual assaults in this population based on affected individual's impaired ability to safely avoid or navigate potentially dangerous situations.

Poor visual acuity is known to be correlated with reduced earning potential and reduced well-being.[8] In a study of 960 homeless adults, 41% reported an unmet need for eyeglasses,[9] with need for eyeglasses in homeless children ranging from 13% to 26%.[10] Studies done in both the United States[11] and Canada[12] show increased risk of ocular morbidity in homeless samples. Despite having access to universal health care, only 14% of homeless Canadian study participants reported visiting an ocular specialist in the last year versus 41% of the general population. Eighty-nine percent of participants stated that if ocular services were brought to them, they would use such services.[13]

The most common eye conditions in persons who are homeless are the same as those in the general population, including macular degeneration, cataracts, diabetic eye disease, glaucoma, dry eyes, and low vision. However, persons who are homeless and struggle with low visual acuity are at increased risk of traumatic injuries due to inability to see an intruder at a campsite or an oncoming vehicle. Poor eyesight can lead to inability to negotiate food and shelter, safe sexual practices, and employment. All of these can lead to further homelessness, criminalization, and victimization.

PULMONARY DISEASES
Pearl

Although smoking is recognized as a significant health threat, focusing on smoking cessation in marginalized populations may erode the therapeutic relationship that providers seek to build with their homeless patients.

According to data published by the Centers for Disease Control and Prevention (CDC), an estimated 900,000 Americans die prematurely every year from 5 causes of death: heart disease, cancer, stroke, lung disease, and unintentional injury. Smoking is implicated as a modifiable risk factor in 4 of these 5 preventable causes of death.[14] Although the overall prevalence of smoking in the United States is estimated at around 20%, the prevalence of smoking among those living below the federal poverty level in 2009 was around 31%.[15] Studies investigating the prevalence of smoking among homeless populations have documented prevalence rates as high as 80%.[16] In 1 study, investigators found rates of obstructive lung disease as high as 15% (95% CI 8%–26%) in a population of urban homeless.[17] A cluster analysis of 2733 homeless veterans found that 1 of 4 unique disease clusters was marked by elevated rates of cardiopulmonary disease, including COPD.[18]

These data beg the question of why smoking, an admittedly expensive habit, is so prevalent among the poorest members of the society. In 1 qualitative study regarding attitudes toward smoking in California family homeless shelters, participants reported that smokers associated relief from stress and boredom and higher levels of social inclusion with cigarette smoking.[19] Given the highly unpredictable and stressful environment of homelessness, it may not be unreasonable to view smoking as having more short-term benefit than long-term cost. Although smoking cessation education is considered a bedrock principle of primary care, in this population, advocacy of smoking cessation without appreciation for the larger content of homeless people's lives may actually erode versus enhance the therapeutic relationships on which all care rests.

Asthma is another pulmonary disease frequently encountered among homeless persons. In 1 small study (N = 67), 24% indicated a previous diagnosis of asthma, with 40% reporting wheezing and 20% affirming dyspnea on exertion.[17] In comparison, the American Lung Association reports asthma prevalence rates in US community-dwelling adults between 6.4 and 12%.[20] Extended exposure to both cold and heat, walking for hours at a time, and elevated levels of stress may all lead to asthma exacerbation.[21] In the authors' experience, the prohibitive cost of multidose albuterol inhalers increases the likelihood of adverse outcomes in this population, and drives the costs of unreimbursed care for asthma and COPD exacerbations. The bulk of portable nebulizers and lack of ready access to electricity make that modality of care impractical in this population. One easily implemented technique that might minimize aerosolized transmission would be arranging beds so that shelter residents slept head to toe versus head to head.[4]

CARDIAC DISEASE
Pearl

Obesity is the leading cause of death in both homeless and nonhomeless persons. Awareness of cardiac risk factors and barriers to obtaining treatment is critical in providing successful preventive management of obesity and hypertension in this vulnerable population.

Every year, approximately 600,000 people will die of heart disease in the United States. It is the leading cause of death for both men and women.[22] Middle-aged homeless men are more likely to die of heart disease than age-matched nonhomeless men, and heart disease is the leading cause of death in older homeless men.[23] Homeless persons have similar cardiac risk factors to the general population, such as smoking, hypertension, and obesity, but they have less ability to combat risk factors. For instance, diet often consists of high fat and cholesterol foods due to affordability and availability. In a study based in Toronto, Canada, 202 homeless adults were assessed for cardiac risk factors. In this study, 78% smoked, 35% had hypertension (with only 33% aware they had hypertension), and 46% were obese (body mass index >25). Approximately 30% of persons used both alcohol and cocaine.[24] This highlights the incredible need for preventive cardiology services for individuals who are homeless.

However, persons who are homeless will often delay seeking care, undergo fewer procedures, decline medications, and obtain less follow-up care. Reasons include lack of transportation, poor understanding of the seriousness of the condition, lack of finances, and often distrust of the medical system.[25] There seems to be an inverse relationship between socioeconomic status and 1-year mortality rate in individuals with cardiac disease.[26] In the authors' opinions, barriers to treating cardiac disease in homeless persons can only be overcome through some of the following mechanisms: mobile vans and clinics (addressing transportation and trust issues), meticulous patient education (addressing the poor understanding of health issues), education to hospital systems about the rates of cardiac disease in homeless persons and the systemic effect it has on hospital admissions (addressing 1 side of the financial barriers), and creative discharge planning that includes a combination of patience, appropriate follow-up care, and medications at bedside (addressing financial and trust issues).

DENTAL CARE
Pearl

Poor dentition can have a negative impact on nutrition, physical health, and on self-efficacy and mental health. There are far too few dental care resources available for homeless people.

Malnutrition, poor dental hygiene, tobacco use, and facial trauma are frequent causes of disfigured, decayed, and missing teeth. Access to dental care is generally difficult due transportation challenges and affordability of procedures. In the General Accounting Office Report to Congress, it was reported that more than half of homeless persons reported not seeking dental care in the preceding 2 years and one-third did not seek dental care in their lifetime.[27] In a Boston shelter, 90% of homeless persons had untreated dental caries.[28] Poor oral hygiene is 10 times higher in homeless children than an age-matched population.[29]

In persons who are homeless, lack of oral hygiene can result in multiple dental caries and periodontal disease that can lead to infection and loss of teeth. Medical conditions that are more common in homeless persons, such as diabetes, human immunodeficiency virus (HIV), or acquired immunodeficiency syndrome (AIDS), can exacerbate oral disease and make healing more difficult. Persons with poor dentition struggle with poor self-esteem and self-worth, which can lead to substance use, depression, and further homelessness.[5]

Even when persons who are homeless would like to receive dental treatment, barriers to receipt of care can be mindboggling. Generally, initial appointments are cost prohibitive. Often, even free clinics will charge for more expensive procedures and, given the level of dental care required by most homeless persons, it is rare that procedures are free of charge. The most successful strategies in treating oral hygiene in homeless persons include mobile dental clinics, community organization affiliation with a dental school, and volunteer dental nights.[30] Most persons who are homeless will not seek out dental care[23] and providers must inquire, encourage, and assist in provision with these important services.

DIABETES MELLITUS
Pearl

Many shelters rely on food donations to serve their participants. Be aware that the nutritional value of donated food is often low, and that careful planning and procurement of food is needed to address the needs of diabetic homeless people.

The CDC estimates that, in 2011, an estimated 25.8 million people, 8.3% of the US population, had a diagnosis of diabetes. An additional 35% of adults older than 20 years of age were diagnosable with prediabetes, defined as a fasting hemoglobin A1C level between 5.7 and 6.4.[31] Data regarding the prevalence of diabetes in homeless populations is sparse; 1 study of homeless citizens of New York City (N = 177) found that 35% of that sample were diabetic.[32]

Challenges to the successful management of diabetes abound in homeless populations. For example, homeless people are often unable to safely store insulin and insulin syringes. Optimal management of insulin in shelters requires access to refrigeration as well as accurate labeling of insulin type and patient name, both of which may wear off of manufacturer labels. A closely related issue is access to glucometers and glucometer strips. Given the array of glucometer manufacturers and models, it would not be possible for any health care system to stock test strips to fit any glucometer. Maintaining a calibrated and regularly tested glucometer and supply of test strips at a shelter may be beyond the scope of services offered by a shelter.

Remember that asking a person to fulfill what may seem to be a simple, straightforward task such as checking and tracking their blood sugar may not be possible in the chaos of homelessness.

Poor management of diabetes among homeless populations can have unexpected, life-threatening, consequences. For example, impaired cognitive and motor function secondary to hypoglycemia may prove fatal for urban homeless people because they spend significant amounts of time navigating traffic-filled roadways. Additionally, the physical manifestations of hypoglycemia may mimic intoxication. People exhibiting dizziness, altered mental status, and nausea may be assumed to be inebriated and left to their own devices. Shelters serving intoxicated homeless people should have ready access to a glucometer to ensure that episodes of hypoglycemia are not overlooked.

Obesity and diabetes are of particular concern in homeless populations because of the extended amount of time homeless people spend walking and their lack of access to properly fitting footwear. Diabetic neuropathy increases the likelihood of tissue damage caused by ill-fitting footwear and this is exacerbated by obesity. Resulting problems, from nonhealing ulcers to Charcot disease, present sometimes unmanageable obstacles for the homeless.

DERMATOLOGIC CONCERNS

Unmanaged chronic diseases cause many of the dermatologic challenges faced by homeless people. Lack of access to bathing facilities and to clean socks leads to higher rates of tinea pedis compared with the general population. One study done in a homeless shelter in Boston, MA, found that 38% of participants had tinea pedis.[33] Maceration of tissue may lead to intradigital fissuring, which may, in turn, lead to bacterial superinfection of open wounds.

Access to clean socks is essential for homeless people. One of the authors of this article started a foot washing clinic at a homeless shelter. Once a week, people signed up for foot washing, nail and callous trimming, and clinical evaluation of comorbidities noted during foot washing. Participants with tinea pedis were given an antifungal cream donated by a local pharmaceutical nonprofit, and all participants received 3 pairs of new socks. This intervention required a minimum level of clinical staffing (1 nurse practitioner); trained volunteers did all of the foot washing and trimming or filing services.

Clothing challenges are not confined to footwear. Ill-fitting, restricting, unwashed clothing anywhere on the body increases the likelihood of cellulitis secondary to abrasion. Cellulitis and tinea in intra-abdominal skin folds are not uncommon in obese homeless people,[33] for whom access to daily bathing facilities is unavailable.

In many cases, interventions to minimize dermatologic disease are within the scope of shelters. The key is recognizing that common shelter practices may need to be adapted to meet new demands. For example, shelters that do not allow daytime occupancy are foregoing an opportunity to provide respite from the damaging effects of chronic sun exposure. Provision for foot washing in shelter settings may be possible, even when showering facilities are not available. Access to washers and dryers in shelters might also be useful interventions.

GENITOURINARY INFECTIONS
Pearl
___

Homeless people may not always be in a position to advocate that their sexual partners use condoms. The presence of STDs may be a marker for abuse and/or depression.

The prevalence of nonsexually transmitted genital-urinary diseases (eg, candida, vaginitis) in homeless people is unknown. It would not be unreasonable for these rates to be elevated relative to the general population, based solely on a relative lack of access to bathing and clothes washing facilities. In addition to programs that stock socks for homeless people, the authors' experiences have led to advocating for making cotton underwear available at all shelters. Cotton fabrics breathe much better than synthetics, thus minimizing the buildup of excess moisture in the genital region, thereby discouraging the growth of candida.

A thorough review of the diagnosis and treatment of sexually transmitted diseases (STDs) is well beyond the scope of this article. Interested readers are referred to the CDC's *2015 Sexually Transmitted Diseases Treatment Guidelines*, available at no cost online. That being said, there are several unique features of homelessness that exacerbate the risk of the transmission and acquisition of STDs. Awareness of these issues can help shelter administrators and staff design and deliver more effective support for safe sex.

In the authors' experiences working with homeless populations in the Southeastern United States, a basic issue for homeless people is lack of access to condoms. This leads to a higher prevalence of unprotected sex among homeless people.[34] Human beings are sexual creatures and the lack of access to condoms does not imply celibacy in homeless shelters. Rather, this lack of access implies higher rates of unprotected sex, leading to higher rates of STDs.

In the authors' opinions, another issued affecting the elevated rate of STDs in homeless populations is that of transactional sex. Anyone who has spent time with homeless persons, both men and women, is aware that sex is used as a commodity in this population to barter for food, shelter, and to achieve companionship.[35] The issue is not that people are sexually active. The issue is that transactional sex is, by definition, based on a marked asymmetry of power between 2 individuals. One of the many problematic aspects of this asymmetrical relationship is that the more powerful person may be able to ignore the less powerful person's request that a condom be used with intercourse. In addition to the obvious increase in the likelihood of transmission of STDs, this behavior only serves to amplify the powerless person's sense of shame, helplessness, and social marginalization.[36]

Shelters are not designed to provide environments for sexual activity but they can serve a powerful role by clearly advocating for an atmosphere of mutual respect among all shelter users. Shelters should strongly consider embracing a culture of inclusion and respect among all shelter users and staff. Bright, visible posters should be used to communicate intolerance for race, gender, or any other discrimination.

SUMMARY

Homelessness is a national and international problem, and the medical problems that persons who are homeless face are serious and unrelenting. Homelessness leads to poor health and poor health leads to homelessness. Common conditions, such as high blood pressure, diabetes, asthma and even a small laceration, can become life-threatening because of inability to obtain medications, unhealthy diet, or lack of access to a clean environment. Successful providers must always be cognizant of the role of structural violence in the lives of their homeless patients. This means that patients experiencing homelessness may find themselves unable to transition into housing and health, despite working 1 or more minimum wage jobs. This, in turn, serves to erode faith in the very institutions from which practitioners strive to offer care. Serving these patients requires time, patience, and a willingness to engage around nontraditional issues in clinical care, including asking about living conditions, medication access and affordability, and transportation. Other keys to care, in the authors' experiences, include a willingness to work with patients on goals that they prioritize as important. It is also helpful to set goals with homeless patients and to empower them toward greater self-efficacy at every encounter. Provision of medical care for homeless persons may require coordination with medical outreach teams, shelters, and free clinics.

REFERENCES

1. Henwood BF, Byrne T, Scriber B. Examining mortality among formerly homeless adults enrolled in Housing First: an observational study. BMC Public Health 2015;15:1209.
2. Sturgis R, Sirgany A, Stoops M, et al. Bringing our neighbors in from the cold. A report from the National Coalition for the Homeless. 2010. Available at: http://www.nationalhomeless.org/publications/winter_weather/report.html. Accessed Feburary 27, 2016.
3. CDC. Hypothermia-related deaths - United States, 1999-2002 and 2005. MMWR Morb Mortal Wkly Rep 2006;55(10):282–4.
4. O'Connell J. The health care of homeless persons: a manual of communicable diseases & common problems in shelters & on the streets. Boston: Boston Health Care for the Homeless Program; 2004.
5. Coalition NHftH. Exposure-related conditions: symptoms and prevention strategies. Nashville (TN): HCH Clinicians' Network; 2007. Available at: https://www.nhchc.org/wp-content/uploads/2012/01/Dec2007HealingHands.pdf.
6. Wright J. Health care for homeless people: evidence from the National Health Care for the Homeless Program. New York: WW Norton & Co; 1990.
7. Bassuk EL, Melnick S, Browne A. Responding to the needs of low-income and homeless women who are survivors of family violence. J Am Med Womens Assoc 1998;53(2):57–64.
8. Tielsch JM, Sommer A, Katz J, et al. Socioeconomic status and visual impairment among urban Americans. Arch Ophthalmol 1991;109(5):637–41.
9. Baggett TP, O'Connell JJ, Singer DE, et al. The unmet health care needs of homeless adults: a national study. Am J Public Health 2010;100(7):1326–33.
10. Berti LC, Zylbert S, Cable G. Comparison of health status of children utilizing a school-based health center for comprehensive care. Pediatr Res 2000;47(4):175A.
11. Ho J, Chang R, Wheeler N, et al. Ophthalmic disorders among the homeless and nonhomeless in Los Angeles. J Am Optom Assoc 1997;68(9):567–73.
12. Nia J, Wong D, Motamedinia D. The visual acuity and social issues of the homeless population in Toronto. Univ Toronto Med J 2003;80(2):84–6.
13. Noel CW, Fung H, Srivastava R, et al. Visual impairment and unmet eye care needs among homeless adults in a Canadian city. JAMA Ophthalmol 2015;133(4):455–60.
14. CDC. Leading causes of death. 2015. Available at: http://www.cdc.gov/nchs/fastats/leading-causes-of-death.htm.
15. CDC. Vital Signs: current cigarette smoking among adults aged greater than or equal to 18 years, United States 2009. MMWR Morb Mortal Wkly Rep 2010;60(35):1207–12. Available at: http://www.cdc.gov/MMWR/preview/mmwrhtml/mm6035a5.htm. Accessed February 3, 2016.

16. Tsai J, Rosenheck RA. Smoking among chronically homeless adults: prevalence and correlates. Psychiatr Serv 2012;63(6):569–76.
17. Snyder LD, Eisner MD. Obstructive lung disease among the urban homeless. Chest 2004;125(5):1719–25.
18. Goldstein G, Luther JF, Jacoby AM, et al. A taxonomy of medical comorbidity for veterans who are homeless. J Health Care Poor Underserved 2008;19(3): 991–1005.
19. Stewart HC, Stevenson TN, Bruce JS, et al. Attitudes toward smoking cessation among sheltered homeless parents. J Community Health 2015;40(6):1140–8.
20. Association AL. Asthma in adults fact sheet. 2016. Available at: http://www.lung.org/lung-health-and-diseases/lung-disease-lookup/asthma/learn-about-asthma/asthma-adults-facts-sheet.html?referrer=https://www.google.com/.
21. Badiaga S, Richet H, Azas P, et al. Contribution of a shelter-based survey for screening respiratory diseases in the homeless. Eur J Public Health 2009; 19(2):157–60.
22. CDC. Heart disease fact sheet. 2015. Available at: http://www.cdc.gov/dhdsp/data_statistics/fact_sheets/fs_heart_disease.htm.
23. Hwang SW, Orav EJ, Oconnell JJ, et al. Causes of death in homeless adults in Boston. Ann Intern Med 1997;126(8):625–8.
24. Lee TC, Hanlon JG, Ben-David J, et al. Risk factors for cardiovascular disease in homeless adults. Circulation 2005;111(20):2629–35.
25. Flaskerud JH, Strehlow AJ. A culture of homelessness? Issues Ment Health Nurs 2008;29(10):1151–4.
26. Alter DA, Naylor CD, Austin P, et al. Effects of socioeconomic status on access to invasive cardiac procedures and on mortality after acute myocardial infarction. N Engl J Med 1999;341(18):1359–67.
27. GAO. Oral health: dental disease is a chronic problem among low-income populations. April, 2000. (HEHS-00–72). Available at: http://www.gao.gov/new.items/he00072.pdf.
28. Kaste LM, Bolden AJ. Dental-caries in homeless adults in Boston. J Public Health Dent 1995;55(1):34–6.
29. Wright J. Children in and out of the streets. Am J Dis Child 1991;145:516–9.
30. Hale A, Allen J, Caughlan J, et al. Healing Hands: filling the gaps in dental care, vol. 3. Nashville (TN): NHC Clinicians' Network; 2003.
31. CDC. National Diabetes Fact Sheet, 2011. 2011. Available at: http://www.cdc.gov/diabetes/pubs/pdf/ndfs_2011.pdf.
32. Asgary R, Sckell B, Alcabes A, et al. Rates and predictors of uncontrolled hypertension among hypertensive homeless adults using New York City shelter-based clinics. Ann Fam Med 2016;14(1):41–6.
33. Stratigos AJ, Stern R, Gonzalez E, et al. Prevalence of skin disease in a cohort of shelter-based homeless men. J Am Acad Dermatol 1999;41(2):197–202.
34. Tucker JS, Wenzel SL, Golinelli D, et al. Understanding heterosexual condom use among homeless men. Aids Behav 2013;17(5):1637–44.
35. Towe VL, Sifakis F, Gindi RM, et al. Prevalence of HIV infection and sexual risk behaviors among individuals having heterosexual sex in low income neighborhoods in Baltimore, MD: The BESURE Study. J Acquire Immune Defic Syndr 2010;53(4):522–8.
36. Dunkle KL, Wingood GM, Camp CM, et al. Economically motivated relationships and transactional sex among unmarried African American and white women: results from a US national telephone survey. Public Health Rep 2010;125:90–100.

Infectious Disease Issues in Underserved Populations

Samuel Neil Grief, MD, FCFP[a],*, John Paul Miller, MD[b]

KEYWORDS

- Infectious disease • Underserved populations • Minorities • Inmates • Homeless
- HIV • Health outcomes • Barriers

KEY POINTS

- Underserved populations are afflicted with infectious diseases at disproportionally higher rates than the general population.
- Underserved populations face many unique barriers to accessing quality health care.
- Although the Affordable Care Act has helped mitigate some of these challenges, significant obstacles remain.
- Primary care physicians are uniquely qualified to deliver high quality, culturally competent care to this important population.

INTRODUCTION

Although underserved populations have many of the same health concerns as the general population, they are disproportionately affected by higher rates of both acute and chronic illness, receive lower quality care, and experience worse health-related outcomes.[1] Although the Affordable Care Act (ACA) has expanded insurance coverage to many Americans, underserved populations continue to face numerous barriers to accessible and quality health care.[2]

Although early identification and treatment of infection have the potential to reduce transmission and improve health outcomes,[3] shortage of primary care physicians; immigration status; difficulties with transportation; communication issues, including health illiteracy, appointment availability, and previous negative experiences with health care, are some of the challenges underserved populations encounter in navigating the complex health care system.[2] Given these and other obstacles, infectious diseases are much more likely to be diagnosed at a late stage.[4,5]

Disclosure Statement: The authors have nothing to disclose.
[a] Department of Family Medicine, University of Illinois at Chicago, 1919 West Taylor Street, Chicago, IL 60612, USA; [b] Bakersfield Memorial Family Medicine Residency Program, Department of Family Medicine, University of California Irvine School of Medicine, 420 34th Street, Bakersfield, CA 93301, USA
* Corresponding author.
E-mail address: sgrief@uic.edu

Prim Care Clin Office Pract 44 (2017) 67–85
http://dx.doi.org/10.1016/j.pop.2016.09.011
0095-4543/17/© 2016 Elsevier Inc. All rights reserved.

A comprehensive and integrated patient-centered approach delivered by providers knowledgeable about the specific needs of underserved populations is imperative. In addition, community-based outreach and collaboration with social support services is vital. Primary care physicians are uniquely qualified and positioned to provide essential care to these vulnerable populations.

THE HOMELESS

In the United States, more than 650,000 American men, women, and children of all ages and ethnicities are homeless at any given time.[6] People facing homelessness often lack adequate health insurance coverage, and struggle with substance use, poor nutrition, mental illness, and chronic medical conditions, including infectious diseases.[7] Competing priorities for shelter, food, and safety mean homeless populations often delay seeking health care.[8] These issues contribute to fragmented care that often takes place in crowded emergency departments and requires frequent acute hospitalizations.[8]

Attempts to alleviate an issue may lead to unintended consequences. Although shelters provide protection from the elements, overcrowding may contribute to increased risk of contracting infectious diseases such as pneumonia, tuberculosis (TB), hepatitis A, and skin infestations.[3] Homeless women and youth are particularly vulnerable to contracting infectious diseases because they are more likely to suffer from mental illness, use drugs, and engage in high-risk sexual practices, such as exchanging sex for drugs, shelter, food, or money.[9]

Human Immunodeficiency Virus–Acquired Immunodeficiency Syndrome

An estimated 3.4% of the homeless population is infected with the human immunodeficiency virus (HIV) compared with 0.4% in the general population.[10] Prevalence rates in homeless men who have sex with men (MSM) and injection drug users are much higher at 30% and 8%, respectively.[11] It is also estimated that 50% of persons living with HIV or acquired immunodeficiency syndrome (AIDS) (PLWHA) are at risk for becoming homeless.[12] The lack of affordable housing, high costs of medical care, and job loss due to discrimination are contributing factors.[13] Risky behaviors, such as needle sharing, unprotected sex, and survival sex (exchanging sex for money or drugs), increase transmission risk.[14]

Due to underlying immunosuppression, homeless individuals with HIV/AIDS may be at increased risk of acquiring other infectious diseases. The prevalence of TB in the HIV-positive population is increased 2-fold in those who stay in shelters compared with those who do not.[12] Evidence shows that homeless or marginally housed PLWHA experience delays in HIV diagnosis[15] and entry into care,[16] as well as lower rates of continuity of care.[17] Adherence to treatment is problematic and is complicated in those with underlying depression and/or substance abuse.[18]

Overall, homeless PLWHA have lower CD4 counts, higher viral loads, are less likely to be prescribed or adhere to treatment regimens,[4,19,20] and have higher mortality rates compared with their nonhomeless counterparts.[21] Conversely, stable housing improves access to care, HIV-related outcomes, and reduces the risk of ongoing transmission.[22]

Hepatitis C

Hepatitis C virus (HCV) is the most common chronic blood-borne viral infection in the United States with an estimated prevalence of 2% in the general population.[17] Prevalence rates in the homeless population were reported as 24% in a recent study[8] and as high as 65% to 69% among those who are HIV-positive.[17] Strikingly, as many as 50% of homeless persons with HCV are unaware that they are infected,[23,24] which puts noninfected contacts at significant risk. Concurrent injection drug use is the strongest risk factor for contracting HCV.[25] Older age, veteran status, having multiple tattoos, and previous incarceration are also risk factors.[26]

Because HCV is asymptomatic until significant complications arise, early screening and detection is paramount.[24] Recent guidelines from the US Preventive Services Task Force and the Centers for Disease Control and Prevention (CDC) recommend routine screening for high-risk individuals.[26,27] The availability of rapid point-of-care testing[28] and more effective, tolerable, and easier to administer treatment regimens hold promise for the future.[29]

Tuberculosis

Despite a declining overall incidence of TB in the United States to a record low,[30] outbreaks of TB in certain populations, including the homeless, continue to be a public health challenge.[3] A prevalence of 6%[31] and incidence 46 times the general population has been estimated for homeless people.[32] Poor nutritional status and concomitant illnesses such as HIV may promote susceptibility to TB and progression to active disease.[33] Poorly ventilated and overcrowded living conditions were responsible for several recent outbreaks.[34]

Early recognition and treatment of disease are imperative to improve health outcomes and limit the spread of TB to others.[33] Unfortunately, issues such as alcohol use, use of illicit drugs, incarceration, and underlying psychiatric illness contribute to difficulties in diagnosis and treatment of TB in the homeless.[30] The transient nature of the homeless population makes contact identification and tracking difficult, and results in delays in diagnosis and treatment.[5] Poor compliance with treatment regimens leads to increased morbidity and mortality compared with the general population.[5]

Interferon-gamma release assays as an alternative to traditional skin testing, chest radiograph screening,[35] incentives,[36] directly observed therapy (DOT),[5] and the use of a simplified 12-dose regimen of isoniazid and rifapentine[37] are some of the strategies used to improve detection and treatment.

Other Infectious Diseases

Scabies and body louse infections are more common in homeless individuals compared with the general population.[38] Transmission occurs through close person-to-person contact or through contaminated clothing or bedding.[38] Louse-borne disease caused by *Bartonella quintana* (trench fever) and *Rickettsia prowazekii* (typhus) is also possible.[39] Frequent scratching of pruritic skin can lead to bacterial superinfections.[38]

Community-acquired pneumonia and influenza are common in the homeless population.[40] Overcrowding, smoking and alcohol use, and chronic lung disease increase risk.[41] Vaccination against pneumococcal pneumonia and influenza is underutilized and recommended.[41] Homelessness is also associated with higher rates of tinea pedis, impetigo, and folliculitis.[39]

INJECTION DRUG USERS

Illicit drug use is a common and growing social problem in the United States, with an estimated prevalence of 9.4%.[42] Minorities, including African Americans and Latinos, are disproportionately affected.[43] Persons who inject drugs, also known as injection drug users (IDUs), are at a substantially increased risk of acquiring and transmitting blood-borne viruses such as HIV, hepatitis B virus (HBV), and HCV.[44,45] In addition, illicit drug use is associated with higher rates of TB and sexually transmitted infections (STIs).[46,47]

Factors that facilitate the transmission of infectious disease in drug users include unstable living conditions,[48] inability to access treatment programs,[49] and fear of criminalization and stigmatization,[48] as well as undiagnosed or untreated mental health disorders.[48] In addition, individuals may be asymptomatic and/or unaware they are actively infected, which puts unaffected partners at risk.

Illicit drug use impairs judgment, which can increase disease transmission through risky sexual behavior,[50] needle sharing, and the use of unsterile drug injection equipment (cookers, cotton, and rinse water).[48]

Finally, women IDUs of childbearing age face unique challenges. They often underutilize family planning and prenatal services.[48] Moreover, actively infected pregnant women who use illicit drugs are at risk of transmitting disease to their children during pregnancy and delivery.[48]

Human Immunodeficiency Virus–Acquired Immunodeficiency Syndrome

Injection drug use is currently the third most common risk factor for contracting HIV and accounted for 8% or 3900 new cases in 2010.[51] HIV transmission also occurs through high-risk sexual behaviors, including but not limited to unprotected sex and engaging in sexual behaviors under the influence of drugs or in exchange for drugs.[52] Coinfection with other infectious diseases, such as HCV and herpes simplex virus (HSV)-2, is common and further increases transmission and progression of disease.[48]

Addressing comorbid conditions, such as mental illness, substance use disorders, and homelessness, improves HIV treatment.[53] Delaying treatment due to concerns about nonadherence is unwarranted,[54] and may contribute to further spread of HIV[55] and lower survival rates.[56] In addition, treatment with antiretroviral therapy (ART) of infected individuals prevents transmission to others.[48] Care should be taken when combining ART with other drugs, such as methadone and buprenorphine, because potentially toxic drug interactions can occur.[57]

Tuberculosis

Similar to other underserved populations, TB prevention, identification, and treatment remain a challenge among illicit drug users.[47] Drug use has been associated with increased prevalence of both latent TB infection (LTBI) and active TB.[58] Several studies report an LTBI prevalence of 10% to 59%.[47] Several factors may contribute to the high prevalence of TB in drug users, including homelessness, prior incarceration,[59] alcohol[60] and tobacco use,[61] and concurrent HIV.[62] Some evidence suggests drug use may have a direct effect on cell-mediated immune response[63,64] but the clinical significance of this remains unclear.[64]

Drug users with TB have higher rates and longer periods of infectivity, which leads to greater likelihood of transmission[65] and extrapulmonary disease.[62] Coinfection with HIV, HBV, and HCV is common.[59] Coinfection with HIV increases progression from latent to active infection[62] and is associated with higher TB-related mortality.[66] Drug users are less likely to get screened or to initiate and complete treatment, resulting in increased transmission, the development of multidrug resistance, and more severe disease.[67]

Hepatitis B and C Viruses

Being an IDU is the most common risk factor in the transmission of HCV in the United States, accounting for 48% of all new infections in 2007.[68] Furthermore, IDUs accounted for 15% of the 43,000 new cases of HBV[68]; 75% to 90% of IDUs are anti-HCV positive.[69] An emerging epidemic of HCV infection is being seen in young adult injection drug users who have transitioned from the use of oral opioids.[70] Coinfection with HBV and HCV is not uncommon.[71] Among HIV-infected persons who inject drugs illicitly, 80% also are infected with HCV.[49] Compared with HIV, HCV is much more infectious[72] and can survive in syringes and on inanimate objects for prolonged periods of time.[73] As a result, environmental contamination and sharing injection preparation equipment are important modes of transmission.[74] Newer, highly effective and tolerated treatment regimens for HCV are available.[29] Administering HCV treatment in concert with medically supervised opioid therapy can increase adherence and treatment success.[29]

Other Infectious Diseases

The reported prevalence rates of STIs among persons who use drugs illicitly are 1% to 6% for syphilis, 1% to 5% for chlamydia, 1% to 3% for gonorrhea, and 38% to 61% for HSV-2 infection.[48] Skin and soft tissue infections, such as cellulitis and abscesses, are common in IDUs and are frequent reasons for hospital admission.[75] Right-sided infective endocarditis, most commonly caused by *Staphylococcus aureus*, can occur.[76] Coinfection with HIV is not infrequent and advanced immunosuppression (CD4 count <200/mm^3) increases mortality.[76] Nonadherence to long inpatient antibiotic treatment regimens is common in IDUs.[76] Shorter courses of antibiotics and the use of oral therapy in the outpatient setting may be appropriate in some cases.[76]

LESBIAN, GAY, BISEXUAL, AND TRANSGENDER

Although some progress has been made in understanding and addressing health disparities in the lesbian, gay, bisexual, and transgender (LGBT) community, it remains a significant national public health issue. LGBT populations, like other marginalized groups, face barriers to culturally competent and quality health care.[77] They are more likely to lack insurance coverage and experience significant societal stigma and discrimination.[77]

Mental illness,[78] substance use,[79] and sexual and physical abuse[80] occur at higher rates compared with the heterosexual population and have negative consequences on general health. In addition to some infectious diseases, studies have found that sexual and gender minorities have more chronic conditions and overall poorer health status.[78] Recent policy and legal changes offering nondiscrimination protections[81] and recognizing same-sex marriage[82,83] may help to mitigate some of these challenges.

Human Immunodeficiency Virus–Acquired Immunodeficiency Syndrome

Although MSM are greatly affected by HIV/AIDS, minority men are disproportionally affected.[77] In 2010, it was estimated that MSM accounted for 56% of all HIV cases and roughly two-thirds of the 50,000 new cases of HIV in the United States.[84] Coinfection with other STIs, including syphilis, among HIV-positive MSM is common.[85]

Transgender women, especially African Americans, are also significantly affected by HIV/AIDS. Prevalence rates of 28% and 56%, respectively, have been reported.[86] However, transgender women are less likely to receive ART[87] and have higher HIV-related morbidity and mortality compared with other populations.[88] Possible interactions between ART and hormone therapy is a concern for many transgender women.[89]

HIV prevalence in transgender men is low (0%–3%)[89] but data are limited.[90] Moreover, although female to female sexual transmission of HIV is rare,[91] lesbian, bisexual, and other women who have sex with women (WSW) are still at risk of HIV primarily through male sexual contact and injection drug use.[92]

Human Papilloma Virus

Transmission of the human papilloma virus (HPV) between female sexual partners is common.[93] Furthermore, most WSW have had sex with men and many continue to do so.[94] Abnormalities have been detected on cervical smear testing, even in women who have not had sex with men,[95] highlighting the importance of adherence to current cervical cancer screening and vaccination guidelines.

The prevalence of HPV is high in MSM, increasing the risk of genital warts and cancers of the penis, oropharynx, and anus.[96] MSM are 17 times more likely to develop anal cancer than heterosexual men,[97] with a much higher rate in those who are coinfected with HIV/AIDS.[98]

Other Infectious Diseases

Primary and secondary syphilis in the United States have continued to increase at an alarming rate in MSM, now accounting for 83% of new cases.[85] MSM transmission accounts for 15% to 25% of all new cases of HBV.[99] In MSM, gonorrheal and chlamydial infections of the rectum and pharynx are common, especially in those with HIV.[100] The prevalence of bacterial vaginosis in WSW is estimated to be nearly 26% compared with 14% in heterosexual populations.[101] The results of several studies suggest female to female sexual transmission is likely.[101,102] Limited data exist on transmission rates of STIs among WSW but probably varies by the type of STI and sexual behavior.[103]

INMATE POPULATION

Individuals who inhabit correctional facilities, both state and federal, are at increased risk for infectious disease.[104] The prevalence of HIV and other infectious diseases is much higher among inmates than among the general population.[104] High-risk sexual behavior and illicit drug use among incarcerated inmates, and a general lack of condoms and sterile needles or syringes, predispose these individuals to greater risk of infectious diseases.[104] The prevalence of ever having an infectious disease among state and federal prisoners and the general population are compared in **Table 1**.[105]

A similar comparison is presented in **Table 2** among jail inmates versus the general population.[105]

Human Immunodeficiency Virus–Acquired Immunodeficiency Syndrome

Contracting HIV for men and women is far more likely in prison.[106] Incarcerated women suffer disproportionately from HIV/AIDS and other infectious diseases.[107] High-risk behavior among prison inmates is likely a significant contributing factor to transmission and acquisition of HIV.[108,109] Unfortunately, prisoners in low- and middle-income countries (LMICs) are at much higher risk for HIV and other infectious diseases. The prisoner prevalence of HIV in 20 LMICs is greater than 10%.[110] Overcrowding, lack of public health initiatives, and inadequate access to clean injecting equipment for intravenous drug users are among the reasons for the continued higher risk for HIV and other infectious diseases among incarcerated prisoners.[111]

Education and enhanced protection from sexually transmitted diseases, along with expanded HIV testing among the US inmate population will likely continue to reduce the rate of HIV among all US incarcerated individuals.[104,112] Awareness of HIV status does affect risk behavior, supporting arguments for increased HIV screening among

Table 1
Prevalence of ever having infectious disease among state and federal prisoners versus general population

	State and Federal Prisoners		General Population	
	Percent (%)	Standard Error	Percent (%)	Standard Error
Ever had an infectious disease[a]	21.0	1.3%	4.8	0.2%
TB	6.0	0.6	0.5	0.1
Hepatitis[b]	10.9	1.0	1.1	0.1
Sexually transmitted diseases[c]	6.0	0.5	3.4	0.1

[a] Excludes HIV or AIDS due to unknown or missing data.
[b] Includes hepatitis B and C for the prison population and all types of hepatitis for the general population.
[c] Excludes HIV or AIDS.
Adapted from The prevalence of ever having an infectious disease among state and federal prisoners and the general population (2011–12). Bureau, National Inmate Survey (NIS), 2011–12; and the Substance Abuse and Mental Health Services Administration, National Survey on Drug Use and Health (NSDUH), 2009–2012.

jail and prison populations.[113] **Fig. 1** reflects the declining rate of HIV or AIDS among US incarcerated individuals.

RACIAL AND ETHNIC MINORITIES

According to the 2010 US Census, approximately 36.3% of the population currently belongs to a racial or ethnic minority group: American Indian or Alaska Native (AI/AN), Asian American, Black or African American, Hispanic or Latino, and Native Hawaiian or other Pacific Islander.[114] Racial and ethnic health disparities are widespread in the United States.[115,116] These disparities are apparent in regard to infectious disease.[117,118] For example, morbidity and mortality rates from HIV/AIDS in the United States are highest among black or African American, Hispanic or Latino, and native Hawaiian or other Pacific Islander racial or ethnic minorities.[119]

Table 2
Prevalence of ever having infectious disease among state and federal jail inmates versus general population

	Jail Inmates		General Population	
	Percent (%)	Standard Error	Percent (%)	Standard Error
Ever had an infectious disease[a]	14.3	0.7%	4.6	0.1%
TB	2.5	0.3	0.4	<0.05
Hepatitis[b]	6.5	0.5	0.9	<0.05
Sexually transmitted diseases[c]	6.1	0.5	3.5	0.1

[a] Excludes HIV or AIDS due to unknown or missing data.
[b] Includes HBV and HCV for the jail population, and all types of hepatitis for the general population.
[c] Excludes HIV or AIDS.
Adapted from The prevalence of ever having an infectious disease among state and federal jail inmates and the general population (2011–12). Bureau, National Inmate Survey (NIS), 2011–12; and the Substance Abuse and Mental Health Services Administration, National Survey on Drug Use and Health (NSDUH), 2009–2012.

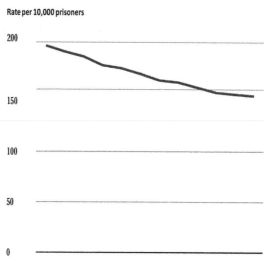

Rate per 10,000 prisoners

2001 2002 2003 2004 2005 2006 2007 2008 2009 2010 2011 2012

Fig. 1. Rate of HIV or AIDS cases among state and federal prisoners, 2001 to 2012. (*Data from* Bureau of Justice Statistics, National Prisoner Statistics Program, 2001–2012. Available at: http://www.bjs.gov/content/pub/pdf/mpsfpji1112.pdf. Accessed March 8, 2016.)

Human Immunodeficiency Virus–Acquired Immunodeficiency Syndrome

The AIDS epidemic disproportionately affects racial and ethnic minorities. In 2007, African Americans made up 13% of the US population but accounted for nearly half of PLWHA. HIV/AIDS rates (cases per 100,000) were 77 among black or African Americans, 35 among Native Hawaiians or other Pacific Islanders, 28 among Hispanics, 13 among AI/AN, 9.2 among whites, and 7.7 among Asian Americans.[120]

Non-Asian racial or ethnic minorities continue to experience higher rates of HIV diagnosis than whites. Compared with whites, a lower percentage of blacks diagnosed with HIV were prescribed ART and a lower percentage of both blacks and Hispanics had suppressed viral loads.[121]

Tuberculosis

TB case rates declined among all racial or ethnic minority groups and among US and foreign-born individuals from 2006 to 2010. However, rates remained higher among racial or ethnic minority groups than among whites in 2010.[122] Case rates of TB in the United States are still highest among the foreign-born who have immigrated from Latin America, Asia, and Africa[122,123] but are also elevated among US born black and AI/AN persons.[124,125] Lower respiratory tract infection morbidity and mortality rates are higher among AI/AN children than US children.[114,126]

There are also substantial racial and ethnic disparities for most, if not all, vaccine-preventable illnesses, most notably including HBV, influenza, and pneumococcal disease.[114] The CDC's Racial and Ethnic Adult Disparities in Immunization Initiative (READII) was a 2-year project aimed to improve immunization rates for influenza and pneumococcal pneumonia among the African-American and Hispanic communities. Results were favorable, and many strategies for bridging the immunization gap were developed and learned.[127,128]

HEALTH LITERACY

Health literacy is the degree to which individuals have the capacity to obtain, process, and understand basic health information and services needed to make appropriate health decisions.[129] Limited health literacy affects all ages, races, incomes, and education levels; however, the impact of limited health literacy disproportionately affects lower socioeconomic and minority groups.[130] It also affects people's ability to search for and use health information, adopt healthy behaviors, and act on important public health alerts. Limited health literacy is also associated with worse health outcomes and higher costs.[131]

Although limited health literacy affects most adults at some point in their lives, there are disparities in prevalence and severity. Some groups are more likely than others to have limited health literacy:

- Adults older than the age of 65 years
- Racial and ethnic groups other than white
- Recent refugees and immigrants
- People with less than a high school or general educational development degree (GED)
- People with incomes at or below the poverty level
- Non-native speakers of English.[132]

Limited health literacy is negatively associated with the use of preventive services (eg, mammograms or flu shots), management of chronic conditions (eg, diabetes, high blood pressure, asthma, and HIV/AIDS), and self-reported health.[132] Recent research has focused on health literacy as one of the critical factors in health disparities.[133–135] The greatest opportunities for reducing health disparities are in empowering individuals and changing the health system to meet their needs.[135] The National Action Plan to Improve Health Literacy, released May 2010 by the US Department of Health and Human Services, seeks to engage organizations, professionals, policymakers, communities, individuals, and families in a linked, multisector effort to improve health literacy.[132] The plan includes 7 broad goals with multiple high-level strategies for various stakeholders and provides a focal point for the field.

What are the 7 Goals in the Plan?

- Goal 1: Develop and disseminate health and safety information that is accurate, accessible, and actionable.
- Goal 2: Promote changes in the health care delivery system that improve information, communication, informed decision-making, and access to health services.
- Goal 3: Incorporate accurate and standards-based health and developmentally appropriate health and science information and curricula into child care and education through the university level.
- Goal 4: Support and expand local efforts to provide adult education, English-language instruction, and culturally and linguistically appropriate health information services in the community.
- Goal 5: Build partnerships, develop guidance, and change policies.
- Goal 6: Increase basic research and the development, implementation, and evaluation of practices and interventions to improve health literacy.
- Goal 7: Increase the dissemination and use of evidence-based health literacy practices and interventions.[132]

BARRIERS TO HEALTH CARE FOR THE UNDERSERVED

The advent of the ACA has made health insurance more accessible for millions of Americans, including underserved populations. It also offers access to preventive services, including screening for HIV, STIs, depression, and substance abuse; the delivery of culturally competent care; coordinated care for chronic conditions; and calls for enhanced data collection and research on health disparities. Despite these advancements, significant barriers to quality medical care still exist **(Box 1)**.[47,77,136–141]

Box 1
Barriers to heath care

Health care delivery system barriers

- Inadequate number of providers
- Location of clinics and hospitals
- Availability (operating hours and long appointment wait times)
- Limited data or research on issues related to underserved
- Inadequate reimbursement for behavioral health services in primary care setting
- Inadequate education, testing, and counseling services
- Restricted access to substance use treatment, mental health, and specialty care (HIV clinics)
- Increased administrative and infrastructure challenges with Medicaid expansion

Provider barriers

- Lack of cultural competency
- Poor attitudes
- Lack awareness and knowledge of specific health needs of underserved populations
- Bias, unwelcoming environment

Individual or population barriers

- Lack insurance coverage
- Lack of primary care provider
- Low education and health literacy
- Language barriers
- Immigration status
- Lack support system
- Comorbid mental illness and/or substance abuse
- Mistrust of health care system due to previous negative experiences
- Difficulty adhering to treatment or medication regimens
- Concerns about confidentiality
- Sexual and physical violence (LGBT community)
- Lack of documentation, such as an identification card

DISEASE PREVENTION AND HARM REDUCTION STRATEGIES

Implementing culturally competent public health strategies in a manner that respects the rights of underserved populations is vital for preventing and treating HIV infection, TB, viral hepatitis, STIs, and other infectious diseases.

Health Care Delivery System Improvement Strategies

Although providing comprehensive, integrated, and accessible care in a safe nondiscriminatory environment free from fear of harassment and/or legal intervention is the first priority,[48,66,141,142] the first task may be assessing health care provider's attitudes and knowledge, and providing the necessary training and education.[136]

Targeted counseling, education, and risk assessment (eg, for drug use and STIs) in concert with timely disease-specific testing[48,136,142,143] is fundamental, along with improving the availability and access to condoms[3,48]; vaccination programs[3,48]; evidence-based interventions, such as ART,[136,142] TB, and pre-exposure prophylaxis[142]; and mental health services.[48,136]

Vital for IDUs are access to sterile injection and drug preparation equipment (ie, needle exchange programs),[48,136,140–143] training in overdose prevention and the provision of naloxone,[144] and improving access to substance abuse treatment programs such as medication-assisted therapy (MAT).[48,66,136,141–143]

Prevention and control strategies in shelters include ensuring adequate ventilation[5] and strict enforcement of screening and education programs for all staff and clients.[5,66] Protocols for identifying high-risk clients (eg, those with HIV) and handling and/or referral of symptomatic clients (eg, cough alert logs) are important.[66] Finally, bed systems to position (head to toe) and track potentially infectious clients can be helpful.

Providing multiple services (testing, diagnosis, and treatment) in one location,[48,66] combining treatment services (DOT for TB, MAT for substance abuse,[66] hormone therapy, and ART)[142] and supervised therapy (DOT, MAT)[66] can improve adherence. Adherence reminders, such as beepers, pill boxes and calendars, and providing incentives also may be useful.[48,66,136]

Support Services Improvement Strategies

Community-based outreach programs aim to engage at-risk populations by providing disease-specific and risk reduction education, materials such as condoms and clean needles, and crisis intervention and referrals to essential support services, including drug treatment programs.[48,66,136,137,141]

Despite health insurance becoming more accessible and affordable for many underserved, the enrollment process can be complicated and confusing.[138] Frontline workers, including case managers, are uniquely positioned to help guide individuals through this complex process.[138] In addition, assistance is needed with transportation (eg, bus tickets),[138] housing, employment services, and legal advice.[142]

Confidential notification of partners who may have been exposed to certain infectious diseases (STIs, HIV, and HCV) through high-risk sexual behavior and/or being an IDU is effective in reducing further transmission.[48] Disease-specific testing, counseling, vaccination, and referral for treatment or other needed services may be necessary.[48]

REFERENCES

1. Focus on health care disparities. Disparities in health and health care: five key questions and answers. Menlo park (CA): The Henry J Kaiser Family Foundation; 2012.

2. Kullgren J, McLaughlin C, Mitra N, et al. Nonfinancial barriers and access to care for U.S. adults. Health Serv Res 2011;47(1pt2):462–85.

3. Badiaga S, Raoult D, Brouqui P. Preventing and controlling emerging and ree-merging transmissible diseases in the homeless. Emerg Infect Dis 2008;14(9): 1353–9.

4. Kidder DP, Wolitski RJ, Campsmith ML, et al. Health status, health care use, medication use, and medication adherence among homeless and housed peo-ple living with HIV/AIDS. Am J Public Health 2007;97(12):2238–45.

5. McAdam JM. Combatting tuberculosis and homelessness: recommendations for policy and practice. Nashville (TN): National Health Care for the Homeless Council; 1994.

6. Sermons MW, Witte P. State of homelessness in America. Washington, DC: Na-tional Alliance to End Homelessness; 2011.

7. Hwang SW, Henderson MJ. Health care utilization in homeless people: trans-lating research into policy and practice. Agency for Healthcare Research and Quality Working Paper No. 10002. 2010. Available at: http://gold.ahrq.gov. Ac-cessed March 8, 2016.

8. Bharel M, Lin W, Zhang J, et al. Health care utilization patterns of homeless in-dividuals in Boston: Preparing for Medicaid expansion under the Affordable Care Act. Am J Public Health 2013;103(S2):S311–7.

9. Moore J. Unaccompanied and homeless youth: review of literature. Greensboro (NC): National Center for Homeless Education; 1995–2005.

10. HIV/AIDS and homelessness. Washington, DC: National Coalition for the Home-less; 2009.

11. Robertson M, Clark R, Charlebois E, et al. HIV seroprevalence among homeless and marginally housed adults in San Francisco. Am J Public Health 2004;94(7): 1207–17.

12. Fact sheet: homelessness and HIV/AIDS. Washington, DC: National Alliance to End Homelessness; 2006.

13. Tomaszewski EP. Human rights update. HIV/AIDS and homelessness. Washing-ton, DC: National Association of Social Workers; 2011.

14. Marshall B, Shannon K, Kerr T, et al. Survival sex work and increased HIV risk among sexual minority street-involved youth. J Acquir Immune Defic Syndr 2010;53(5):661–4.

15. Aidala A, Cross J, Stall R, et al. Housing status and HIV risk behaviors: Implica-tions for prevention and policy. AIDS Behav 2005;9(3):251–65.

16. Aidala A, Lee G, Abramson D, et al. Housing need, housing assistance, and connection to HIV medical care. AIDS Behav 2007;11(S2):101–15.

17. Chak E, Talal A, Sherman K, et al. Hepatitis C virus infection in USA: An estimate of true prevalence. Liver Int 2011;31(8):1090–101.

18. Royal S, Kidder D, Patrabansh S, et al. Factors associated with adherence to highly active antiretroviral therapy in homeless or unstably housed adults living with HIV. AIDS Care 2009;21(4):448–55.

19. Schwarcz S, Hsu L, Vittinghoff E, et al. Impact of housing on the survival of per-sons with AIDS. BMC Public Health 2009;9(1):220.

20. Nelson K, Thiede H, Hawes S, et al. Why the wait? Delayed diagnosis among men who have sex with men. J Urban Health 2010;87(4):642–55.

21. Milloy M, Marshall B, Montaner J, et al. Housing status and the health of people living with HIV/AIDS. Curr HIV/AIDS Rep 2012;9(4):364–74.

22. Audain G, Bookhardt-Murray LJ, Fogg CJ, et al, editors. Adapting your practice: treatment and recommendations for unstably housed patients with HIV/AIDS.

Nashville (TN): Health Care for the Homeless Clinicians' Network, National Health Care for the Homeless Council, Inc; 2013.

23. Gelberg L, Robertson MJ, Arangua L. Prevalence, distribution, and correlates of Hepatitis C virus infection among homeless adults in Los Angeles. Public Health Rep 2012;127:407–21.

24. Strehlow A, Robertson M, Zerger S, et al. Hepatitis C among clients of health care for the homeless primary care clinics. J Health Care Poor Underserved 2012;23(2):811–33.

25. Hayes B, Briceno A, Asher A, et al. Preference, acceptability and implications of the rapid hepatitis C screening test among high-risk young people who inject drugs. BMC Public Health 2014;14(1):645.

26. Moyer V. Screening for Hepatitis C virus infection in adults: U.S. Preventive Services Task Force recommendation statement. Ann Intern Med 2013;159(5):349.

27. Centers for Disease Control and Prevention. Testing for HCV infection: an update of guidance for clinicians and laboratorians. MMWR Morb Mortal Wkly Rep 2013;62:362–5.

28. Shivkumar S, Peeling R, Jafari Y, et al. Accuracy of rapid and point-of-care screening tests for Hepatitis C. Ann Intern Med 2012;157(8):558.

29. McCance-Katz E, Valdiserri R. Hepatitis C virus treatment and injection drug users: it is time to separate fact from fiction. Ann Intern Med 2015;163(3):224.

30. Centers for Disease Control and Prevention. Trends in Tuberculosis – United States, 2012. MMWR Morb Mortal Wkly Rep 2013;62:201–5.

31. Bamrah S, Yelk Woodruff R, Powell K, et al. Tuberculosis among the homeless, United States, 1994–2010. Int J Tuberc Lung Dis 2013;17(11):1414–9.

32. Beijer U, Wolf A, Fazel S. Prevalence of tuberculosis, hepatitis C virus, and HIV in homeless people: a systematic review and meta-analysis. Lancet Infect Dis 2012;12(11):859–70.

33. Tan de Bibiana J, Rossi C, Rivest P, et al. Tuberculosis and homelessness in Montreal: a retrospective cohort study. BMC Public Health 2011;11(1):833.

34. Centers for Disease Control and Prevention. Reported tuberculosis in the United States, 2013. 2014.

35. Paquette K, Cheng M, Kadatz M, et al. Chest radiography for active tuberculosis case finding in the homeless: a systematic review and meta-analysis. Int J Tuberc Lung Dis 2014;18(10):1231–6.

36. Lutge E, Wiysonge C, Knight S, et al. Material incentives and enablers in the management of tuberculosis. Cochrane Database Syst Rev 2012;(1):CD007952.

37. Sterling T, Villarino M, Borisov A, et al. Three months of rifapentine and isoniazid for latent tuberculosis infection. N Engl J Med 2011;365(23):2155–66.

38. Badiaga S, Menard A, Tissot Dupont H, et al. Prevalence of skin infections in sheltered homeless. Eur J Dermatol 2005;15:382–6.

39. Raoult D, Foucault C, Brouqui P. Infections in the homeless. Lancet Infect Dis 2001;1(2):77–84.

40. Roncarati J, Bernardo J. Community acquired pneumonia. The health care of homeless persons - Part I. In: the health care of homeless persons: a manual of communicable diseases and common problems in shelters and on the streets. Boston: The Boston Health Care for the Homeless Program; 2004.

41. Wrezel O. Respiratory infections in the homeless. UWO Med J 2009;78(2):61–5.

42. National Institute on Drug Abuse. Nationwide trends. Available at: http://www.drugabuse.gov/publications/drugfacts/nationwide-trends. Accessed January 20, 2016.

43. Estrada A. Epidemiology of HIV/AIDS, hepatitis B, hepatitis C, and tuberculosis among minority injection drug users. Public Health Rep 2002;117(Suppl 1): S126–34.
44. Lansky A, Books J, DiNenno E, et al. Epidemiology of HIV in the United States. J Acquir Immune Defic Syndr 2010;55(Suppl 2):S64–8.
45. Nelson P, Mathers B, Cowie B, et al. Global epidemiology of hepatitis B and hepatitis C in people who inject drugs: Results of systematic reviews. Lancet 2011; 378(9791):571–83.
46. Des Jarlais D, Semaan S, Arasteh K. At 30 years: HIV/AIDS and other STDs among persons who use psychoactive drugs. In: Hall B, Hall J, Cockerell C, editors. HIV/AIDS in the post-HAART Era: manifestations, treatment, and epidemiology. Shelton (CT): People's Medical Publishing House; 2011. p. 753–78.
47. Deiss R, Rodwell T, Garfein R. Tuberculosis and illicit drug use: Review and update. Clin Infect Dis 2009;48(1):72–82.
48. Centers for Disease Control and Prevention. Integrated prevention services for HIV infection, viral hepatitis, sexually transmitted diseases, and tuberculosis for persons who use drugs illicitly: summary guidance from CDC and the U.S. Department of Health and Human Services. MMWR Morb Mortal Wkly Rep 2012;61(RR-5):1–46.
49. Tempalski B, Cleland C, Pouget E, et al. Persistence of low drug treatment coverage for injection drug users in large metropolitan areas. Subst Abuse Treat Prev Policy 2010;5:23.
50. Des Jarlais D, Semaan S. HIV and other sexually transmitted infections in injection drug users and crack cocaine smokers. In: Holmes KK, Sparling PF, Stamm WE, et al, editors. Sexually transmitted diseases. 4th edition. New York: McGraw-Hill; 2008. p. 237–55.
51. Centers for Disease Control and Prevention. Estimated HIV incidence in the United States, 2007–2010. HIV Surveillance Supplemental Report 2012;17(4).
52. Kral A, Bluthenthal R, Lorvick J, et al. Sexual transmission of HIV-1 among injection drug users in San Francisco, USA: Risk-factor analysis. Lancet 2001; 357(9266):1397–401.
53. Altice F, Kamarulzaman A, Soriano V, et al. Treatment of medical, psychiatric, and substance-use comorbidities in people infected with HIV who use drugs. Lancet 2010;376(9738):367–87.
54. Malta M, Magnanini M, Strathdee S, et al. Adherence to antiretroviral therapy among HIV-infected drug users: a meta-analysis. AIDS Behav 2008;14(4): 731–47.
55. Cohen M, Chen Y, McCauley M, et al. Prevention of HIV-infection with early antiretroviral therapy. N Engl J Med 2011;365(6):493–505.
56. Kitahata M, Gange S, Abraham A, et al. Effect of early versus deferred antiretroviral therapy for HIV on survival. N Engl J Med 2009;360(18):1815–26.
57. McCance-Katz EF, Sullivan L, Nallani S. Drug Interactions of clinical importance among the opioids, methadone and buprenorphine, and other frequently prescribed medications: a review. Am J Addict 2010;19(1):4–16.
58. Mamani M, Majzoobi M, Torabian S, et al. Latent and active tuberculosis: Evaluation of injecting drug users. Iran Red Crescent Med J 2013;15(9):775–9.
59. Getahun H, Gunneberg C, Sculier D, et al. Tuberculosis and HIV in people who inject drugs: Evidence for action for TB, HIV, prison and harm reduction services. Curr Opin HIV AIDS 2012;7(4):345–53.
60. Getahun H, Baddeley A, Raviglione M. Managing tuberculosis in people who use and inject illicit drugs. Bull World Health Organ 2013;91(2):154–6.

61. Altet-Gomez MN, Alcaide J, Godoy P, et al. Clinical and epidemiological aspects of smoking and tuberculosis: a study of 13,038 cases. Int J Tuberc Lung Dis 2005;9:430–6.

62. Selwyn P, Hartel D, Lewis V, et al. A prospective study of the risk of tuberculosis among intravenous drug users with human immunodeficiency virus infection. N Engl J Med 1989;320(9):545–50.

63. Wei G, Moss J, Yuan C. Opioid-induced immunosuppression: Is it centrally mediated or peripherally mediated? Biochem Pharmacol 2003;65(11):1761–6.

64. Kapadia F, Vlahov D, Donahoe R, et al. The role of substance abuse in HIV disease progression: reconciling differences from laboratory and epidemiologic investigations. Clin Infect Dis 2005;41(7):1027–34.

65. Oeltmann J, Kammerer J, Pevzner E, et al. Tuberculosis and substance abuse in the United States, 1997-2006. Arch Intern Med 2009;169(2):189.

66. World Health Organization (WHO). Policy Guidelines for Collaborative TB and HIV Services for injecting and other drug users an integrated approach. 2008.

67. Golub JE, Bur S, Cronin WA, et al. Delayed tuberculosis diagnosis and tuberculosis transmission. Int J Tuberc Lung Dis 2006;10:24–30.

68. Daniels D, Grytdal S, Wasley A. Surveillance for acute viral hepatitis—United States, 2007. MMWR Surveill Summ 2009;58(SS-3):1–27.

69. Amon J, Garfein R, Ahdieh-Grant L, et al. Prevalence of hepatitis C virus infection among injection drug users in the United States, 1994–2004. Clin Infect Dis 2008;46(12):1852–8.

70. Page K, Morris M, Hahn J, et al. Injection drug use and hepatitis C virus infection in young adult injectors: Using evidence to inform comprehensive prevention. Clin Infect Dis 2013;57(Suppl 2):S32–8.

71. Chu C, Lee S. Hepatitis B virus/hepatitis C virus coinfection: epidemiology, clinical features, viral interactions and treatment. J Gastroenterol Hepatol 2008; 23(4):512–20.

72. Wicker S, Cinatl J, Berger A, et al. Determination of risk of infection with blood-borne pathogens following a needlestick injury in hospital workers. Ann Occup Hyg 2008;52(7):615–22.

73. Doerrbecker J, Friesland M, Ciesek S, et al. Inactivation and survival of hepatitis C virus on inanimate surfaces. J Infect Dis 2011;204(12):1830–8.

74. Pouget E, Hagan H, Des Jarlais D. Meta-analysis of hepatitis C seroconversion in relation to shared syringes and drug preparation equipment. Addiction 2012; 107(6):1057–65.

75. Ebright J, Pieper B. Skin and soft tissue infections in injection drug users. Infect Dis Clin North Am 2002;16(3):697–712.

76. Moss R, Munt B. Injection drug use and right sided endocarditis. Heart 2003; 89(5):577–81.

77. Kates J, Ranji U, Beamesderfer A, et al. Health and access to care and coverage for lesbian, gay, bisexual, and transgender individuals in the US. Menlo Park (CA): The Henry J. Kaiser Family Foundation; 2015. Issue Brief.

78. Lick D, Durso L, Johnson K. Minority stress and physical health among sexual minorities. Perspect Psychol Sci 2013;8(5):521–48.

79. Ostrow D, Stall R. Alcohol, tobacco, and drug use among gay and bisexual men. In: Wolitski R, Stall R, Valdiserri R, editors. Unequal opportunity: health disparities affecting gay and bisexual men in the United States. New York: Oxford University Press; 2008. p. 1–60.

80. Centers for Disease Control and Prevention. The National Intimate Partner and Sexual Violence Survey: 2010 findings on victimization by sexual orientation. 2013.

81. Department of Health and Human Services. Patient Protection and Affordable Care Act; standards related to essential health benefits, actuarial value and accreditation. Final rule. Fed Reg 2013;78(37):12833–72.

82. Supreme Court of the United States, United States v. Windsor, June 26, 2013.

83. Supreme Court of the United States, Obergefell v. Hodges, June 26, 2015.

84. Centers for Disease Control and Prevention. HIV among gay, bisexual, and other men who have sex with men. 2013.

85. Centers for Disease Control and Prevention. Sexually transmitted disease surveillance 2014. Atlanta (GA): U.S. Department of Health and Human Services; 2015.

86. Centers for Disease Control and Prevention. HIV among transgender people. 2013.

87. Melendez R, Pinto R. HIV prevention and primary care for transgender women in a community-based clinic. J Assoc Nurses AIDS Care 2009;20(5):387–97.

88. San Francisco Department of Public Health. HIV/AIDS epidemiology annual report. San Francisco (CA): HIV Epidemiology Section; 2010.

89. Sevelius J. Transgender issues in HIV. HIV Specialist December 2013.

90. Bauer G, Redman N, Bradley K, et al. Sexual health of trans men who are gay, bisexual, or who have sex with men: results from Ontario, Canada. Int J Transgend 2013;14(2):66–74.

91. Kwakwa H, Ghobrial M. Female-to-female transmission of human immunodeficiency virus. Clin Infect Dis 2003;36(3):e40–1.

92. Chan S, Lupita R, Thornton K, et al. Likely female-to-female sexual transmission of HIV — Texas, 2012. MMWR Morb Mortal Wkly Rep 2014;63(10):209–12.

93. Marrazzo J, Stine K, Koutsky L. Genital human papillomavirus infection in women who have sex with women: a review. Am J Obstet Gynecol 2000; 183(3):770–4.

94. Diamant A, Schuster M, McGuigan K, et al. Lesbians' sexual history with men. Arch Intern Med 1999;159(22):2730.

95. Marrazzo J, Koutsky L, Kiviat N, et al. Papanicolaou test screening and prevalence of genital human papillomavirus among women who have sex with women. J Low Genit Tract Dis 2002;6(1):61–2.

96. Goldstone S, Palefsky J, Giuliano A, et al. Prevalence of and risk factors for human papillomavirus (HPV) infection among HIV-seronegative men who have sex with men. J Infect Dis 2011;203(1):66–74.

97. Frisch M. Cancer in a population-based cohort of men and women in registered homosexual partnerships. Am J Epidemiol 2003;157(11):966–72.

98. Frisch M. Human papillomavirus-associated cancers in patients with human immunodeficiency virus infection and acquired immunodeficiency syndrome. J Natl Cancer Inst 2000;92(18):1500–10.

99. Centers for Disease Control and Prevention. Viral hepatitis and men who have sex with men. 2012.

100. Scott K, Philip S, Ahrens K, et al. High prevalence of gonococcal and chlamydial infection in men who have sex with men with newly diagnosed HIV infection. J Acquir Immune Defic Syndr 2008;48(1):109–12.

101. Evans A, Scally A, Wellard S, et al. Prevalence of bacterial vaginosis in lesbians and heterosexual women in a community setting. Sex Transm Infect 2007;83(6):470–5.

102. Vodstrcil L, Walker S, Hocking J, et al. Incident bacterial vaginosis (BV) in women who have sex with women is associated with behaviors that suggest sexual transmission of BV. Clin Infect Dis 2015;60(7):1042–53.

103. Fethers K. Sexually transmitted infections and risk behaviours in women who have sex with women. Sex Transm Infect 2000;76(5):345–9.

104. Hammett TM. HIV/AIDS and other infectious diseases among correctional facilities: Transmission, burden, and an appropriate response. Am J Public Health 2006;96(6):974–8.

105. Bureau, National Inmate Survey (NIS), 2011-12; and the Substance Abuse and Mental Health Services Administration, National Survey on Drug Use and Health (NSDUH). The prevalence of ever having an infectious disease among state and federal prisoners and the general population (2011-12). 2009-2012.

106. Chandler C. Death and dying in America: The prison industrial complex's impact on women's health. Berkeley Womens Law J 2003;18:40–60.

107. Acoca L. Defusing the time bomb: understanding and meeting the growing health care needs of incarcerated women in America. Crime & Delinquency. Sage Publications 1998;49–69. Available at: http://cad.sagepub.com/content/44/1/49.Crime & Delinquency 44.1.

108. Choopanya K, Des Jarlais DC, Vanichseni S, et al. Incarceration and risk for HIV infection among injection drug users in Bangkok. J Acquir Immune Defic Syndr 2002;29:86–94.

109. Buavirat A, Page-Shaffer K, van Griensven GJP, et al. Risk of prevalent HIV infection associated with incarceration among injecting drug users in Bangkok: case-control study. BMJ 2003;326:308.

110. Dolan K, Kite B, Black E, et al. HIV in prison in low-income and middle-income countries. Lancet Infect Dis 2007;7:32–41.

111. Simooya OO. Infections in prison in low and middle income countries: Prevalence and prevention strategies. Open Infect Dis J 2010;4:33–7.

112. Gough E, Kempf MC, Graham L, et al. HIV and hepatitis B and C incidence rates in U.S. correctional populations and high risk groups: A systematic review and meta-analysis. BMC Public Health 2010;10:777.

113. Marks G, Crepaz N, Senterfitt JW, et al. Meta-analysis of high-risk sexual behavior in persons aware and unaware they are infected with HIV in the United States. J Acquir Immune Defic Syndr 2005;39:446–53.

114. National Foundation for Infectious Diseases and the National Coalition for Adult Immunization. A report on reaching underserved ethnic and minority populations to improve adolescent and adult immunization rates. October 2002.

115. Braveman PA, Cubbin C, Egerter S, et al. Socioeconomic disparities in health in the United States: What the patterns tell us. Am J Public Health 2010;100(Suppl 1):S186–96.

116. Richardus JH, Kunst AE. Black-white differences in infectious disease mortality in the United States. Am J Public Health 2001;91(8):1251–3.

117. Adekoya N. Medicaid/state children's health insurance program patients and infectious diseases treated in emergency departments: U.S., 2003. Public Health Rep 2007;122(4):513–20. Available at: http://www.ncbi.nlm.nih.gov/pubmed/17639655. Accessed January 19, 2016.

118. Centers for Disease Control and Prevention. HIV surveillance report. Diagnosis of HIV Infection and AIDS in the United States and Dependent Areas. 2009.

119. Available at: https://report.nih.gov/nihfactsheets/viewfactsheet.aspx?csid=124. Accessed January 29, 2016.

120. Available at: http://stacks.cdc.gov/view/cdc/20865/cdc_20865_DS1.pdf. Accessed January 29, 2016.
121. Cain KP, Benoit SR, Winston CA, et al. Tuberculosis among foreign-born persons in the United States. JAMA 2008;300(4):405–12.
122. Cain KP, Haley CA, Armstrong LR, et al. Tuberculosis among foreign-born persons in the United States: achieving tuberculosis elimination. Am J Respir Crit Care Med 2007;175(1):75–9.
123. Bloss E, Holtz TH, Jereb J, et al. Tuberculosis in indigenous peoples in the U.S., 2003-2008. Public Health Rep 2011;126(5):677–89. Centers for Disease Control and Prevention, 2012. Available at: http://www.ncbi.nlm.nih.gov/pubmed/21886328. Accessed February 3, 2016.
124. Centers for Disease Control and Prevention (CDC). Trends in tuberculosis - United States, 2011. MMWR Morb Mortal Wkly Rep 2012;61(11):181–5. Available at: http://www.ncbi.nlm.nih.gov/pubmed/22437911. Accessed January 12, 2016.
125. Peck AJ, Holman RC, Curns AT, et al. Lower respiratory tract infections among American Indian and Alaska native children and the general population of U.S. Children. Pediatr Infect Dis J 2005;24(4):342–51.
126. Singleton RJ, Holman RC, Folkema AM, et al. Trends in lower respiratory tract infection hospitalizations among American Indian/Alaska native children and the general U.S. child population. J Pediatr 2012;161(2):296–302.e2.
127. Kicera TJ, Douglas M, Guerra FA. Best-practice models that work: The CDC's Racial and Ethnic Adult Disparities Immunization Initiative (READII) Programs. Ethn Dis 2005;15(2 Suppl 3). S3-17–20.
128. Morita J. Addressing racial and ethnic disparities in adult immunization, Chicago. J Public Health Manag Pract 2006;12(4):321–9.
129. U.S. Department of Health and Human Services. Healthy People 2010 (2nd ed.) [with understanding and improving health (vol. 1) and objectives for improving health (vol. 2)]. Washington, DC: U.S. Government Printing Office; 2000.
130. Kutner M, Greenberg E, Jin Y, et al. The health literacy of America's adults: results from the 2003 National Assessment of Adult Literacy (NCES 2006-483). Washington, DC: U.S. Department of Education, National Center for Education Statistics; 2006.
131. Berkman ND, DeWalt DA, Pignone MP, et al. Literacy and health outcomes (AHRQ Publication No. 04-E007-2). Rockville (MD): Agency for Healthcare Research and Quality; 2004.
132. Available at: http://health.gov/communication/hlactionplan/pdf/Health_Literacy_Action_Plan.pdf. Accessed February 2, 2016.
133. Kelly PA, Haidet P. Physician overestimation of patient literacy: A potential source of health care disparities. Patient Educ Couns 2007;66(1):119–22.
134. Osborn CY, Paasche-Orlow MK, Davis TC, et al. Health literacy: an overlooked factor in understanding HIV health disparities. Am J Prev Med 2007;33(5):374–8.
135. Sentell TL, Halpin HA. Importance of adult literacy in understanding health disparities. J Gen Intern Med 2006;21(8):862–6.
136. Song J. HIV/AIDS and homelessness: recommendations for clinical practice and public policy. Nashville (TN): National Health Care for the Homeless Council, Health Care for the Homeless Clinician's Network; 1999. p. 14. Available at: www.nhchc.org/Publications/HIV.pdf.

137. Zlotnick C, Zerger S, Wolfe P. Health care for the homeless: what we have learned in the past 30 years and what's next. Am J Public Health 2013; 103(S2):S199–205.

138. Medicaid and the uninsured. Medicaid coverage and care for the homeless population: key lessons to consider for the 2014 Medicaid expansion. Washington, DC: The Henry J Kaiser Family Foundation; 2012.

139. Rabiner M, Weiner A. Health care for homeless and unstably housed: Overcoming barriers. Mt Sinai J Med 2012;79(5):586–92.

140. Inungu J, Beach E, Skeel R. Challenges facing health professionals caring for HIV-infected drug users. AIDS Patient Care STDs 2003;17(7):333–43.

141. Comprehensive HIV prevention for people who inject drugs, Revised guidance. Washington, DC: The U.S. President's Emergency Plan for AIDS Relief (PEPFAR); 2010.

142. Poteat T, Keatley J. Transgender people and HIV: policy brief. Geneva (Switzerland): World Health Organization (WHO); 2015.

143. Valdiserri R, Khalsa J, Dan C, et al. Confronting the emerging epidemic of HCV infection among young injection drug users. Am J Public Health 2014;104(5): 816–21.

144. Piper T, Rudenstine S, Stancliff S, et al. Overdose prevention for injection drug users: Lessons learned from naloxone training and distribution programs in New York City. Harm Reduct J 2007;4:3.

Cancer in the Medically Underserved Population

Oluwadamilola O. Olaku, MD, MPH[a,b,]*, Emmanuel A. Taylor, MSc, DrPH[c]

KEYWORDS

- Cancer • Incidence • Mortality • Underserved • Screening • Prevention
- Health disparities • Global health

KEY POINTS

- In the United States, the lifetime risk of developing cancer is about 1 in 2 in men and 1 in 3 in women. Liver cancer is increasing among all population groups.
- The World Cancer Research Fund estimates that about 20% of all cancers diagnosed in the United States are related to body fatness, physical inactivity, excess alcohol consumption, and/or poor nutrition.
- There was a decline in breast and cervical cancer screening between 2008 and 2013. However, there was significant increase in colorectal cancer screening during the same period.
- Disparities in cancer incidence and mortality are not fully explained by correlations of race and lower socioeconomic status, or minority race and insurance status.
- The incidence and mortality of cancer is decreasing in Western countries through decreasing prevalence of known risk factors, early detection, and improved treatment.

INTRODUCTION

Cancer is a group of diseases characterized by uncontrolled growth and spread of abnormal cells. If the spread is not controlled it can result in death.[1] Cancer is the second most common cause of death in the United States. It accounts for nearly 1 in 4 deaths. In the United States, the lifetime risk of developing cancer is 1 in 2 in men (42%) and 1 in 3 in women (38%). According to the American Cancer Society (ACS), 1,685,210 new cases of cancer will be diagnosed in 2016 and an estimated 595,690 deaths will occur as a result of cancer. A significant proportion of cancer can be prevented. In 2016, about 188,800 of the estimated 595,690 cancer deaths

[a] Office of Cancer Complementary and Alternative Medicine, National Cancer Institute, 9609 Medical Center Drive, 5-W622, MSC 9743, Bethesda, MD 20892-9743, USA; [b] Kelly Services, Kelly Government Solutions, 6101 Executive Boulevard, Suite 392, Rockville, MD 20852, USA; [c] Center to Reduce Cancer Health Disparities, National Cancer Institute, 9609 Medical Center Drive, 6-W104, MSC 9746, Rockville, MD 20850-9746, USA
* Corresponding author. Office of Cancer Complementary and Alternative Medicine, National Cancer Institute, 9609 Medical Center Drive, 5-W622, MSC 9743, Bethesda, MD 20892-9743.
E-mail address: Olakuo@mail.nih.gov

Prim Care Clin Office Pract 44 (2017) 87–97
http://dx.doi.org/10.1016/j.pop.2016.09.020
0095-4543/17/Published by Elsevier Inc.
primarycare.theclinics.com

in the United States will be caused by cigarette smoking, according to a recent study by ACS epidemiologists. In addition, the World Cancer Research Fund (WCRF) estimates that about 20% of all cancers diagnosed in the United States are related to body fatness, physical inactivity, excess alcohol consumption, and/or poor nutrition, and thus could also be prevented.[2] Cancers that are related to infectious agents, such as human papillomavirus (HPV), hepatitis B virus (HBV), hepatitis C virus (HCV), human immunodeficiency virus (HIV), and *Helicobacter pylori* could be avoided by preventing these infections through behavioral changes or vaccination, or by treating the infection.[1]

An Institute of Medicine report titled "Unequal Treatment: Confronting Racial and Ethnic Disparities in Health Care" mentioned that one of the core aims of health care is the provision of care that does not vary in quality because of race, ethnicity, sex, socioeconomic status, and geographic considerations. This report showed compelling evidence of significant variation in the rates of medical procedures by race, even when insurance status, income, age, and severity of conditions are comparable.[3] This report revealed that underrepresented and underserved populations are less likely to receive routine medical procedures and experience a lower quality of health services. As defined by Vincent Morelli in the introduction of this issue, medically underserved areas and medically underserved populations are determined by the Health Resources and Services Administration by measuring 4 variables: (1) ratio of primary care physicians per 1000 population; (2) infant mortality; (3) percentage of the population below the poverty level; and (4) percentage of the population age 65 years or older. It has been estimated that more than 100 million Americans are medically underserved.[4]

Otis Brawley,[5] Chief Medical and Scientific Officer and Executive Vice President of the ACS, observed in his study on colorectal cancer that there were similar age-adjusted mortalities in black and white people in the 1970s. Significant disparities in mortality began in the early 1980s. This disparity coincided with the advent of large-scale screening programs and coverage for colonoscopies. Although overall mortalities have declined for all racial/ethnic populations and socioeconomic levels, the rate of decrease among white people was faster, thus exacerbating the disparity over time.[4,5]

There are 2 predominant hypotheses that have formed the basis for why inequities exist. Current data do not support or refute either one. Genomic sequencing has not supported a definite biological construct on which to base disparities. However, there is some evidence that raise questions about possible differences in treatment response, and the need to consider interaction of tumor and host biology.[6]

Others have attributed disparities solely to societal and health care system factors as they relate to unequal access to care. Observed disparities are not fully explained by the correlations between minority race and lower socioeconomic status, or minority race and insurance status (uninsured or publicly insured).[7] It seems that underserved patients with Medicaid or no insurance present with more advanced cancer and are less likely to receive definitive cancer-directed surgery and/or radiation therapy. In addition, these patients have far worse survival rates.[8]

There is growing evidence to support different outcomes as a result of inequities in the structure of the health care system.[9] Patients from disadvantaged populations tend to receive care in settings that differ in terms of quality. For example, patients with breast and colon cancer treated at hospitals with large minority populations had higher mortality regardless of race.[10] Patient preferences in treatment and other clinical management options should be considered by providers; however, providers must distinguish between deeply rooted values and transient beliefs that may be amenable to information and intervention.[4]

CAUSES OF CANCER

Factors associated with increased risk for cancer include:

1. Genetics: some types of cancer run in certain families, but most causes are not clearly linked to genes that people inherit from their parents.
2. Tobacco smoke: there are more than 70 carcinogens in tobacco smoke.
3. Diet and physical activity: poor diet and not being active are key factors that can increase a person's cancer risk. WCRF International guidelines for cancer prevention include being physically active for at least 30 minutes every day; limiting consumption of energy-dense foods; eating a variety of vegetables, fruits, and wholegrains; and limiting consumption of red and processed meats.[2]
4. Sun and ultraviolet (UV) ray exposure: exposure to UV light from the sun has been shown to have a carcinogenic effect. Low skin exposure to UVB radiation from the sun or caused by specific individual behavior may also have a negative effect.[11]
5. Radiation: exposure to ionizing radiation increases the risk of cancer throughout the lifespan. Cancer risk increases after exposure to moderate and high doses of radiation (0.1–0.2 Gy).[12] The largest number of radiotherapy-related second cancers are lung, esophageal, and female breast cancer. The highest percentages of second cancers related to radiotherapy are among survivors of Hodgkin disease and cancers of the oral cavity, pharynx, and cervix uteri.[13]
6. Other carcinogens (environmental [eg, asbestos] and infectious agents [eg, herpes simplex virus]): the global burden of cancer attributable to infectious agents is estimated to be about 18%. The main infectious agents responsible for the global cancer burden are *H pylori*, HPV, HBV, HIV, and human herpes virus.[14]

EPIDEMIOLOGY

Overall, the age-adjusted cancer incidence rate for all cancers combined decreased by 0.5% per year for both sexes from 2002 to 2011 ($P<.001$) (**Fig. 1**). This finding is based on trend analysis of the surveillance epidemiology and end result (SEER)-13 data. Among men, cancer incidence rates decreased on average by 1.8% annually from 2007 to 2011 ($P = .003$). Overall cancer incidence rates among women increased 0.8% annually from 1992 to 1998 ($P = .003$), but were stable from 1998 to 2011. Among children aged 0 to 14 and 0 to 19 years, rates have increased by 0.8% per year over the past decade, continuing a trend dating from 1992 ($P<.001$).[15]

The observed rates of all cancers combined in all racial groups were lower among women than among men between 2007 and 2011 (412.8 vs 526.1 per 100,000). Black men had the overall highest incidence of cancer among men of any racial/ethnic group (587.7 per 100,000). Among women, white women had the overall highest incidence of cancer (418.6 per 100,000). In each of the racial/ethnic groups, prostate cancer remains the most common cancer among men, followed by lung and colorectal cancer among all racial/ethnic groups respectively. However, these ranks are reversed in Hispanic men. Among women, breast cancer is the most common cancer among all racial/ethnic groups. Lung and colorectal cancer are the second and third most common cancers among all racial/ethnic groups, except among Asian people and Pacific Islanders (API) and Hispanic people, among whom the ranks are reversed again.[15]

The cancer death rate for all cancer sites combined (2007–2011) was higher for men than for women (211.6 vs 147.4 deaths per 100,000). Of all racial or ethnic groups, black men had the highest cancer death rate (269.3 deaths per 100,000 men). Lung cancer was the leading cause of death in both men and women. Among men, lung, prostate, and colorectal cancers were the leading causes of cancer death in every

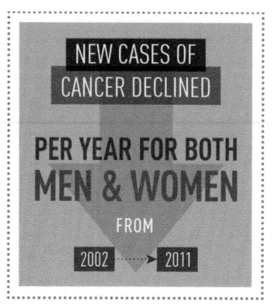

Fig. 1. Cancer incidence 2002 to 2011. (*From* National Cancer Institute. Cancer Incidence 2002 to 2011. Available at: https://www.cancer.gov/. Accessed February 17, 2016.)

racial and ethnic group except API men, for whom lung, liver, and colorectal cancers ranked highest. The leading causes of cancer death in women were lung, breast, and colorectal cancers, although the rank order of these top 3 cancers varied for American Indian/Alaska Native and Hispanic women.[15]

The 2015 report to the nation on the status of cancer used national data to determine the incidence of the 4 major molecular subtypes of breast cancer by age, race/ethnicity, poverty level, and other factors. The 4 molecular subtypes, which can be approximated by their hormone receptor (HR) status and expression of the HER2 gene are: luminal A (HR+/HER2−), Luminal B (HR+/HER2+), HER2-enriched (HR−/HER2+), and triple negative (HR−/HER2−). The 4 subtypes respond differently to treatment and have different survival rates. Non-Hispanic black people had the highest rates of late-stage disease and of poorly differentiated/undifferentiated disorder among all the subtypes. All of these factors are associated with lower survival among black people; resulting in the highest rates of breast cancer deaths[16] (**Fig. 2**).

SCREENING

The Healthy People (HP) initiative was initiated in 1979 as a Surgeon General's report. It tracks 10-year national objectives for improving the health of all Americans.[17] One of the goals of HP is a reduction in cancer deaths and a reduction in the incidence of late-stage cancers that may be reduced by screening (cervical, breast, colorectal, and prostate).[18] Brown and colleagues[18] observed marked disparities in cancer screening and provider counseling rates for certain population subgroups, including the uninsured and those with low income or no usual source of health care. The access to care of Hispanic people and those below the 200% federal poverty level were the most compromised as measured by not having health insurance and not having a usual source of care.[18]

BREAST CANCER IN WOMEN:
KNOW THE SUBTYPE

It's important for guiding treatment and predicting survival.

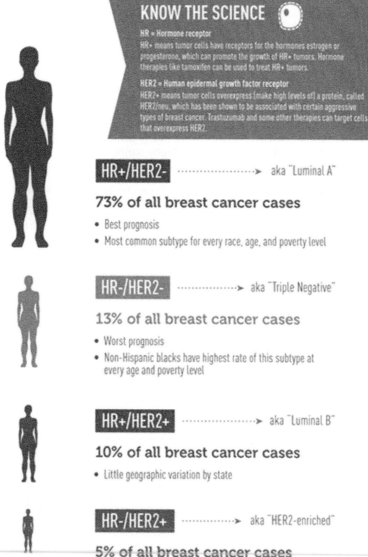

KNOW THE SCIENCE

HR = Hormone receptor
HR+ means tumor cells have receptors for the hormones estrogen or progesterone, which can promote the growth of HR+ tumors. Hormone therapies like tamoxifen can be used to treat HR+ tumors.

HER2 = Human epidermal growth factor receptor
HER2+ means tumor cells overexpress (make high levels of) a protein, called HER2/neu, which has been shown to be associated with certain aggressive types of breast cancer. Trastuzumab and some other therapies can target cells that overexpress HER2.

HR+/HER2- ·····················➤ aka "Luminal A"

73% of all breast cancer cases

- Best prognosis
- Most common subtype for every race, age, and poverty level

HR-/HER2- ·················➤ aka "Triple Negative"

13% of all breast cancer cases

- Worst prognosis
- Non-Hispanic blacks have highest rate of this subtype at every age and poverty level

HR+/HER2+ ·····················➤ aka "Luminal B"

10% of all breast cancer cases

- Little geographic variation by state

HR-/HER2+ ···············➤ aka "HER2-enriched"

5% of all breast cancer cases

- Lowest rates for all races and ethnicities

Fig. 2. Breast cancer subtypes. (*From* National Cancer Institute. Available at: https://www.cancer.gov/. Accessed February 17, 2016.)

From 2008 to 2013, self-reported cervical cancer screening overall declined by 3.8 percentage points, and breast cancer screening declined by 1.5 percentage points overall. The reason for the decrease is not certain. However, it could have been caused by the economic recession between 2008 and 2010. There is a link between economic recession and decreased health care coverage.[19] There was a significant increase of 6.1 percentage points for colorectal cancer screening in the overall population from 2008 to 2013 (**Table 1**). The evidence is insufficient to determine whether screening for prostate cancer with Prostate-specific antigen (PSA) or digital rectal examination reduces mortality from prostate cancer.[20]

Barriers to Screening

Ogedegbe and colleagues[21] identified 3 categories of barriers to screening in low-income minority women in community health centers. The categories are:

1. Patients' attitude and beliefs: examples are competing priorities, loss of privacy, lack of cancer screening knowledge, perception of good health, fear of pain and of cancer diagnosis.
2. Social network experience: this includes family discouragement, lack of medical recommendation, and knowledge of someone harmed by test.
3. Accessibility: this includes cost of test, lack of transportation, and language barrier.

United States Preventive Services Task Force Screening Recommendations

Breast cancer: biennial screening mammography for women age 50 to 74 years. The decision to start screening mammography before age 50 years should be an individual one.

Cervical cancer: screening recommended in women aged 21 to 65 years, with cytology every 3 years. Women aged 30 to 65 years who want to lengthen the screening interval are required to have a combination of cytology and HPV testing every 5 years.

Colorectal cancer: fecal occult blood testing, sigmoidoscopy, or colonoscopy in adults beginning at age 50 to 75 years.

Lung cancer: for adults aged 55 to 80 years with a history of smoking, the United States Preventive Services Task Force (USPSTF) recommends annual screening for lung cancer with low-dose computed tomography (CT) in adults aged 55 to 80 years who have a 30-pack-year smoking history and currently smoke or have quit within the past 15 years. Screening should be discontinued once a person has not smoked for

Table 1
Cervical, breast, and colorectal cancer screening 2008 to 2013

| | Cancer Type | | | | | |
| | Breast (%) | | Cervix (%) | | Colorectal (%) | |
Race/Ethnicity	2008	2013	2008	2013	2008	2013
Total	73.7	72.6	84.5	80.7	52.1	58.2
Asian	76.2	72.2	71.5	70.5	47.5	50.6
Black or African American	76.5	72.9	86.1	82.2	48.0	59.1
White	73.3	72.6	85.1	81.4	53.3	58.6
Hispanic or Latino	68.3	66.7	81.3	77.1	34.9	43.0

Data from National Health Interview Survey (NHIS), Centers for Disease Control and Prevention, National Center for Health Statistics (CDC/NCHS).

15 years or develops a health problem that substantially limits life expectancy or the ability or willingness to have curative lung surgery.

Prostate cancer: the USPSTF recommends against PSA-based screening for prostate cancer.[22]

PREVENTION

The second edition of *The Cancer Atlas* released by the ACS and the International Agency for Research on Cancer argues that many cancers are largely preventable and prevention is cost-effective.[23] There is evidence to suggest that a diagnosis or suspicion of cancer can be a financial stressor. In a population-based study in western Washington, 197,840 patients with cancer were matched with an equal number of controls by age, sex, and zip code. Patients with cancer were 2.6 times more likely to file for bankruptcy than cancer-free controls ($P<.05$).[24]

Observational epidemiologic studies have shown associations between the following modifiable lifestyle factors or environmental exposures and specific cancers.

Cigarette Smoking/Tobacco Use

Research has consistently shown the association between tobacco use and cancers of many sites. Specifically, cigarette smoking has been established as a cause of cancers of the lung, oral cavity, esophagus, bladder, kidney, pancreas, stomach, and cervix, and also acute myelogenous leukemia. It is estimated that cigarette smoking causes 30% of all cancer deaths in the United States. Smoking avoidance and cessation result in decreased incidence and mortality from cancer.[25] In addition, Andersen and colleagues[26] found that meeting ACS cancer prevention guidelines, especially regarding tobacco and alcohol consumption, was associated with a lower cancer risk in underserved populations.

Infections

Infectious agents have been estimated to cause 18% of all cancers globally.[14] The burden of cancers caused by infections is much greater in developing nations (26%) than in developed nations (8%). Infection with an oncogenic strain of HPV is considered a necessary event for subsequent cervical cancer. Immunity conferred by vaccines results in a marked decrease in precancerous lesions. Oncogenic strains of HPV are also linked with cancers of the penis, vagina, anus, and oropharynx. Other examples of infectious agents that cause cancer are HBV and HCV (liver cancer), and *H pylori* (gastric cancer).[14]

Radiation

Exposure to UV radiation and ionizing radiation are established causes of cancer. Nonmelanoma skin cancers are caused by exposure to solar UV radiation.[27] There is extensive epidemiologic and biological evidence that links exposure to ionizing radiation with the development of cancer, especially those that involve the hematological system, breast, lungs, and thyroid. The National Research Council of the National Academies, Committee to Assess the Health Risks from Exposure to Low Levels of Ionizing Radiation, the Biologic Effects of Ionizing Radiation VII report concluded that no dose of radiation should be considered completely safe.[28] The major sources of population exposure to ionizing radiation are medical radiation (including x-rays, CT, fluoroscopy) and naturally occurring radon gas in the basements of homes. There is a significant and negative correlation between income and radon levels.[29] Reducing radiation exposure and limiting unnecessary CT scans and other diagnostic studies are important prevention strategies.[30,31]

Diet

The WCRF/American Institute for Cancer Research (AICR) concluded that both fruits and nonstarchy vegetables were associated with probable decreased risk for cancers of the mouth, esophagus, and stomach. Fruits were also associated with probable decreased risk of lung cancer.[32,33]

Alcohol

The WCRF/AICR report judged the evidence to be convincing that drinking alcohol increased the risks of cancers of the mouth, esophagus, breast, and colorectum. Further, the evidence was judged to be probable that drinking alcohol increased the risk of liver cancer, and colorectal cancer in women.[32,33]

Physical Activity

In the WCRF/AICR report, the evidence was judged convincing that increased physical activity protects against colorectal cancer. The evidence was probable that physical activity was associated with lower risk of postmenopausal breast and endometrial cancer. As with dietary factors, physical activity seems to play a role in selected malignancies.[32,33]

Obesity

The WCRF/AICR report concluded that obesity is convincingly linked to postmenopausal breast cancer and cancers of the esophagus, pancreas, colorectum, endometrium, and kidney.

Chemoprevention

Chemoprevention refers to the use of natural or synthetic compounds to interfere with early stages of carcinogenesis before invasive cancer appears.[34] Daily use of selective estrogen receptor modulators (tamoxifen or raloxifene) for up to 5 years reduces the incidence of breast cancer by about 50% in high-risk women. Dutasteride (alpha-reductase inhibitor) has been shown to reduce the incidence of prostate cancer.[35] Other chemopreventive candidates include cyclooxygenase-2 inhibitors and aspirin. Secondary analyses from pooled data whose primary end points were vascular events showed that aspirin taken daily for 4 years was associated with an 18% reduction in overall cancer death.[36]

Vitamin and dietary supplement use

The evidence is insufficient to support the use of multivitamin and mineral supplements or single vitamins or minerals to prevent cancer.[37]

GLOBAL HEALTH

Cancer is a leading cause of death worldwide. The numbers of cases and deaths are expected to grow as populations grow, age, and adopt lifestyle behaviors that increase cancer risk.[38] In 2012, an estimated 14.1 million new cases and 8.2 million cancer deaths occurred worldwide.[39] The highest rates are in North America, Oceania, and Europe for both sexes. Prostate cancer is the most commonly diagnosed cancer among men in North and South America; northern, western, and southern Europe; and Oceania. In Eastern Europe, lung cancer is the most common. The leading cancers among men in Africa include prostate, lung, colorectum, liver, esophagus, Kaposi sarcoma, leukemia, stomach, and non-Hodgkin lymphoma. However, in Asia, they include lung, lip, oral cavity, liver, stomach, colorectal and prostate cancers.

Breast cancer is the most common cancer among women in North America, Europe, and Oceania. Breast and cervical cancers are the most frequently diagnosed cancers in Latin America and the Caribbean, Africa, and most of Asia. In addition, common female cancers in Asia include lung (China, Korea), liver (Mongolia), and thyroid (South Korea).[39]

Eight major cancers account for more than 60% of total global cases and deaths: lung and bronchus, colon and rectum, female breast, prostate, stomach, liver, esophagus, and cervix uteri.[39]

The incidence and mortality of cancer are decreasing in Western countries through decreasing prevalence of known risk factors, early detection, and improved treatment. However, rates of lung, breast, and colorectal cancers are increasing in low-income and middle-income countries. This increase is caused by increased risk of smoking, excess body weight, physical inactivity, and changing reproductive patterns. In addition, these countries also bear a disproportionate burden of infection-related cancers, such as cervix, liver, and stomach.[39]

SUMMARY

The incidence and mortality of cancer in the United States have been decreasing over the last few years, largely because of appropriate and timely screening, prevention, and better treatment. Despite this downward trend, disparities persist among the various ethnic and racial groups in the United States. The disparities can be minimized or eliminated by encouraging equitable distribution and use of resources. A sincere commitment by individual governments, international agencies, donors, and the private sector is required to reduce the burden of cancer globally.

REFERENCES

1. ACS. Cancer facts and figures 2016. Atlanta (GA): American Cancer Society; 2016.
2. WCRF, AIRC. Diet, nutrition, physical activity and prostate cancer. Washington, DC: AIRC; 2014.
3. Institute of Medicine. Unequal treatment confronting racial and ethnic disparities in health care. Washington, DC: National Academies Press; 2003.
4. Wong S. Medically underserved populations: disparities in quality and outcomes. J Oncol Pract 2015;11:193–4.
5. Brawley OW. Colorectal cancer control: providing adequate care to those who need it. J Natl Cancer Inst 2014;106:ju075.
6. Fine MJ, Ibrahim SA, Thomas SB. The role of race and genetics in health disparities research. Am J Public Health 2005;95:2125–8.
7. Haider AH, Scott VK, Rehman KA, et al. Racial disparities in surgical care and outcomes in the United States: a comprehensive review of the patient, provider, and systemic factors. J Am Coll Surg 2013;216:482–92.
8. Walker GV, Grant SR, Guadagnolo BA, et al. Disparities in stage at diagnosis, treatment and survival in non-elderly adult patients with cancer according to insurance status. J Clin Oncol 2014;27:3945–50.
9. Birkmayer NJ, Gu N, Baser O, et al. Socioeconomic status and surgical mortality in the elderly. Med Care 2008;46:893–9.
10. Breslin TM, Morris AM, Gu N, et al. Hospital factors and racial disparities in mortality after surgery for breast and colon cancer. J Clin Oncol 2009;27:3945–50.

11. Elwood JM, Jopson J. Melanoma and sun exposure: an overview of published studies. Int J Cancer 1997;73:198–203.

12. Kamiya K, Ozasa K, Akiba S, et al. Long term effects of radiation exposure on health. Lancet 2015;386:469–78.

13. Intidher Labidi-Galy S, Tassy L, Blay JY. Radiation induced soft tissue sarcoma. Available at: http://sarcomahelp.org/radiation-induced-sarcoma.html. Accessed February 8, 2016.

14. Parkin DM. The global health burden of infection-associated cancers in the year 2002. Int J Cancer 2006;118:3030–44.

15. Kohler BA, Sherman RL, Howlader N, et al. Annual report to the nation on the status of cancer, 1975-2011, featuring incidence of breast cancer subtypes by race/ethnicity, poverty and state. J Natl Cancer Inst 2015;107:djv048.

16. New analysis of breast cancer subtypes could lead to better risk stratifications; annual report to the nation shows that mortality and incidence for most cancers continue to decline. Available at: http://cancer.gov/news-events/press-releases/2015/report-nation-march-2015-press-release. Accessed February 17, 2016.

17. Department of Health, Education and Welfare, Public Health Service. Healthy People: the Surgeon General's report on health promotion and disease prevention. Washington, DC: Government Printing Office; 1979.

18. Brown ML, Klabunde CN, Cronin K, et al. Challenges in meeting Healthy People 2020 objective for cancer related preventive services, NHIS 2008 and 2010. Prev Chronic Dis 2014;11:E29.

19. William DR. Race, socioeconomic status and health. The added effect of racism and discrimination. Ann N Y Acad Sci 1999;896:173–88.

20. Prostate cancer screening for health professionals (PDQ). Available at: www.cancer.gov/types/prostate/hp/prostate-screening-pdq. Accessed February 29, 2016.

21. Ogedegbe G, Cassells AN, Robinson CM, et al. Perceptions of barriers and facilitators of cancer early development among low income minority women in community health centers. J Natl Med Assoc 2005;97:162–70.

22. US Preventive Services Task Force. Published recommendations. Available at: http://www.uspreventiveservicestaskforce.org/BrowseRec/Index/browse-recommendations. Accessed June 18, 2016.

23. Jemal A, Vineis P, Bray F, et al. The cancer atlas 2nd edition. Atlanta (GA): American Cancer Society; 2014.

24. Ramsey S, Blough D, Kirchhoff A, et al. Washington State cancer patients found to be at greater risk for bankruptcy than people without a cancer diagnosis. Health Aff (Millwood) 2013;32:1143–52.

25. National Cancer Institute. PDQ® Cancer Prevention overview. Bethesda (MD): National Cancer Institute; 2016. Available at: http://www.cancer.gov/about-cancer/causes-prevention/hp-prevention-overview-pdq. Accessed March 1, 2016.

26. Andersen SW, Blot WJ, Shu X, et al. Adherence to cancer prevention guidelines and cancer risk in low-income and African American populations. Cancer Epidemiol Biomarkers Prev 2016;25(5):846–53.

27. Scotto J, Fears TR, Fraumeni JF Jr. Solar radiation. In: Schottenfeld D, Fraumeni JF Jr, editors. Cancer epidemiology and prevention. 2nd edition. New York: Oxford University Press; 1996. p. 355–72.

28. National Research Council (US), Committee to Assess Health Risks from Exposure to Low Levels of Ionizing Radiation. Health risks from exposure to low levels of ionizing radiation: BEIR VII phase 2. Washington, DC: National Academy Press; 2006.

29. National Council on Radiation Protection and Measurements. Ionizing radiation exposure of the population of the United States. Bethesda (MD): National Council on Radiation Protection and Measurement; 2009.
30. Reddy NK, Bhutani MS. Racial disparities in pancreatic cancer and radon exposure: a correlation study. Pancreas 2009;38:391–5.
31. Mettler FA Jr, Thomadsen BR, Bhargavan M, et al. Medical radiation exposure in the U.S. in 2006: preliminary results. Health Phys 2008;95:502–7.
32. World Cancer Research Fund/American Institute for Cancer Research. Food, Nutrition, Physical Activity, and Prevention of Cancer: a Global Perspective. Washington, DC: AICR; 2007.
33. Norat T, Aune D, Chan D, et al. Fruits and vegetables: updating the epidemiologic evidence for the WCRF/AICR lifestyle recommendations for cancer prevention. Cancer Treat Res 2014;159:35–50.
34. William WN Jr, Heymach JV, Kim ES, et al. Molecular targets for cancer chemoprevention. Nat Rev Drug Discov 2009;8:213–25.
35. Andriole GL, Bostwick DG, Brawley OW, et al. Effect of dutasteride on the risk of prostate cancer. N Engl J Med 2010;362:1192–202.
36. Rothwell PM, Fowkes FG, Belch JF, et al. Effect of daily aspirin on long term risk of death due to cancer: analysis of individual patient data from randomized trials. Lancet 2011;377:31–41.
37. Fortmann SP, Burda BU, Senger CA, et al. Vitamin and mineral supplements in the primary prevention of cardiovascular disease and cancer: an updated systematic evidence review for the US preventive services task force. Ann Intern Med 2013;159:824–34.
38. Torre LA, Siegel RL, Ward EM, et al. Global cancer incidence and mortality rates and trends. An update. Cancer Epidemiol Biomarkers Prev 2016;25(1):16–27.
39. Ferlay J, Soerjomataram I, Ervik M, et al. Cancer incidence and mortality worldwide: sources, methods and major patterns in GLOBOCAN 2012. Int J Cancer 2015;136:359–86.

Psychological Issues in Medically Underserved Patients

Mathew Devine, DO[a,b,*], Lauren DeCaporale-Ryan, PhD[c,d,e],
Magdalene Lim, PsyD[f,g], Juliana Berenyi, DO[h]

KEYWORDS

- Underserved • Psychosocial • Mental health • Depression • Primary care • Suicide

KEY POINTS

- Multiple populations in the United States face increased social and environmental stressors. These populations often seek mental health care from their primary care physician. Recommendations are outlined to improve their care experience.
- Recognize that subgroups of underserved populations that face additional stigma are at increased risked psychosocially (eg, based on race, age, and SES). Culturally sensitive programs help patients feel supported by their treatment team.
- Increase comfort using behavioral screening tools, such as Patient Health Questionnaire–9, to assess for mood disorders in underserved populations to more effectively identify and provide help for mental health conditions.
- Identify ways to support engagement in behavioral health (eg, having colocated care, ability to conduct a warm hand-off).
- Identify a team member who can support practical needs (eg, completion of paperwork, referrals to community resources), such as a social worker or care manager.

Disclosure: The authors of this article report no direct financial interest in the subject matter or any material discussed in this article.

[a] Department of Family Medicine, University of Rochester, 777 South Clinton Avenue, Rochester, NY 14620, USA; [b] Accountable Health Partners, 135 Corporate Woods Suite 320, Rochester, NY 14623, USA; [c] Department of Psychiatry, University of Rochester Medical Center, 300 Crittenden Boulevard, Box Psych, Rochester, NY 14642, USA; [d] Department of Medicine, University of Rochester Medical Center, 300 Crittenden Boulevard, Box Psych, Rochester, NY 14642, USA; [e] Department of Surgery, University of Rochester Medical Center, 300 Crittenden Boulevard, Box Psych, Rochester, NY 14642, USA; [f] Department of Psychiatry, University of Rochester Medical Center, 300 Crittenden Boulevard, Rochester, NY 14642, USA; [g] Department of Medicine, University of Rochester Medical Center, 300 Crittenden Boulevard, Rochester, NY 14642, USA; [h] Department of Family Medicine, University of Rochester Family Medicine Resident, 777 South Clinton Avenue, Rochester, NY 14620, USA
* Corresponding author.
E-mail address: Mathew_devine@urmc.rochester.edu

INTRODUCTION

Improving the health of underserved populations is an ongoing focus of many medical industries including the US government. One critical problem with underserved populations is their potential for increased suffering from psychosocial stressors/mental health disorders. Practicing family physicians have many day-to-day interactions with psychosocial issues as part of their primary care practice workload. It has been identified that about half of the care for common mental disorders is delivered in general medical settings, leading Nordquist and Regier[1] to describe general medical settings as the "de facto mental health care system" in the United States. This article describes categories of underserved populations, including racially and culturally diverse; pediatric; geriatric; refugee; rural; and lesbian, gay, bisexual, or transgender (LGBT) individuals. Each section defines the population is being presented, identifies the mental health problems each is likely to encounter, explores the barriers that prevent access to care, and identifies potential methods to minimize such barriers. The following sections differentiate the ways in which psychiatric issues vary in underserved settings compared with the general population. Recommendations are offered for primary care physicians (PCP) to support improved recognition and management of psychosocial stressors and psychiatric illness among the underserved, who frequently present to primary care settings for such care.

Prevalence of Mental Health Diagnoses Identified in Primary Care

Recent analyses suggest that approximately 8% of adults in the United States suffer from current depressive symptoms. Prevalence rates for a lifetime diagnosis of depression suggest that nearly 16% of adults have suffered from depressive symptoms. Additionally, 4% endorse having suffered from a lifetime diagnosis of anxiety without evidence of depressive symptoms.[2] These rates are significantly influenced by patient demographic factors, including age, sex, race and ethnicity, education, employment status, and place of living. It is in this context that understanding the unique needs of the underserved is important to best care for the populations described next.

UNDERSERVED POPULATIONS IN THE UNITED STATES
Racially and Culturally Diverse Individuals

Racial minorities in the United States include Hispanics (12.5%), African Americans (12.3%), and Asians (3.6%), and account for one-third of the US population.[3] Racial minorities often suffer from poorer health and are overrepresented in drug-induced death, infant mortality, preterm birth, homicide rates, periodontitis, tuberculosis, obesity, and human immunodeficiency virus.[4] Racial health disparities are influenced by several other factors, including cultural identity, psychosocial stressors (eg, poverty), environmental factors (eg, violence), and unmet health needs.[5,6] The higher prevalence of mental health problems among racial minority individuals is largely accounted for by social determinants.[5]

Research to create and improve effective therapeutic interventions for racial minatory groups emphasizes understanding mental health stigma and the impact of perceived discrimination among these individuals.[7,8] Each individual has a different life experience rooted in culture and history, and different perceptions of his or her care needs. For example, barriers to care include "self-reliance and self-silence" coping among African American women,[9] and low perceived need despite significant psychosocial trauma among subgroups of immigrant Latinos.[10] Research on racial matching and culturally sensitive treatments highlights the need to consider how racial and cultural experiences influence interest and engagement in care.[11]

Individuals with Deprived Socioeconomic Status

More than 46 million people live below the poverty line in the United States.[12] Lower socioeconomic status (SES) frequently places people in unsafe environments and vulnerable positions.[13] Lower SES results in food insecurity, and reduced access to education, employment, and community resources.[14] Chronic adversity, exposure to trauma and loss, and discrimination[15,16] attribute to higher rates of homelessness, crime, incarceration, and substance abuse. Such predisposing vulnerabilities increase risk for poor health behaviors, chronic disease, and psychiatric disorders,[13] and limit personal resources, such as mastery and coping strategies.[17]

Diagnoses of depression, anxiety, posttraumatic stress disorder (PTSD), substance abuse, and schizophrenia have all been shown to have higher prevalence in impoverished, urban neighborhoods.[17–20] These patients tend to receive less specialty care for mental health. Instead, patients rely on acute hospital care[21] for medical and psychiatric needs, especially schizophrenia and substance abuse.[19] Multiple obstacles prevent those with low SES from engaging in specialty care including long wait times for service, limited health insurance benefits, limited clinicians willing or able to provide services at lower rates of reimbursement, and multicultural barriers (perceived bias, cultural mistrust).[13]

A case example (**Fig. 1**) is presented demonstrating how psychosocial barriers preclude patients from adequately accessing care. This case outlines the experience of a 25-year-old African American woman, and the adversity she faced from an early age Recommendations for interventions outlined in the case are also included in **Fig. 1**.

Children and Adolescents

Children younger than age 18 experiencing psychosocial stressors sometimes create increased challenges for families as a result of their dependence on their parent or guardian. The leading mental health burdens for children younger than 10 and their families are developmental disabilities, emotional disorders, and disruptive behavioral disorders.[22] Pediatric behavioral health specialists are in an even smaller supply than those working with the adult population. However, there are school-based services and community programs that can offer some assistance to this population.

In the United States, barriers to care in the underserved pediatric population include cost of care, inconvenience of access, poorly integrated systems of care, and inadequate insurance coverage.[22] Through the use of developmental and mental health screening tools and general screenings, PCPs can help to identify and work with school-based and behavioral health teams for ongoing treatment. Because of the shortage of specialty care it is important that PCPs are well educated and trained to work with minor to moderate psychosocial disturbances in children. For severe needs it is important that there is appropriate access for consultation and assistance because rectifying these problems early on provides health benefits throughout that child's life and development. According to the Centers for Disease Control and Prevention's National Health and Nutrition Examination Survey, which includes prevalence data for children ages 8 to 15, the three most prevalent mental health issues for children are (1) attention-deficit/hyperactivity disorder, (2) mood disorders, and (3) major depression disorders. Screening for these mental health conditions should be considered during outpatient visits including sports physical and well child visits (**Table 1** for screening details).[23]

Older Adults

Older adults have unique clinical needs and face multiple transitions. Estimates suggest that about 6 to 8 million (nearly 1 in 5) of those older than 65 have a mental health

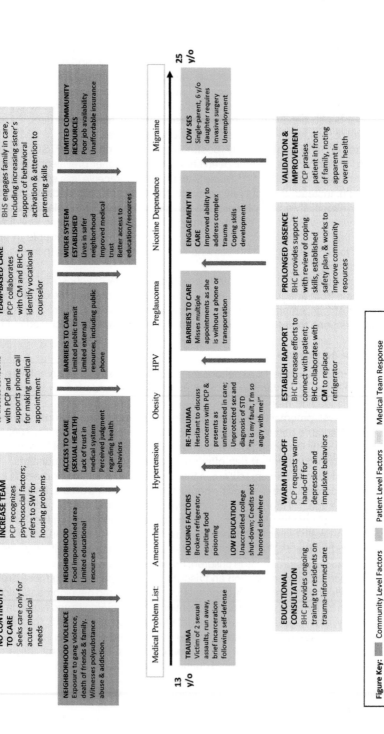

Figure Key: ▮ Community Level Factors ▮ Patient Level Factors ▮ Medical Team Response

or substance use disorder, and as the population doubles by 2030, so too will the number who suffer from such diagnoses.[24] Older adults with mental health conditions often experience poorer health behaviors and outcomes, and account for a disproportionate amount of health care costs.[25] Despite such prevalence rates, older adults less frequently engage in behavioral health care because of limited financial resources, difficulty accessing care due to chronic medical illness, lack of transportation, and the perceived stigma associated with treatment.[25] These limiting factors are further exacerbated by a significant shortage of specialty-trained workforce; currently, there is less than one geriatric psychiatrist per every 6000 older adults in need.[24,25]

Subsequently, care is most often sought in brief visits with PCPs, who are less likely to screen for mood symptoms and to refer older adults to specialty mental health care.[25,26] Anxiety and mood disorders are often undetected, as is suicide risk. Older adults account for nearly 18% of completed suicides in the United States,[27] with an average of 58% having seen their PCP within the month before their death.[28] Diagnosis of behavioral health concerns and risk of self-harm is often complicated by patients' presentation of somatic complaints and the complexity of differentiating between mood symptoms, medical problems, and dementia processes.[29] Moreover, PCPs generally have insufficient time to provide the necessary follow-up for improved outcomes (see **Table 1** for screening details).[30]

Refugee Individuals and Families

Refugees are given legal status and entry into the United States based on demonstration that they have been persecuted or have fear of persecution because of race, religion, nationality, political opinion, or membership in a particular social group.[31] In 2014, approximately 70,000 refugees entered the United States primarily hailing from Afghanistan, Iraq, Somali, Democratic Republic of Congo, Myanmar, Colombia, Sudan, Vietnam, Eritrea, China, and Syria.[32]

Leaving one's home and resettling in a new place creates significant distress and places refugees at risk for a variety of mental health concerns. Experiences of fleeing one's home are most often traumatic. Refugees suffer hardships, such as imprisonment, torture, loss of property, malnutrition, physical and sexual assault, and separation from family. These traumatic experiences can lead to PTSD, anxiety, and depressive disorders, such as major depression and adjustment disorder. The prevalence of these conditions in refugee populations varies greatly and can range anywhere from 4% to 86% for PTSD and 5% to 31% for depression.[33] The manifestations of these diseases differ on a case-by-case basis, with acute and chronic presentation, and symptoms may include psychosis and somatization.

Once refugees resettle in a new country, although their lives are often safer, the stress they experience is great. Frequently their family and friends remain in the countries they have fled or are still fleeing and the worry for their well-being can be extreme.

◄——

Fig. 1. Timeline depicting the experiences of a 25-year-old, underserved African American woman, single parent to 6-year-old daughter, and victim of domestic violence, referred to a psychologist for management of depression and anxiety. Timelines, developed collaboratively with patients can help clinicians understand the patient-level factors and sociocultural/environmental context that influence overall health. By working with an integrated team, the environmental factors, although still troublesome, are mitigated and patients are able to begin pursuing improved health and meet other personal goals for a more optimal lifestyle. BHC, Behavioral Health Clinician; CM, Care Manager; HPV, human papilloma virus; PCP, Primary Care Physician; STD, sexually transmitted disease; SW, Social Worker.

Table 1
Point of care screening tools for PCPs

Patient Population	Modify Direct Patient Experience	Collaborate with Others About	Seek Continued Education About
To improve access to care, PCPs can…			
All	Use tools, such as a timeline and/or genogram, to understand psychosocial experiences and their impact on health	Seek supportive consultation and consider warm hand-off to improve patient comfort with specialty care	Please review specific education examples below
Racially/ethnically diverse	Inquire about and understand an individual's perception regarding mental health treatment, rooted in family and cultural history, including their past experiences with the mental health system and experiences of stigma and discrimination Communicate respect to patients regarding their cultural perspective of illness and value their partnership throughout the treatment process Offer patient education materials tailored to race, education level, and language	Patient culture-specific concerns (eg, stigma about mental health treatment)	Diversity training, and training for Trauma-Informed Medical Care[51] for clinicians and staff
Low SES individuals/ families	Address patients' functional needs using supportive inquiry focused on patients' safety, including: • Whether their basic needs of food, shelter, and utilities are met, • What exposure to risk and violence they encounter, and • What types of relationships (supportive and deleterious) exist Ensure availability of transportation, eliminating potential barriers to care	Identify ways to support engagement in behavioral health (eg, having co-located care, ability to conduct a warm hand-off) Identify a team member who can support practical needs (eg, completion of paperwork, referrals to community resources, such as a social worker or care manager	Community resources (eg, churches, local organizations) that support access to housing, clothing, food, and hygiene products

Pediatrics	Screen for risk of abuse or neglect and make appropriate referrals to reduce risk of harm Be able to screen for development, and intellectual disabilities and behavioral health disorders If case is severe to identify specialty care clinicians for medication management and therapeutic interventions	Be informed about alternative means of care, including home visits and tele health services Unique presentation of clinical symptoms and how to work best with parents/guardians and school-based professionals
Older adults	Screen all older adults for depression and risk of suicide Identify specialty care clinicians for medication management and therapeutic interventions Recognize the family as "patient," attending to caregiver needs Work with depression care managers to facilitate access to and use of interventions Screen for risk of abuse or neglect and make appropriate referrals to reduce risk of harm	Unique presentation of clinical symptoms Community resources, such as churches, respite programs, and support groups for patients and caregivers Be informed about alternative means of care, including home visits and tele health services
Refugees	Use of screening tools (eg, Harvard Trauma Questionnaire, Resettlement Stressor Scale, War Trauma Scale) to help initiate dialogue about trauma experiences while overcoming some of the cultural and communication barriers that exist[52] Ensure collaboration with social work/care management for maintenance of insurance benefits Because of their traumatic experiences, refugees can be fearful and hesitant to provide the truth Extra care and awareness must be given in assessing this population Consider interpreter services available	Understand how language can be stigmatizing (eg, "depression" or "mental health" may have negative connotations") Learn how to frame questions (eg, do not ask, "Are you depressed?" but instead ask "How are you sleeping?" Be informed about community resources available for resettlement

(continued on next page)

Table 1
(continued)

Patient Population	Modify Direct Patient Experience	Collaborate with Others About	Seek Continued Education About
Rural populations	Use behavioral screening tools, such as Patient Health Questionnaire-9, to access for depression in rural populations specifically farmers to identify and provide help for mental health conditions Improve access to medical centers with improved communication methods (telemedicine, and/or geographic location)		Increase in trained community workers/personnel to come to the homes of this population
LGBT individuals	Create a safe environment that allows patients to trust clinicians and staff, thereby building rapport and opportunity for information sharing about sexual orientation and psychosocial experiences Routinely screen critical health behaviors, including substance use and safe sex practices, and of mood disorders, risk for suicide and self-harm behaviors Allow time for discussion about patients' coming out experience and/or plans to do so; provide support and resources available in your community		Subgroups of this population and the additional stigma they face because of increased risked psychosocially (eg, based on race, age, and SES) Culturally sensitive programs help patients feel supported by their treatment team

Family and friends abroad depend financially on refugees. More than $1 billion in remittance was sent from the United States in 2012, making up a significant percent of the household income of recipients.[34] Refugees often must restart their careers, because professional degrees do not transfer; former professionals are forced to work in manual labor or minimum wage jobs. Assimilating into a new culture and learning a new language also has challenges and feelings of isolation, confusion, and frustration are common. These stressors not only put refugees at higher risk for mental health concerns but can also exacerbate existing chronic medical conditions.

Rural Populations

Multiple studies have evaluated the prevalence of mental health conditions in urban versus rural environments. These studies conclude that in general the prevalence of overall mental health disorders seems higher in urban settings. Despite the lower prevalence in rural communities there is an appreciable decrease in access to mental health services. Moreover, there is some evidence that certain conditions, such as functional psychosis and manic-depressive psychosis, are higher in rural areas.[35]

Additionally, there is an increased rate of suicides in rural populations specifically among farmers (which is just under twice the rate of the US adult suicide rate).[36] The rates of suicide in most rural communities are 17.14 per 100,000 versus 11.51 per 100,000 in most urban areas.[37] Studies also show suicide rates are higher with those individuals taking antidepressant medications.[37]

To bridge this gap, Federally Qualified Health Centers (CHCs) continue to grow as a delivery medical network in rural communities. A recent study identified that treatment of mental health and substance abuse are some of the most common reasons that individuals visit CHCs. These centers use a treatment model that includes housing other specialties to work within these practices to increase access to all forms of medical care not just from their PCPs. However, with the visit demand high for addressing mental health needs there is a shortage of behavioral health specialists to provide this care even though most centers have rooms to have them working in their facilities. Based on this shortage only 6.5% of these encounters are with on-site behavioral health specialists at rural CHCs. The lack of these services again identifies that the opportunities for having mental health professionals directly involved with care in rural communities is less than urban communities.

Lesbian/Gay/Bisexual/Transgender Individuals

Estimates suggest that 3.5% of individuals identify as LGBT in the United States.[38] LGBT individuals face multiple stressors: discrimination, disproportionate poverty rates compared with the general population,[39] and increased chronic medical conditions. Subgroups of the LGBT population encounter higher rates of asthma, headaches, allergies, osteoarthritis, gastrointestinal problems, and human immunodeficiency virus/AIDS.[40] Lesbians, gay men, and bisexual individuals are more likely to smoke than heterosexual peers. Tobacco, alcohol, and illicit drug use vary significantly as a result of age, affiliation with LGBT culture, stressful life events, and emotional regulation.[41]

Often, LGBT individuals face rejection by their communities, resulting in inequality in the workplace and in access to medical care,[40] and increased exposure to physical and sexual violence.[42] Individuals frequently report a lack of familial support, which correlates to increased rates of mental illness and substance abuse.[43] Discrimination and higher levels of day-to-day stress create greater risk for psychiatric disease. A study of women found that lesbians had higher frequency of depression, PTSD, and phobias compared with heterosexual women.[44] Similarly, gay men tend to experience higher rates of depression and anxiety.[45] Research supports that similar mood disturbances are common among bisexual and transgender individuals; however, data pertaining to the mental health needs among these groups are presently limited.[46]

LGBT individuals are at increased risk of suicidal ideation. Bisexuals are more likely to report higher levels of self-harm, thoughts of suicide, and suicidal attempts compared with heterosexual, gay men, and lesbians; rates increase for lesbian and bisexual women who are not "out."[47] Research indicates that among transgender individuals, suicidal ideation has been reported from 38% to 65% of the time; 16% to 32% of transgender patients have reported a history of suicide attempt.[48]

Despite the need for medical and mental health intervention, in 2011, the Institute of Medicine noted that LGBT patients face barriers to care because of a lack of understanding about their treatment needs. Studies show that lesbian and bisexual women frequently consult PCPs for emotional support if their PCP is aware of their sexual orientation; however, not all want or choose to disclose this information.

METHODS TO RESOLUTION AND IMPROVING MENTAL HEALTH CARE IN THE UNDERSERVED

Meeting the mental health needs of the underserved requires many changes be made to improve access to care. Establishing a system to improve accessibility to trained PCPs or specialty providers is critical. This section focuses on the methods (previously evaluated or currently under consideration) in various settings across the United States to improve mental health care for the general population and the underserved. **Table 2** provides information on how to maximize care in the various underserved populations discussed previously.

Because of the ongoing shortage of PCPs and behavior health service (BHS) providers emerging technologies may increase flexibility to reaching the underserved, although research on efficacy of such technology use is still needed. Health information technologies, such as smart phones, smart televisions, handheld apps, and desktop software, and the Internet can improve patient education and access to care for those previously underserved populations.[49] These technologies offer a wide range of possibilities for treatment remotely of underserved populations. Because of the early stages of these technologies data on their usefulness are limited. Such technology requires upfront costs to practices and patients (eg, having necessary devices). However, technology offers flexibility of coding, allowing for customizable software that adapts for different languages and visual technologies for the consumer. Mass screenings can be done using online forms, which can be scored and delivered to health professionals to identify high-risk patients in need of care. Video capabilities can link mental health and PCPs to patients from far distances to save on travel and compensate for barriers (eg, chronic illness, inability to drive). Such interventions do not currently have as much oversight, and the efficacy, and ethical nature of these interventions are still being evaluated.[49] In our opinion the oversight of this sector will certainly help to improve evaluation and dissemination of these well-intentioned efforts.

Increased education and specialty training should be offered by health systems or medical educators for mental health providers and physicians to recognize symptoms and know when and how to treat and when to refer. These ongoing issues can better be addressed if practices are able have designated BHS providers involved in underserved primary care practices. Because there are not enough BHS professionals, many rural practices have begun to use evidence-based community partnerships models. These models are still being researched and they are used to provide remote

Table 2
How to maximize care provided for populations of the underserved

	Depression and Mood Disorders	Anxiety	Substance Use	Other
Children and adolescents	• Beck Depression Inventory for Youth • Children's Depression Inventory • Center for Epidemiologic Studies–Depression Scale for Children • Reynolds Child Depression Scale • Reynolds Adolescent Depression Scale	• Beck Anxiety Inventory for Youth • Multidimensional Anxiety Scale for Children	• CRAFFT Screener • Drug Abuse Screen Test –10 (for older youth) • Teen Addiction Severity Index	• Autism Behavior Checklist • Child Behavior Checklist • Conners' Rating Scales–Revised • Vanderbilt ADHD Rating Scales
Adults	• Beck Depression Inventory–II • Beck Depression Inventory–Primary Care[a] • Center for Epidemiologic Studies Depression • Center for Epidemiologic Studies–Depression Revised • Mood Disorder Questionnaire (Bipolar Disorder) • Patient Health Questionnaire–2/9	• Abbreviated PTSD Checklist–Civilian[a] • Generalized Anxiety Disorder-7[a] • Harvard Trauma Questionnaire • Primary Care–PTSD[a] • Life Event Checklist • War Trauma Scale	• Alcohol Use Disorders Identification Test • Alcohol Use Disorders Identification Test–PC[a] • CAGE AID • Drug Abuse Screen Test-10	• Resettlement Stressor Scale
Older adults	• Cornell Scale for Depression in Dementia[a] • Geriatric Depression Scale[a] • Geriatric Depression Scale–Short • Hamilton Depression Scale (see "Adults" section)	• Geriatric Anxiety Inventory • Geriatric Anxiety Scale	• CAGE AID • T-ACE	• Katz Index of Independence in Activities of Daily Living • Lawton Instrumental Activities of Daily Living

Screening should be an ongoing process and means of assessing symptom severity, effectiveness of intervention.
These are designed to be brief and can be implemented in primary care settings.
[a] Denotes measures specifically assessed for use in primary care settings.

training and mental health education and screening for primary care offices.[50] This quality improvement initiative gives clinicians opportunities to provide point-of-care tools to their patients that can help with their treatment. These initiatives are still being studied and if effective these community-based partnerships can be used across the country to help underserved communities improve access to their patients.

SUMMARY

The underserved have a significantly greater prevalence of mental health problems and face significantly greater barriers to care. PCPs serve on the front line in their roles with the underserved populations. They need to continue to be aware of the needs of those with mental health conditions, and to know how to address them until the barriers have been solved with future promising interventions.

REFERENCES

1. Norquist GS, Regier DA. The epidemiology of psychiatric disorders and the de facto mental health care system 1. Annu Rev Med 1996;47:473–9.
2. Strine TW, Mokdad AH, Balluz LS, et al. Depression and anxiety in the United States: findings from the 2006 behavioral risk factor surveillance system. Psychiatr Serv 2008;59:1383–90.
3. Centers for Disease Control and Prevention. Disparities analytics. 2013. Available at: http://www.cdc.gov/disparitiesanalytics/. Accessed February 10, 2016.
4. U.S. Census Bureau. 2010 census redistricting data (Public Law 94-171) summary file. Available at: http://www.census.gov/prod/cen2010/doc/pl94-171.pdf. Accessed June 1, 2016.
5. Chang TE, Weiss AP, Marques L, et al. Race/ethnicity and other social determinants of psychological well-being and functioning in mental health clinics. J Health Care Poor Underserved 2014;25:1418–31.
6. Parrish MM, Miller L, Peltekof B. Addressing depression and accumulated trauma in urban primary care: challenges and opportunities. J Health Care Poor Underserved 2011;22(4):1292–301.
7. Barry CL, McGinty EE, Pescosolido BA, et al. Stigma, discrimination, treatment effectiveness, and policy: public views about drug addiction and mental illness. Psychiatr Serv 2014;65(10):1269–72.
8. Pedersen ER, Paves AP. Comparing perceived public stigma and personal stigma of mental health treatment seeking in a young adult sample. Psychiatry Res 2014;219(1):143–50.
9. Watson NN, Hunter CD. Anxiety and depression among African American women: the costs of strength and negative attitudes toward psychological help-seeking. Cultur Divers Ethnic Minor Psychol 2015;21(4):604.
10. Fortuna LR, Porche MV, Alegria M. Political violence, psychosocial trauma, and the context of mental health services use among immigrant Latinos in the united states. Ethn Health 2008;13(5):435–63.
11. Chen FM, Fryer GE Jr, Phillips RL Jr, et al. Patients' beliefs about racism, preferences for physician race, and satisfaction with care. Ann Fam Med 2005;3(2):138–43.
12. DeNavas-Walt C, Proctor BD. U.S. Census Bureau, current population reports, P60–252, Income and poverty in the United States: 2014. 2015.
13. Groh C. Poverty, mental health, and women: implications for psychiatric nurses in primary care settings. J Am Psychiatr Nurses Assoc 2007;13(5):267–74.

14. Stafford M, Marmot M. Neighbourhood deprivation and health: does it affect us all equally? Int J Epidemiol 2003;32(3):357–66.
15. Myers HF, Wyatt GE, Ullman JB, et al. Cumulative burden of lifetime adversities: trauma and mental health in low-SES African Americans and Latino/as. Psychol Trauma 2015;7(3):243–51.
16. Glover DA, Williams JK, Kissler KA. Using novel methods to examine stress among HIV-positive African American men who have sex with men and women. J Behav Med 2012;36:283–94.
17. Lorant V, Deliège D, Eaton W, et al. Socioeconomic inequalities in depression: a meta-analysis. Am J Epidemiol 2003;157(2):98–112.
18. Chow JC, Jaffee K, Snowden L. Racial/ethnic disparities in the use of mental health services in poverty areas. Am J Public Health 2003;93(5):792–7.
19. Curtis S, Copeland A, Fagg J, et al. The ecological relationship between deprivation, social isolation and rates of hospital admission for acute psychiatric care: a comparison of London and New York city. Health Place 2006;12(1):19–37.
20. Fryers T, Melzer D, Jenkins R. Social inequalities and the common mental disorders: a systematic review of the evidence. Soc Psychiatry Psychiatr Epidemiol 2003;38(5):229–37.
21. Kangovi S, Barg F, Carter T, et al. Understanding why patients of low socioeconomic status prefer hospitals over ambulatory care. Health Aff 2013;32(7):1196–203.
22. Patel V, Kieling C, Maulik PK, et al. Improving access to care for children with mental disorders: a global perspective. Arch Dis Child 2013;98(5):323–7.
23. National Institute of Mental Health. Any disorder among children. Available at: http://www.nimh.nih.gov/health/statistics/prevalence/any-disorder-among-children.shtml. 2016. Accessed June 2, 2016.
24. Committee on the Mental Health Workforce for Geriatric Populations. In: Eden J, Maslow K, Le M, Board on Health Care Services, Institute of Medicine, et al, editors. The mental health and substance use workforce for older adults: in whose hands? Washington, DC: National Academies; 2012.
25. Bartels SJ, Gill L, Naslund JA. The affordable care act, accountable care organizations, and mental health care for older adults: implications and opportunities. Harv Rev Psychiatry 2015;23(5):304–19.
26. Klap R, Unroe KT, Unützer J. Caring for mental illness in the United States: a focus on older adults. Am J Geriatr Psychiatry 2003;11:517–24.
27. Drapeau CW, McIntosh JL. U.S.A. suicide: 2013 official final data. 2015. Available at: http://www.suicidology.org/Portals/14/docs/Resources/FactSheet. Accessed December 12, 2015.
28. Luoma JB, Martin CE, Pearson JL. Contact with mental health and primary care providers before suicide: a review of the evidence. Am J Psychiatry 2002;159(6):909–16.
29. Unützer J, Schoenbaum M, Druss BG, et al. Transforming mental health care at the interface with general medicine: report for the president's commission. Psychiatr Serv 2006;57(1):37–47.
30. Arean PA, Ayalon L, Hunkeler E, et al. Improving depression care for older, minority patients in primary care. Med Care 2005;43(4):381–90.
31. US Citizenship & Immigration Services. Refugees. 2015. Available at: http://www.uscis.gov/humanitarian/refugees-asylum/refugees. Accessed February 10, 2016.
32. Centers for Disease Control and Prevention. About refugees. 2012. Available at: www.cdc.gov/immigrantrefugeehealth/about-refugees.html. Accessed February 10, 2016.

33. Hollifield M, Warner TD, Lian N, et al. Measuring trauma and health status in refugees: a critical review. JAMA 2002;288(5):611–21.

34. Pew Research Center. Remittance flows worldwide in 2012. 2014. Available at: http://www.pewsocialtrends.org/2014/02/20/remittance-map/. Accessed February 10, 2016.

35. Peen J, Schoevers RA, Beekman AT, et al. The current status of urban-rural differences in psychiatric disorders. Acta Psychiatr Scand 2010;121:84–93.

36. Spoont M, Minneapolis V. Rural vs. urban ambulatory health care: a systematic review. Minneapolis (MN): Department of Veterans Affairs Health Services Research & Development Service; 2011.

37. Gregoire A. The mental health of farmers. Occup Med (Lond) 2002;52(8):471–6.

38. Gallup Politics. Special report: 3.4% of U.S. adults identify as LGBT. 2012. Available at: http://www.gallup.com/poll/158066/special-report-adults-identify-lgbt.aspx. Accessed January 6, 2016.

39. Badgett M, Durso L, Schneebaum A. New patterns of poverty in the lesbian, gay, and bisexual community. Los Angeles (CA): The Williams Institute; 2013.

40. Ranji U, Beamesderfer A, Kates J, et al. Health and access to care and coverage for lesbian, gay, bisexual, and transgender individuals in the US. Menlo Park (CA): Kaiser Foundation Issue Brief; 2015.

41. Centers for Disease Control and Prevention. CDC fact sheet, substance abuse among gay and bisexual men. Atlanta (GA): Author; 2010.

42. Lick D, Durso L, Johnson K. Minority stress and physical health among sexual minorities. Perspect Psychol Sci 2013;8(5):521–48.

43. Ryan C, Huebner D, Diaz RM, et al. Family rejection as a predictor of negative health outcomes in white and Latino lesbian, gay, and bisexual young adults. Pediatrics 2009;23(1):346–52.

44. Gilman SE, Cochran SD, Mays VM, et al. Risk of psychiatric disorders among individuals reporting same-sex sexual partners in the national comorbidity survey. Am J Public Health 2001;91:933–9.

45. Berg MB, Mimiaga MJ, Safren SA. Mental health concerns of gay and bisexual men seeking mental health services. J Homosex 2008;54(3):293–306.

46. Institute of Medicine. The health of lesbian, gay, bisexual, and transgender people: building a foundation for better understanding. Washington, DC: National Academies Press; 2011.

47. Koh AS, Ross LK. Mental health issues: a comparison of lesbian, bisexual and heterosexual women. J Homosex 2006;51(1):33–57.

48. Clements-Nolle K, Marx R, Katz M. Attempted suicide among transgender persons: the influence of gender-based discrimination and victimization. J Homosex 2006;51(3):53–69.

49. Clarke G, Yarborough BJ. Evaluating the promise of health IT to enhance/expand the reach of mental health services. Gen Hosp Psychiatry 2013;35(4):339–44.

50. Hunt JB, Curran G, Kramer T, et al. Partnership for implementation of evidence-based mental health practices in rural federally qualified health centers: theory and methods. Prog Community Health Partnersh 2012;6(3):389–98.

51. Green BL, Saunders PA, Power E, et al. Trauma-informed medical care: CME communication training for primary care providers. Fam Med 2015;47(1):7–14.

52. Bolton E. PTSD in refugees. 2015. Available at: http://www.ptsd.va.gov/professional/trauma/other/ptsd-refugees.asp. Accessed February 10, 2016.

Substance Use Issues Among the Underserved
United States and International Perspectives

Alicia Ann Kowalchuk, DO*, Sandra J. Gonzalez, MSSW, LCSW,
Roger J. Zoorob, MD, MPH

KEYWORDS

- Alcohol • Drugs • Illicit drugs • Substance use • Substance use disorders
- Substance abuse • Tobacco

KEY POINTS

- Substance use and substance use disorders (SUDs) have a disproportionate impact on the underserved, with tobacco use most prevalent worldwide and causing the greatest morbidity and mortality.
- Trauma, which has a disproportionate impact on underserved populations, is a strong risk factor for the development of SUDs.
- Integration of substance use screening and SUD treatment into primary care is a promising solution for increasing access and engagement in care.

GLOBAL SCOPE OF SUBSTANCE USE

The most commonly used substance worldwide is tobacco: 21% of the world's population 15 years old and older smokes tobacco products. Approximately 80% of the world's 1 billion smokers live in low-income and middle-income countries. Tobacco kills approximately half its users and 6 million people globally every year, 90% of whom are direct users; 10% of these deaths are due to second-hand exposure. Rates of use vary by country and region and are inversely related to education level attainment, socioeconomic status, and the consumer price of tobacco products, which is strongly tied to tax rates. Tobacco use rates are directly related to the marketing of tobacco products in a society. Globally, tobacco smoking prevalence rates are 5 times higher in men (37%) than women (7%), with that gap narrowest in Europe, where approximately 20% of women smoke tobacco products.[1]

Department of Family and Community Medicine, Baylor College of Medicine, 3701 Kirby Drive, Suite 600, Houston, TX 77098, USA
* Corresponding author.
E-mail address: aliciak@bcm.edu

Prim Care Clin Office Pract 44 (2017) 113–125
http://dx.doi.org/10.1016/j.pop.2016.09.013
0095-4543/17/© 2016 Elsevier Inc. All rights reserved.

primarycare.theclinics.com

Alcohol, the second most commonly used substance, is the third leading cause of disability and disease worldwide and the leading cause in middle-income countries, although per capita alcohol consumption and binge drinking are highest among high-income countries. Alcohol consumption causes more than 3 million deaths worldwide annually. Although the highest rates of alcohol abstinence are found in the lowest socioeconomic strata in societies around the world, the burdens of alcohol-related disability, disease, and mortality are disproportionately borne by those of lower socioeconomic status and less developed countries. This discrepancy has been attributed to a variety of factors, including poorer access to health care; smaller support networks to help individuals address their alcohol problems; higher rates of manual labor employment (in which on-the-job alcohol impairment injuries are more likely); poorly maintained roads and less safe and reliable vehicles, contributing to higher alcohol-impaired driving fatalities; and nutritional deficiencies. There are also substantial gender differences in alcohol consumption and associated mortality, with male drinkers consuming on average approximately 2.5 times more alcohol than female drinkers worldwide and suffering approximately double the mortality rate of alcohol-attributable deaths.[2]

Worldwide, drug use rates have remained stable since 2010; however, up to 7%, or 300 million, of the world's population between 15 and 64 years of age have used an illicit drug in the past year. It is estimated that 16 to 39 million people are regular users and/or have an SUD, and 12.7 million inject drugs. Annually, there are 183,000 drug-related deaths, accounting for a mortality rate of 40 deaths per million. Cannabis, used by 2.5% of the world's population, is the most widely used substance after tobacco and alcohol and is associated with the most arrests for drug offenses globally. Opiates are used by 0.2% of the global population yet are responsible for the largest disease burden and highest number of drug-related deaths worldwide, primarily from injection drug use–related infectious diseases, such as HIV and hepatitis C virus, and overdoses. Cocaine is also consumed by 0.2% of the world's population, although, unlike tobacco, alcohol, cannabis, and opiates, cocaine use is less widespread, concentrated primarily in the Americas and Europe. As seen with tobacco and alcohol, illicit drug use is more prevalent in men than women.[3]

SCOPE OF SUBSTANCE USE IN THE UNITED STATES

Among US adults, 18% use tobacco products, a decrease of more than 50% in the past 50 years. Despite this public health achievement, tobacco products kill half a million US adults annually, and tobacco use remains the leading preventable cause of premature disability and death. Tobacco use is not evenly distributed across US society. As seen globally, tobacco use rates are inversely related to educational level attainment and socioeconomic status. The tobacco smoking rate in the Medicaid population is double that of the general population, with tobacco-related diseases accounting for 15%, or $40 billion, of total Medicaid spending. Geographically, tobacco use is highest in the southern and western states and lowest in the west coast and northeastern states. Of all US ethnic and racial groups, non-Latino whites and Native Americans have the highest tobacco use rates. The gender gap for tobacco use is small in the United States, with female tobacco use rates approximately 80% of male tobacco use rates. Persons with mental illness are a group particularly vulnerable to tobacco use effects in the United States due to high prevalence of use and low rates of successful quit attempts. The picture for the general US population is brighter, with former tobacco users now outnumbering current tobacco users.[4]

Among US adults, 88% report consuming alcohol during their lifetime, with 72% reporting use within the past year and 57% within the past month. Past-month binge drinking (5 or more drinks on any 1 occasion) prevalence is 25%, and 7% of US adults report heavy drinking (5 or more binge drinking episodes) in the past month. Among US adults, 7% have an alcohol use disorder (AUD).[5] Alcohol use is the third leading preventable cause of death in the United States, after tobacco use and obesity, with approximately 88,000 deaths from alcohol-related causes reported annually.[6] Alcohol is involved in approximately a third of all motor vehicle accident fatalities, and alcohol misuse costs are estimated at more than $224 billion annually, primarily due to binge drinking.[7,8] As with tobacco use, alcohol consumption is unevenly distributed across US society, with binge drinking rates highest in Alaska, the upper Midwest, and New England states.[9] Although AUD rates are highest in non-Latino whites and Native Americans, African Americans and Latinos have higher rates of persistent and recurrent AUDs, and the consequences of alcohol misuse remain greater for African Americans, Latinos, and Native Americans compared with Asian Americans and non-Latino whites, which is at least partially attributable to socioeconomic disparities.[10]

Barriers to care, such as lack of access to and availability of treatment in underserved areas, lack of transportation and/or child care, being uninsured or underinsured, and stigma, are all associated with poor engagement and retention in AUD treatment. Minority groups may be less likely to seek or receive specialty care, making the primary care encounter vitally important in the early identification of problematic alcohol consumption in underserved communities.[11] Avoiding stigmatizing language in their practices can be an easy and low-cost practice change intervention for decreasing that barrier to care across underserved populations with SUDs. Stigmatizing language has been eliminated in the *Diagnostic and Statistical Manual of Mental Disorders* (Fifth Edition), and addiction medicine experts are encouraging rapid adoption of this newer terminology.[12–14]

Approximately half (49%) of the US population age 12 and older has used an illicit drug in their lifetime, 17% in the past year, and 10% in the past month. As seen globally, cannabis use accounts for most illicit drug use, with nonmedical use of prescription drugs a distant second.[5] Unintentional prescription drug overdose, however, primarily involving opioids, has become the leading cause of accidental death in US working age adults since 2011.[15] From 1997 to 2007, the milligram-per-person use of prescription opioids in the United States increased 402%, and retail pharmacies dispensed 48% more opiate prescriptions in 2009 than in 2000.[16,17] The rates of opiate prescribing and nonmedical use of prescription opiates have leveled off since 2012, but opiate overdose deaths have continued to increase, and heroin use is on the rise. Rates of other illicit drug use, except cannabis (which has been increasing), have been stable or declining.[18] As with tobacco and alcohol, illicit drug use is unevenly distributed across US society. Prevalence of use of an illicit substance in a community is directly tied to its availability in that community, which is linked primarily to routes of distribution of the illicit drug trade. Overall, most underserved populations in the United States, including adolescents and children, the elderly, minority racial and ethnic groups, and those in the lower socioeconomic strata, have lower rates of illicit drug use than the general population.[17] The homeless and incarcerated populations, however, have higher rates. Women use fewer illicit drugs overall and across all drug classes compared with men except for sedative-hypnotics, such as benzodiazepines and zolpidem.[18]

EFFECTS/COSTS TO FAMILIES/SOCIETY

The economic and societal costs of substance use are astounding. In the United States, more than $700 billion per year in costs related to health care, lost work productivity, and crime can be attributed to the misuse of alcohol, tobacco, and illicit drugs.[19] Risky alcohol use alone cost the country $249 billion in 2010.[20] SUDs have been noted to significantly increase the health care costs in Medicaid beneficiaries with coexisting mental or physical illnesses.[21] Based on global prevalence rates, it is estimated that $250 billion (or approximately 0.3%–0.4% of the world's gross domestic product) would be needed to treat individuals for conditions related to the use of substances, placing a significant financial burden on families and society as a whole.[22]

Although the economic costs associated with substance use are substantial, it is also important to note the societal and personal costs to families. The effects of SUDs are experienced by every member of a family. In addition to higher prevalence of abuse, emotional and physical neglect, legal problems, and difficulties with attachment, children growing up in the care of an adult or adults with SUDs are also at an increased risk of developing an SUD themselves.[23] According to the Substance Abuse and Mental Health Services Administration, 2 in 5 children (40%) live with at least 1 adult with an SUD during their childhood/adolescence and 1 in 4 is exposed to alcohol problems in their family.[24]

Worldwide, the burden for families is great, particularly for those who are socioeconomically disadvantaged. In many countries, when the primary income earner is unable to work or maintain employment due to substance use, the responsibility of ensuring that the family's needs are met falls solely on the nonusing adult partner.[25]

ACCESS TO TREATMENT — GLOBAL PERSPECTIVE

Studies in the United States and other countries have shown that SUD treatment is cost effective, saving a society 7 times the cost of the treatment provided.[26] Globally, although 66% of countries have a government unit or official responsible for SUD treatment services, less than half have a dedicated budget for SUD treatment. Consequently, there is a median of 1.7 beds for SUD treatment per 100,000 people worldwide, illustrating the discrepancy between treatment need and available resources. Inpatient detoxification is the most prevalent acute treatment service available; however, longer-term, longitudinal care of this chronic medical illness is less prevalent. Treatment access within a society is most limited for the underserved of a given society.[26] Retention in SUD treatment has been consistently linked to improved outcomes; however, access to the continuum of care is often limited.

Evidence-based pharmacologic treatment of SUDs, also called medication management or medication-assisted treatment (MAT), is available primarily for alcohol and opiate use disorders (OUDs). Medication managed withdrawal from alcohol or alcohol detoxification is the most widely available MAT worldwide, and benzodiazepines remain the most commonly used medication for that indication and are considered the safest and most effective medications for alcohol withdrawal.[27] There are worrisomely high rates of use of chlorpromazine use in lower-income countries for alcohol withdrawal, because chlorpromazine, which lowers seizure threshold, is not recommended for treatment of alcohol withdrawal.[28] Other MATs for AUD focus on relapse prevention and include acamprosate, naltrexone, and gabapentin, which are all used most frequently in higher-income countries.[29–31]

Three primary medications are available for MAT of OUDs: buprenorphine, methadone, and naltrexone. Buprenorphine and methadone, used as partial and full agonist maintenance medications, respectively, have been shown to decrease injection drug use, increase retention in treatment, and decrease relapse rates in individuals with OUD.[32] Naltrexone, an opioid receptor blocker, has shown the most success in relapse prevention of OUD in populations and societies in which full or partial agonist medications are not available, such as in Russia, where agonist treatment of OUD remains illegal.[33] Methadone is the most widely available MAT for OUD worldwide, with buprenorphine access essentially limited to high income countries.[26]

Although not formally considered an SUD treatment, mutual aid societies or self-help groups, such as Alcoholics Anonymous and Narcotics Anonymous, are active sources of support for individuals with SUDs in approximately 3 of 4 countries worldwide with larger presence in higher income countries. Nongovernmental organizations provide a significant amount of SUD treatment in many countries, with involvement of traditional healers and peers in recovery in formal SUD treatment settings common, especially in lower-income countries and lower-resourced areas. Engagement in helping peers has been shown to have a positive impact on individuals in recovery from SUDs.[26]

ACCESS TO TREATMENT IN THE UNITED STATES

Only 1 in 9 of the more than 23 million people with an SUD enter treatment in the United States. More than 90% of those not entering treatment do not actively seek out treatment because they do not feel they need it. Stigma associated with SUDs and SUD treatment remains a significant barrier as does the lack of knowledge, understanding, and acceptance of the SUD as a chronic disease.[34] Approximately all medications available around the globe for SUD treatment are also available in the United States; however, access to MAT for SUDs is limited by health insurance status and coverage. Mutual aid societies and peer recovery–based services remain widely used resources for underserved persons with SUDs in this country.[35]

TRAUMA AND SUBSTANCE USE

A trauma is an upsetting and frightening event that an individual experiences or witnesses in which there is a threat to the safety of themselves or someone else. The experience of trauma is common throughout the globe, with exposure estimated higher in lower-income countries compared with higher-income countries.[36] It is estimated that approximately 60% of men and 50% of women experience a traumatic event at least once in their lives.[37] In the United States, the lifetime prevalence rate of posttraumatic stress disorder (PTSD) is estimated to be between 6.8% and 8.0%. Among the underserved, however, the rate is at least triple.[38] Risk factors, such as poverty, low levels of social support, and low social capital, are associated with greater rates of PTSD in urban communities.[38,39] Primary care providers practicing in these areas are likely to encounter individuals with PTSD and posttraumatic stress symptoms, making the primary care setting ideal for identification and treatment.[40] Unfortunately, PTSD and posttraumatic stress symptoms often go unrecognized, contributing to greater health care costs and poorer outcomes.[41,42] Adopting a trauma-informed approach, as discussed later, is one method by which providers can better address the impact of trauma in their patients.

The relationship between trauma and substance use is well established in the literature.[38] PTSD and SUDs are often comorbid and associated with increased chronic medical conditions, poor social and occupational functioning, more legal troubles, and higher incidences of intimate partner violence and suicide.[43–45] Sexual assault has been shown associated with a higher risk of drug use and risky drinking in women.[46] Adverse childhood experiences, such as abuse and neglect, have been shown to increase the risk of developing SUDs in adulthood.[47] Traumatized persons, especially those with childhood trauma, are higher utilizers of health care services but may be less likely to effectively engage in care plans because they can be more distrustful of institutions of care and perceived authority figures such as medical providers.[39,48]

The rates of comorbid SUD and PTSD among veterans are also significant. In a study of 456,502 Iraq and Afghanistan veterans, researchers found that 82% to 93% of soldiers with a diagnosis of either AUD or other SUD also had a comorbid mental health disorder. Of these disorders, PTSD was the most commonly diagnosed in Veterans Affairs health care centers and accounted for up to a 4-fold increase in the diagnosis of AUD and a 3-fold increase in the diagnosis of other SUDs.[49]

AUD prevalence rates are much lower in foreign-born individuals than in US-born adolescents and adults. The risk of developing an SUD after the experience of a traumatic event, however, was higher for foreign-born than for US-born individuals.[50]

WOMEN AS AN UNDERSERVED POPULATION (SEE LUZ M. FERNANDEZ AND JONATHAN A. BECKER'S ARTICLE, "WOMEN'S SELECT HEALTH ISSUES IN UNDERSERVED POPULATIONS," IN THIS ISSUE)

Overall, global prevalence rates show that women use substances at a much lower rate than their male counterparts. In developed countries, where there is greater gender equality and more fluidity when it comes to gender roles, particularly in the workforce, attention is paid to the diminishing difference in drinking patterns between men and women.[51] Additionally, although SUDs are more prevalent in men, the gender gap in rates of SUDs has narrowed over the past 30 years.[52] When examining gender differences, women experience the progression from first use to development of an SUD at a much faster rate and may exhibit more severe symptoms than men even though they may have used for a shorter period of time or used less of the substance.[53,54] Women are initiating alcohol use at a much younger age than in the past and their drinking patterns and rates of SUDs are becoming more similar to those of men.[55]

In 2014, 15.8 million women reported that they used illicit drugs in the past year and an additional 4.6 million women reported misuse of prescription drugs. Given the high rate of unplanned pregnancies, the use of substances for women of childbearing age poses an additional concern. Substance use during pregnancy has many short-term and long-term effects for women and their children. Women of childbearing age who drink and are not using effective and consistent contraception may be at risk for an alcohol-exposed pregnancy.[56] If a woman uses substances on a regular basis during pregnancy, her baby may experience withdrawal symptoms at birth, a condition known as neonatal abstinence syndrome, which can occur if a woman uses caffeine, alcohol, opioids, or sedatives.[57] Recently published data from the Behavioral Risk Factor Surveillance System describe drinking patterns in both pregnant and nonpregnant women from 2011 to 2013. Among nonpregnant women, 53.6% reported any use in the past 30 days whereas approximately 1 in 5 women (18.2%) reported binge drinking. Among pregnant women, 1 in 10 reported drinking alcohol in the past 30 days and 3.1% reported binge drinking in the past 30 days.[58] Alcohol consumption during pregnancy has been associated with the development of fetal alcohol spectrum disorders, a group of conditions that may produce physical and neurodevelopmental problems in children whose mothers drank while pregnant.[59]

A particularly vulnerable group of women are those who are engaged in commercial sex work. In the United States and worldwide, commercial sex workers use illicit drugs at a much higher rate compared with women in the general population, placing this group at high risk of HIV infection, sexually transmitted infections, and violence.[60–62] Primary care providers working in underserved communities where commercial sex work may be more prevalent can provide more effective care if they are aware of the complex needs of these women, including the relationship between trauma and substance use.

RACIAL AND ETHNIC MINORITIES

In 2014, it was estimated that 10.2% of the US population had used an illicit drug in the past month. Rates were 12.4% among African Americans ages 12 and up; 14.9% for American Indians and Alaska Natives; 4.1% for Asian Americans; 15.6% among Native Hawaiians or Pacific Islanders; 8.9% for Hispanics/Latinos; and 10.4% for non-Latino whites.[63] Rates of heavy alcohol use tend to be higher among Native Americans compared with other groups.[10]

Underserved populations, including some racial and ethnic groups, often experience greater negative health effects from substance use than other groups.[64,65] African Americans and Latinos are at a greater risk of developing alcohol-related liver disease than whites and have higher rates of deaths from alcohol-related illnesses, including cirrhosis. This may be, in part, attributable to the drinking patterns of those considered heavy drinkers. Among all heavy drinkers, Hispanics and African Americans drink larger quantities of alcohol over a longer period of time than non-Latino whites.[66] Diverse communities often disproportionately experience the weight of SUDs due to cultural and socioeconomic factors, including environmental stress and poor access to or quality of medical care.[67] Once in treatment, studies have shown that African Americans and Latinos are less likely to complete treatment as a result of socioeconomic factors.[68,69] It is important for primary care providers to be aware of the impact of these and other social determinants of health when working with underserved communities.

OLDER ADULTS AS AN UNDERSERVED POPULATION

Historically, the prevalence of illicit drug use by older adults has been significantly lower than that of younger age groups. Moreover, the lifetime rates of drug use for people ages 65 and up are approximately half compared with all other age groups, from 19 to 64.[63] Recent studies, however, point to an increase in SUDs among older adults in the United States and Europe.[70] Of particular public health interest is the impact of the large baby-boomer generation (Americans born between 1946 and 1964), whose substance use is higher than previous cohorts. Researchers recently projected that past-year SUD in adults ages 50 to 59 will increase from 1.9 million in 2002 to 2006 to 3.1 million in 2020 whereas those ages 60 to 69 will increase from 0.6 million to 1.9 million.[71]

ADOLESCENTS

Substance use remains a significant contributor to the death and disease burden of adolescents in many societies.[72] In 2014, 5% of all US adolescents had an SUD.[63] Risk factors, such as increased availability of drugs and alcohol, parental substance use, exposure to violence and trauma, and poverty, all contribute to the incidence of drug and AUDs by adolescents. Overall rates of past-month illicit drug use by adolescents (youth ages 12–17) decreased from 11.6% in 2002 to 8.8% in 2013. The most commonly used substance was cannabis (7.1%) followed by psychotherapeutics, such as benzodiazepines and amphetamines (2.2%), hallucinogens (0.6%), inhalants (0.5%), cocaine (0.2%), and heroin (0.1%). Compared with 2002, past-month alcohol use declined from 28.8% to 22.7% and binge drinking declined from 19.3% to 14.2% in 2013. Although the rates of tobacco use have significantly decreased over the past decade (13.0% in 2002 to 5.6% in 2013), there has been an increase in the use of nicotine products, such as e-cigarettes.[5] Worldwide, there seems to be a discrepancy in the use patterns when it comes to cannabis. A recent study in 30 European and North American countries found that the use of cannabis by adolescents seems to be decreasing in Western Europe and the United States and increasing in Eastern European countries.[73]

RESOURCES AND SOLUTIONS

Several innovative solutions to substance use and SUD problems in the underserved have been developed. Housing First is one such solution and focuses on homeless individuals with co-occurring mental health disorders and SUDs. In the more traditional, treatment-first, stepped approach to housing of the homeless, homeless individuals qualify for increasingly stable and independent housing options as they engage in treatment services. Engagement in treatment, substance use abstinence, and mental health stability are required to move from shelter-based group housing to individual, independent-living housing units. Housing First provides independent living units first, with on-site robust social services and sometimes mental health care, SUD treatment, and health care services on site as well. Housing First residents are encouraged to engage these services but are not required to do so to remain in their homes. Housing First initiatives, pioneered in inner cities across the United States and now being implemented in Canada, Australia, and Europe, have reduced homelessness in the chronically homeless population with co-occurring mental health disorders and SUDs while increasing linkages to care and decreasing substance use.[74]

A second solution also increasingly promoted to increase SUD treatment access and engagement in the United States and around the globe is integration of SUD treatment and primary care services in a chronic care model.[26,34,75] These efforts recognize and address several barriers to SUD treatment, including too few SUD treatment providers, the stigma associated with engaging with traditional SUD treatment settings, and lack of insight by individuals with SUDs that they have an SUD and need treatment.[34] For primary care providers in underserved communities who are working with persons affected by SUDs, more information on chronic care models may be found at http://www.ihi.org/Pages/default.aspx.

Addressing risky substance use behaviors with all preadolescent and adult patients is essential to providing comprehensive care to the underserved. Primary care screening for tobacco use and risky alcohol use in adults and offering a brief intervention are grade B recommendations from the US Preventive Services Task Force.[76] There are numerous resources available for incorporating tobacco screening and cessation counseling as well as alcohol screening and brief intervention into primary care practices.[77]

Beyond screening and brief intervention for alcohol and tobacco use, OUD treatment integration into primary care settings is one of the primary desired outcomes of the US Drug Addiction Treatment Act of 2000 (DATA 2000), which allows physicians to prescribe Food and Drug Administration (FDA)–approved schedule III, IV, or V medications for the treatment of OUDs outside of a licensed methadone facility.[78] Currently, buprenorphine and buprenorphine/naloxone products are the only schedule III medications FDA approved for OUD treatment. Primary care physicians may prescribe buprenorphine products to their patients with OUDs by obtaining a DATA 2000 waiver from the Drug Enforcement Administration after completing 8 hours of training on buprenorphine and OUD treatment and ensuring ability to refer their patients to counseling services.[78] More than 32,000 US physicians have obtained a DATA 2000 waiver, and more than a quarter of waivered physicians are also approved to treat more than 30 patients for OUDs with buprenorphine medications in their practice.[79] Further access to OUD treatment is critical to stemming the ongoing opiate overdose crisis in the United States and many resources are available to help primary care physicians incorporate OUD treatment into their practices.[80]

A third solution to increase SUD treatment retention and effectiveness specifically for traumatized individuals is trauma-informed care. In addition to evidence-based counseling interventions, including Addiction and Trauma Recovery Integration Model and Seeking Safety, which are often delivered in specialized SUD treatment settings, the National Center for Trauma Informed Care lists 4 central themes that any individual, organization, or system can embrace to provide a trauma-informed approach to service delivery:

1. Understand the widespread impact of trauma and paths toward recovery.
2. Recognize signs and symptoms of trauma in clients/patients/consumers, families, and staff/providers.
3. Respond with full integration of knowledge of trauma in policies, procedures, and practices.
4. Actively avoid retraumatization.

Six principles (safety, trustworthiness and transparency, peer support, collaboration, empowerment, and cultural and gender relevancy) underpin these themes. Following these general principles, trauma-informed care can be applied in many settings, including primary care.[79]

REFERENCES

1. World Health Organization. WHO global report on trends in prevalence of tobacco smoking 2015. Geneva (Switzerland): World Health Organization; 2015.

2. World Health Organization. Global status report on alcohol and health, 2014. Geneva (Switzerland): World Health Organization; 2014.

3. United Nations Office on Drugs and Crime. World Drug Report 2014. Available at: http://www.unodc.org/wdr2014/. Accessed February 22, 2016.

4. US Department of Health and Human Services. The health consequences of smoking—50 years of progress: a report of the Surgeon General. Atlanta (GA): US Department of Health and Human Services; Centers for Disease Control and Prevention; National Center for Chronic Disease Prevention and Health Promotion; Office on Smoking and Health; 2014. p. 17.

5. Substance Abuse and Mental Health Services Administration, results from the 2013 National Survey on Drug Use and Health: summary of national findings, NSDUH Series H-48, HHS Publication No. (SMA) 14-4863. Rockville (MD): Substance Abuse and Mental Health Services Administration; 2014.

6. US Centers for Disease Control and Prevention. Alcohol use and health. Available at: http://www.cdc.gov/alcohol/fact-sheets/alcohol-use.htm. Accessed February 22, 2016.

7. National Highway Traffic Safety Administration. 2013 motor vehicle crashes: Overview.

8. Centers for Disease Control and Prevention. Excessive drinking costs U.S. $223.5 billion. Available at: http://www.cdc.gov/features/alcoholconsumption/. Accessed February 12, 2016.

9. US Centers for Disease Control and Prevention. Behavioral Risk Factor Surveillance System. survey data. Atlanta (GA): US Department of Health and Human Services, Centers for Disease Control and Prevention; 2014.

10. Chartier K, Caetano R. Ethnicity and health disparities in alcohol research. Alcohol Res Health 2010;33(1–2):152–60.

11. Schmidt L, Greenfield T, Mulia N. Unequal treatment: racial and ethnic disparities in alcoholism treatment services. Alcohol Res Health 2006;29(1):49.

12. American Psychiatric Association. Diagnostic and statistical manual of mental disorders (DSM-5®). Arlington (VA): American Psychiatric Pub; 2013.

13. Saitz R. Things that Work, Things that Don't Work, and Things that Matter—Including Words. J Addict Med 2015;9(6):429–30.

14. Saitz R. International Statement Recommending Against the Use of Terminology That Can Stigmatize People. J Addict Med 2016;10(1):1–2.

15. National Safety Council Injury Facts Book. 2014.

16. Laxmaiah Manchikanti M, Bert Fellows M, Hary Ailinani M. Therapeutic use, abuse, and nonmedical use of opioids: a ten-year perspective. Pain Physician 2010;13:401–35.

17. United States Food and Drug Administration. Joint Meeting of the anesthetic and life support drugs advisory committee and the drug safety and risk management advisory committee. 2010. Available at: http://www.fda.gov/downloads/AdvisoryCommittees/CommitteesMeetingMaterials/Drugs/AnestheticAndLifeSupport%20DrugsAdvisoryCommittee/UCM217510.pdf. Accessed March 29, 2016.

18. Center for Behavioral Health Statistics and Quality. Behavioral health trends in the United States: results from the 2014 National Survey on Drug Use and Health (HHS Publication No. SMA 15–4927, NSDUH Series H-50). 2015. Available at: http://www.samhsa.gov/data/. Accessed January 29, 2016.

19. National Institute on Drug Abuse. Costs of Substance Abuse. Available at: https://www.drugabuse.gov/related-topics/trends-statistics. Accessed February 29, 2016.

20. Sacks JJ, Gonzales KR, Bouchery EE, et al. 2010 national and state costs of excessive alcohol consumption. Am J Prev Med 2015;49(5):e73–9.

21. Clark RE, Samnaliev M, McGovern MP. Impact of substance disorders on medical expenditures for medicaid beneficiaries with behavioral health disorders. Psychiatr Serv 2009;60(1):35–42.

22. Murray CJ, Lopez AD. Measuring the global burden of disease. N Engl J Med 2013;369(5):448–57.

23. Lander L, Howsare J, Byrne M. The Impact of Substance Use Disorders on Families and Children: From Theory to Practice. Soc Work Public Health 2013;28(3–4):194–205.

24. Substance Abuse and Mental Health Services Administration. Data Spotlight: Over 7 million children live with a parent with alcohol problems. 2012. Available at: http://media.samhsa.gov/data/spotlight/Spot061ChildrenOfAlcoholics2012.pdf. Accessed March 29, 2016.

25. World Health Organization. Global status report on alcohol 2004. Geneva (Switzerland): World Health Organization; 2004.

26. World Health Organization. Atlas on substance use (2010): resources for the prevention and treatment of substance use disorders. Geneva (Switzerland): World Health Organization; 2010.

27. Amato L, Minozzi S, Vecchi S, et al. Benzodiazepines for alcohol withdrawal. Cochrane Database Syst Rev 2010;(3):CD005063.

28. Hedges D, Jeppson K, Whitehead P. Antipsychotic medication and seizures: a review. Drugs Today (Barc) 2003;39(7):551–7.

29. Mason BJ, Goodman AM, Chabac S, et al. Effect of oral acamprosate on abstinence in patients with alcohol dependence in a double-blind, placebo-controlled trial: The role of patient motivation. J Psychiatr Res 2006;40(5):383–93.

30. Garbutt JC, Kranzler HR, O'Malley SS, et al. Efficacy and tolerability of long-acting injectable naltrexone for alcohol dependence: a randomized controlled trial. JAMA 2005;293(13):1617–25.

31. Furieri FA, Nakamura-Palacios EM. Gabapentin reduces alcohol consumption and craving: a randomized, double-blind, placebo-controlled trial. J Clin Psychiatry 2007;68(11):1691–700.

32. Soyka M, Zingg C, Koller G, et al. Retention rate and substance use in methadone and buprenorphine maintenance therapy and predictors of outcome: results from a randomized study. Int J Neuropsychopharmacol 2008;11(5):641–53.

33. Krupitsky E, Zvartau E, Woody G. Use of Naltrexone to Treat Opioid Addiction in a Country in Which Methadone and Buprenorphine Are Not Available. Curr Psychiatry Rep 2010;12(5):448–53.

34. Padwa H, Urada D, Antonini VP, et al. Integrating substance use disorder services with primary care: The experience in California. J Psychoactive Drugs 2012;44(4):299–306.

35. Huebner RB, Kantor LW. Advances in alcoholism treatment. Alcohol Res Health 2011;33(4):295–9.

36. Atwoli L, Stein DJ, Koenen KC, et al. Epidemiology of posttraumatic stress disorder: prevalence, correlates and consequences. Curr Opin Psychiatry 2015;28(4):307.

37. Gradus JL. Epidemiology of PTSD. Washington, DC: National Center for PTSD (United States Department of Veterans Affairs); 2007.

38. Liebschutz J, Saitz R, Brower V, et al. PTSD in urban primary care: high prevalence and low physician recognition. J Gen Intern Med 2007;22(6):719–26.

39. Gapen M, Cross D, Ortigo K, et al. Perceived neighborhood disorder, community cohesion, and PTSD symptoms among low-income African Americans in an urban health setting. Am J Orthopsychiatry 2011;81(1):31–7.

40. Erickson LD, Hedges DW, Call VR, et al. Prevalence of and factors associated with subclinical posttraumatic stress symptoms and PTSD in urban and rural areas of Montana: a cross-sectional study. J Rural Health 2013;29(4):403–12.

41. Klassen BJ, Porcerelli JH, Markova T. The effects of PTSD symptoms on health care resource utilization in a low-income, urban primary care setting. J Trauma Stress 2013;26(5):636–9.

42. Hall Brown T, Mellman TA. The influence of PTSD, sleep fears, and neighborhood stress on insomnia and short sleep duration in urban, young adult, African Americans. Behav Sleep Med 2014;12(3):198–206.

43. Smith PH, Homish GG, Leonard KE, et al. Intimate partner violence and specific substance use disorders: findings from the National Epidemiologic Survey on Alcohol and Related Conditions. Psychol Addict Behav 2012;26(2):236–45.

44. Devries KM, Child JC, Bacchus LJ, et al. Intimate partner violence victimization and alcohol consumption in women: a systematic review and meta-analysis. Addiction 2014;109(3):379–91.

45. Kartha A, Brower V, Saitz R, et al. The impact of trauma exposure and post-traumatic stress disorder on healthcare utilization among primary care patients. Med Care 2008;46(4):388–93.

46. Ullman SE, Starzynski LL, Long SM, et al. Exploring the relationships of women's sexual assault disclosure, social reactions, and problem drinking. J Interpers Violence 2008;23(9):1235–57.

47. Khoury L, Tang YL, Bradley B, et al. Substance use, childhood traumatic experience, and Posttraumatic Stress Disorder in an urban civilian population. Depress Anxiety 2010;27(12):1077–86.

48. Chartier MJ, Walker JR, Naimark B. Separate and cumulative effects of adverse childhood experiences in predicting adult health and health care utilization. Child Abuse Negl 2010;34(6):454–64.

49. Seal KH, Cohen G, Waldrop A, et al. Substance use disorders in Iraq and Afghanistan veterans in VA healthcare, 2001–2010: Implications for screening, diagnosis and treatment. Drug Alcohol Depend 2011;116(1–3):93–101.

50. Szaflarski M, Cubbins LA, Ying J. Epidemiology of alcohol abuse among US immigrant populations. J immigrant Minor Health 2011;13(4):647–58.

51. Obot IS, Room R. Alcohol, gender and drinking problems: perspectives from low and middle income countries. Geneva (Switzerland): World Health Organization; 2005.

52. Greenfield SF, Back SE, Lawson K, et al. Substance abuse in women. Psychiatr Clin North Am 2010;33(2):339–55.

53. Greenfield SF, Brooks AJ, Gordon SM, et al. Substance abuse treatment entry, retention, and outcome in women: a review of the literature. Drug Alcohol Depend 2007;86(1):1–21.

54. Hernandez-Avila CA, Rounsaville BJ, Kranzler HR. Opioid-, cannabis- and alcohol-dependent women show more rapid progression to substance abuse treatment. Drug Alcohol Depend 2004;74(3):265–72.

55. Keyes KM, Martins SS, Blanco C, et al. Telescoping and gender differences in alcohol dependence: new evidence from two national surveys. Am J Psychiatry 2010;167(8):969–76.

56. Floyd RL, Sobell M, Velasquez MM, et al. Preventing alcohol-exposed pregnancies: a randomized controlled trial. Am J Prev Med 2007;32(1):1–10.

57. Muhuri PK, Gfroerer JC. Substance use among women: associations with pregnancy, parenting, and race/ethnicity. Matern Child Health J 2008;13(3):376–85.

58. Tan CH, Denny CH, Cheal NE, et al. Alcohol use and binge drinking among women of childbearing age-United States, 2011-2013. MMWR Morb Mortal Wkly Rep 2015;64(37):1042–6.

59. US Centers for Disease Control and Prevention. Fetal alcohol spectrum disorders (FASDs). Available at: https://www.cdc.gov/ncbddd/fasd/facts.html. Accessed February 12, 2016.

60. Shannon K, Kerr T, Strathdee SA, et al. Prevalence and structural correlates of gender based violence among a prospective cohort of female sex workers. BMJ 2009;339:b2939.

61. Strathdee SA, Philbin MM, Semple SJ, et al. Correlates of injection drug use among female sex workers in two Mexico–U.S. border cities. Drug Alcohol Depend 2008;92(1–3):132–40.

62. Wechsberg WM, Luseno WK, Lam WK, et al. Substance use, sexual risk, and violence: HIV prevention intervention with sex workers in Pretoria. AIDS Behav 2006;10(2):131–7.

63. Substance Abuse and Mental Health Services Administration, results from the 2011 national survey on drug use and health: summary of national findings, NSDUH Series H-44, HHS Publication No (SMA) 12-4713. Rockville (MD): Substance Abuse and Mental Health Services Administration; 2012.

64. Alegria M, Carson NJ, Goncalves M, et al. Disparities in treatment for substance use disorders and co-occurring disorders for ethnic/racial minority youth. J Am Acad Child Adolesc Psychiatry 2011;50(1):22–31.

65. Breslau J, Kendler KS, Su M, et al. Lifetime risk and persistence of psychiatric disorders across ethnic groups in the United States. Psychol Med 2005;35(3): 317–27.

66. Carrion AF, Ghanta R, Carrasquillo O, et al. Chronic liver disease in the Hispanic population of the United States. Clin Gastroenterol Hepatol 2011;9(10):834–41 [quiz: e109–10].

67. Buka SL. Disparities in health status and substance use: ethnicity and socioeconomic factors. Public Health Rep 2002;117(Suppl 1):S118–25.

68. Cook BL, Alegria M. Racial-ethnic disparities in substance abuse treatment: the role of criminal history and socioeconomic status. Psychiatr Serv 2011;62(11): 1273–81.

69. Daley MC. Race, managed care, and the quality of substance abuse treatment. Adm Policy Ment Health 2005;32(4):457–76.

70. Wang Y-P, Andrade LH. Epidemiology of alcohol and drug use in the elderly. Curr Opin Psychiatry 2013;26(4):343–8.

71. Han B, Gfroerer JC, Colliver JD, et al. Substance use disorder among older adults in the United States in 2020. Addiction 2009;104(1):88–96.

72. Toumbourou JW, Stockwell T, Neighbors C, et al. Interventions to reduce harm associated with adolescent substance use. Lancet 2007;369(9570):1391–401.

73. ter Bogt TFM, de Looze M, Molcho M, et al. Do societal wealth, family affluence and gender account for trends in adolescent cannabis use? A 30 country cross-national study. Addiction 2014;109(2):273–83.

74. Padgett DK, Stanhope V, Henwood BF, et al. Substance use outcomes among homeless clients with serious mental illness: comparing housing first with treatment first programs. Community Ment Health J 2011;47(2):227–32.

75. McLellan AT, Starrels JL, Tai B, et al. Can substance use disorders be managed using the chronic care model? Review and recommendations from a NIDA Consensus Group. Public Health Rev 2014;35(2):1–12.

76. United States Preventive Services Task Force. Published Recommendations. Available at: http://www.uspreventiveservicestaskforce.org/BrowseRec/Index. Accessed March 11, 2016.

77. National Institute on Drug Abuse. NIDA/SAMHSA Blending Initiative. Available at: https://www.drugabuse.gov/nidasamhsa-blending-initiative. Accessed March 11, 2016.

78. Public Law 106-310-106th Congress-An Act. Drug Addiction Treatment Act of 2000.

79. Substance Abuse and Mental Health Services Administration. Trauma-informed approach and trauma-specific interventions. Available at: www.samhsa.gov/nctic/trauma-interventions. Accessed March 11, 2016.

80. Substance Abuse and Mental Health Services Administration. TIP 40: clinical guidelines for the use of Buprenorphine in the treatment of opioid addiction. 2004. Available at: http://store.samhsa.gov/product/TIP-40-Clinical-Guidelines-for-the-Use-of-Buprenorphine-in-the-Treatment-of-Opioid-Addiction/SMA07-3939. Accessed March 11, 2016.

Diet and Obesity Issues in the Underserved

Maria C. Mejia de Grubb, MD, MPH*, Robert S. Levine, MD, Roger J. Zoorob, MD, MPH

KEYWORDS

- Obesity • Diet • Underserved populations • Epidemic • Healthy lifestyle
- Socioeconomically vulnerable • Primary care

KEY POINTS

- The obesity epidemic remains an unchecked threat to the health of the United States and the world, particularly among socioeconomically vulnerable communities.
- Identifying successful models that integrate primary care, public health, and community-based efforts is important for accelerating progress in preventing and treating obesity.
- Primary care providers can help, not only as clinicians but also as role models, educators, and leaders of community-based interventions.

INTRODUCTION

The goal of this article is to inform new directions for addressing inequalities associated with obesity by reviewing current issues about diet and obesity among socioeconomically vulnerable and underserved populations. It highlights recent interventions in selected high-risk populations, as well as gaps in the knowledge base. It then identifies future directions in policy and programmatic interventions to expand the role of primary care providers, with an emphasis on those aimed at preventing obesity and promoting healthy weight. Except as noted, obesity among adults in this article is defined as a body mass index (BMI) of greater than 30.0 and overweight as a BMI of 25.0 to 29.0.[1] For children and teens, overweight is defined as a BMI at or above the 85th percentile and below the 95th percentile for children and teens of the same age and sex. Obesity is defined as a BMI at or above the 95th percentile for children and teens of the same age and sex.[2]

The authors have nothing to disclose.
Department of Family and Community Medicine, Baylor College of Medicine, 3701 Kirby Drive, Suite 600, Houston, TX 77098, USA
* Corresponding author.
E-mail address: Maria.Mejiadegrubb@bcm.edu

Prim Care Clin Office Pract 44 (2017) 127–140
http://dx.doi.org/10.1016/j.pop.2016.09.014
0095-4543/17/© 2016 Elsevier Inc. All rights reserved.

primarycare.theclinics.com

EPIDEMIOLOGY IN THE GENERAL POPULATION
Childhood and Adolescence: United States

Estimates from the United States (US) National Health and Examination Survey (NHANES) in 2011 to 2012 showed that, although there was not a significant overall change in high weight for recumbent length ($\geq$95th percentile) among infants and toddlers or obesity in 2- to 19-year-olds between 2003 to 2004 and 2011 to 2012, there was a significant decrease in obesity among 2- to 5-year-olds, from 13.9% to 8.4%, $P = .03$.[3] In addition, about 32% of US young people ages 2 to 19 years were either overweight or obese with 17% being obese in 2011 to 2012 (**Table 1**).[3] This comprised about 33% of boys and 30% of girls. About 1 in 3 boys were considered to be overweight or obese (19% obese) compared with 30.4% of girls (15% obese). The prevalence of overweight and obesity was lower among 2- to 5-year-olds (for whom overweight plus obesity was about 27% and obesity about 8%) than 6-to 11-year-olds (when the corresponding figures were 33% and 18%). Young people aged 12 to 19 years, at 34% and 20%, respectively, were similar to 6-to 11-year-olds.[4]

Adulthood: United States

Estimates of obesity among US adults vary somewhat between different national samples. NHANES (2011–2012) found that more than one-third of US adults ages 20 years or older (34.9%, about 78.6 million people) were obese and noted that this was similar to NHANES data for 2003.[3] The 2014 obesity rankings in the State of American Well-Being report included self-reported data from a national sample of 176,702 interviews conducted from January 2 to December 30, 2014, across all US states.[5] The percentage of people aged 18 years and older who were obese was 27.7%, or about 2% points higher than results from a similar survey taken in 2008.[4] The United Health Foundation's survey (America's Health Rankings), which is also based on self-reports, estimated 29.4% adult obesity for 2014 and 29.6% for 2015.[6]

The Effect of Race, Ethnicity, Gender, and Socioeconomic Status: United States

According to NHANES (2009–2010), 29% of white youth were overweight or obese, with 15.2% being obese. Among black youth, 41.8% were overweight or obese, and 25.7% were obese. Among Hispanic youth, 41.2% were overweight or obese, and 22.9% were obese. Across youth ages 6 to 19 of all races, 33.2% were overweight or obese, and 18.2% were obese.[7]

Among adults (NHANES 2011–2012) 47.8% of non-Hispanic blacks, 42.5% of Hispanics, 32.6% of non-Hispanic whites, and 10.8% of non-Hispanic Asians were found to be obese.[8] The prevalence of obesity was also higher among middle-aged adults,

Table 1 Prevalence of obesity 2011-2012			
Age Range (year-old)	Total (%)	Boys (%)	Girls (%)
0–2 y/o	8.1	—	—
2–19 y/o	16.9	18.6	15
2–5 y/o	8.4	9.5	7.2
6–11 y/o	17.7	16.4	19.1
12–19 y/o	20.5	20.3	20.7

Data from Ogden CL, Carroll MD, Kit BK, et al. Prevalence of childhood and adult obesity in the United States, 2011-2012. JAMA 2014;311(8):806–14.

40 to 59 years old (39.5%), than among adults ages 20 to 39 (30.3%) or older than 60 years (35.4%).[8] Among non-Hispanic black and Mexican-American men, those with higher incomes were more likely to be obese than those with low incomes.[8] The same was true for Mexican-American men; however, among non-Hispanic white men, no statistically significant relationship was found with poverty.[8] In contrast, women with higher incomes were less likely to be obese than women with lower incomes, be they non-Hispanic white, non-Hispanic black, or Mexican-American.[8] These trends only reached statistical significance, however, for non-Hispanic white women. Such variations reflect the complex nature of relationships between socioeconomic status (SES) and obesity. Low-income and food insecure populations in the US, for example, face a multitude of barriers that may direct purchases toward inexpensive, energy-dense, nutritionally poor food. These populations may also be subject to cycles of food deprivation and overeating; high levels of stress, anxiety, or depression; have fewer opportunities for physical activity; and be subject to greater exposure to the marketing of obesity-promoting products.[9] Still, as previously noted,[8] obesity is not universally associated with low SES. A full understanding has not been reached, nor is this likely to happen without a better understanding of differences in motivations and the meaning of excess weight in different socioeconomic groups.[10]

The role of education also seems to be different between men and women. There is no significant relationship between obesity and education among men and an inverse relationship (lower obesity with a college education) among women.[8] Although longitudinal data linking community context to health are sparse, researchers using data from electronic health records of 163,473 children ages 3 to 18 years residing in 1288 communities in Pennsylvania whose weight and height were measured longitudinally observed that social deprivation at birth was associated with higher BMI at 10.7 years of age and with more rapid growth of BMI over time.[11] Children born into the poorest communities displayed sustained and accelerated BMI growth. Community-level deprivation remained associated with BMI trajectories after adjustment for household socioeconomic deprivation. By way of explanation, the investigators hypothesized that the effect of community socioeconomic deprivation on BMI growth may be mediated by parental behaviors related to food purchases and physical activity.[11] They concluded that individual-level intervention programs that ignore the effect of community context may be less efficient.[11]

Obesity in Special Populations

Incarcerated
Rising obesity rates in the US may affect the imprisoned population, thereby increasing the prevalence of obesity-related diseases and the cost and performance of correctional health care. Leddy and colleagues[12] note that as rates of obesity increased in the US so did the US prison population, which nearly tripled between 1987 and 2007, and judged that the frequencies of obesity-related comorbidities are comparable among inmates the general US population. For example, hypertension is 18.3% among inmates and 24.5% for the US, respiratory illness is at 8.5% for inmates and 7.8% for the US, and diabetes is at 4.8% among inmates and 7.0% for the US. They predict that the combination of rising rates of obesity and imprisonment may, therefore, increase the number and proportion of obese inmates.[12]

Some research has found women prisoners to be particularly vulnerable to weight gain, although higher average weekly gains were reported for those incarcerated for 2 weeks or less at the time of study enrollment than those incarcerated longer than 2 weeks (1.7 pounds vs 0.8 pounds).[13] Evidence from Japan suggests that restricted diets and enforced physical activity can improve inmate health.[13]

Homeless

Researchers have noted a food insecurity-obesity paradox, whereby food insecurity, often associated with insufficient resources to purchase food, is associated with over-consumption of food and consequent obesity.[12–14] Many theories have been pro-posed to explain this correlation, including the low cost of energy-dense foods, binge eating habits as an adaptive physiologic response to food scarcity, and child-hood poverty leading to obesity in adulthood.[14] In a study of 436 chronically homeless adults across 11 US cities, 57% were found to be overweight or obese, with the prev-alence being highest among women and Hispanics.[14] The investigators concluded that there was a greater need for attention to obesity in chronically homeless adults and for a better understanding of the seemingly paradoxic nature of relationships be-tween food insecurity, poverty, and obesity.

Military

The US military has long been concerned that increased obesity and poor physical fitness among civilian youth may tend to produce soldiers who are, in the words of some worried military retirees, "Too fat to fight."[15] Military organizations have been quicker to respond to the burgeoning US epidemic than their civilian counterparts, implementing an upgraded Physical Fitness and Weight Control Program (Army Regu-lation 600-9) in 1976.[16] Millions of Americans have been able to maintain a healthy weight and meet physical performance requirements while in military service and, even though it has been found that weight gain is associated with return to civilian life, there is evidence that the health consequences of obesity may be partly mitigated by those who maintain physical fitness.[16]

Global and international issues

The World Health Organization (WHO) estimates that at least 2.8 million people die globally each year from being overweight or obese.[17] Moreover, the worldwide prev-alence more than doubled between 1980 and 2014, at which point 11% of men and 15% of women in the world 18 years of age and older were obese (as defined by a BMI of >30 kg/m^2) versus 5% of men and 8% of women in 1980.[17,18] The higher prev-alence among women was found in all WHO regions, translating to obesity among more than 600 million people.[17,18] Significantly, 42 million children younger than the age of 5 years worldwide were also obese or overweight (defined as a BMI >25). Global obesity presents a double burden of disease, in part, because it is now emerging as a problem in lower and middle income countries, especially in urban centers.[18]

COEXISTENCE OF FOOD INSECURITY AND OBESITY

In addition to the homeless, food insecurity, and obesity may coexist in other disad-vantaged populations. Food insecure households are defined as those which, at some or all times during a year, are uncertain of having or unable to acquire enough food to meet the needs of all their members because they had insufficient money or other resources for food.[19] Current research into this association has resulted in mixed findings.[18–23] Overall, there is only consistent evidence for a higher risk of obesity among food insecure women.[21–23] However, the coexistence of food insecurity and obesity has been reported as expected considering that both are associated with so-cioeconomic disadvantage.[22]

Both food insecurity and obesity may be independent consequences of low income and the resulting lack of access and/or utilization of enough nutritious food (eg, fresh, frozen, canned, in prepared sauces or dishes), stresses of poverty, and a sedentary lifestyle. The ability to afford healthy food and get the right amount of exercise, the 2 factors critical to maintaining a healthy weight, can be challenging for people living in low-income communities. According to the US Department of Agriculture (USDA), 14.0% (17.4 million) of US households were food insecure at some time during 2014.[19] Members of food insecure households use various coping strategies that may contribute to weight gain.

For example, families with limited resources may select lower-quality diets, including high-calorie, energy-dense foods to maintain adequate energy intake. These foods are traditionally the least expensive, are easy to overconsume, have been shown to promote weight gain, and have been found to be more prevalent in low-income communities compared with healthier food options.[23] Research suggests that low-income, minority, and rural communities have fewer supermarkets compared with more affluent areas.[24] The lack of convenient access to supermarkets and full-service grocery stores that offer a larger selection of healthy and more affordable food (eg, fruits and vegetables) in both urban and rural low-income neighborhoods is an obstacle for attaining a healthy diet.

In addition, low-income communities have greater availability of fast food restaurants, especially near schools.[23] Fast food consumption is associated with a diet high in calories and low in nutrients, and frequent consumption may lead to weight gain.[21] Interestingly, McDermott and Stephens,[25] found that, on a per-calorie basis, a fast-food, or convenience diet for a single parent raising 1 child in Baltimore, MD, without government support was more expensive than a diet based on generic brand or frozen foods, even though dairy and vegetables cost more than other food groups. They concluded that, "It is difficult to meet current dietary recommendations without income assistance."[25] Programs that currently help low-income families (incomes <185% of the poverty line) include the Women, Infant, and Children (WIC) Program, the Free and Reduced Meal (FARM) program, or the Commodity Supplemental Food Program (CSFP).[25]

Food Deserts

The USDA defines a food desert as a census tract in a low-income community in which at least one-third of the population lives more than 1 mile from the nearest large supermarket or grocery store in an urban area, and more than 10 miles in a rural area (low-access communities).[19] Food equity is only achieved when the residents of a neighborhood have easy access to affordable nutritious food. The location of the store in relationship to the resident, individual travel patterns characteristics (eg, income, car ownership, disability status), and neighborhood characteristics (eg, the availability of public transportation, availability of sidewalks, crime patterns in the area) are key factors to ensure equitable access to affordable, healthy foods.[26]

Higher Exposure to Marketing of Less Nutritious Foods and Media Influences

Research suggests that minority and low-income populations have poor nutrition that is not simply due to independent personal choice. Instead, food-marketing influences the preferences and consumption of unhealthy food choices.[27–29] Targeted marketing has influenced the increased availability and lower cost of processed, high-calorie foods relative to healthier options, increased portion sizes, food advertising, and fast-food promotion, which are all contributors to the obesity epidemic.[30]

In the US, it has been suggested that future policy recommendations should include setting standards to limit the amount of advertising of foods and beverages of low nutritional value, particularly advertising targeting socioeconomically vulnerable children, via television, radio, new digital and social media, outdoor advertisement, and point-of-sale product placements.[31]

Limited Access to Safe Places to Be Physically Active

Many low-income neighborhoods offer inadequate opportunities for safe exercise, and they lack community recreation areas with free or low-cost access. This limited access is associated with decreased physical activity and increased obesity rates.[32] In fact, communities with lower and medium SES often display fewer public resources, such as parks, trails, and playgrounds, compared with communities with higher SES.[32,33] Data show that improving certain features of the built environment supports physical activity, especially among underserved populations.[33] Recommended implementation strategies include improved access to places for physical activity such as recreation areas and parks,[34] improved infrastructure to support bicycling and walking, locating schools closer to residential areas to encourage nonmotorized travel to and from school, zoning to allow mixed-use areas that combine residential with commercial and institutional uses, improving access to public transportation, and improving personal and traffic safety in areas where persons are or could be physically active.[33–35]

High Levels of Stress and Poor Mental Health

Associations between food insecurity and stress and poor mental health (eg, depression, psychological distress, anxiety) have been reported.[36,37] The financial and emotional burden of food insecurity, in addition to other socioeconomic factors, such as low-wage employment, lack of access to health care, inadequate transportation, poor housing, and neighborhood violence, pose additional constraints in underserved populations. Stress and poor mental health may lead to weight gain through stress-induced hormonal and metabolic changes, as well as unhealthy eating behaviors and physical inactivity.[38] Specifically, chronic stress can promote visceral fat accumulation by dysregulating the hypothalamic-pituitary-adrenal (HPA) axis. Reciprocally, obesity may promote a state of systemic low-grade inflammation mediated by increased adipokine secretion, which can also chronically stimulate and disturb the HPA axis, leading to a vicious cycle with multiple adverse health effects.[38] The pathophysiology of these interactions is exceedingly complex and is reviewed elsewhere.[38–40] Both stress and poor mental health have been linked to obesity in children and adults.[23] For example, low-income mothers suffering with depression or food insecurity may use obesogenic child feeding practices and unfavorable parenting practices that could influence child weight status.[23] In addition, data show that food-insecure people, especially mothers, struggle with cycles of food deprivation and overeating. They adopt strategies such as eating less, cutting the size of meals, skipping meals, and waiting to eat later in the day to spare their children from the impact of hunger, which results in chronic ups and downs in food intake that can contribute to weight gain.[22,23]

HEALTH CONSEQUENCES

Higher body weights are associated with higher incidence of many other health problems, including type 2 diabetes, cardiovascular disease, stroke, nonalcoholic fatty liver disease, gallstones, osteoarthritis, asthma, obstructive sleep apnea, female infertility, and increased risk of disability.[29,41–43] In addition, certain cancers have been linked to obesity, including colon, gall bladder, female breast (postmenopausal), endometrium, renal cell carcinoma, and adenocarcinoma of the esophagus. Higher body weight is also associated with social stigmatization and mental illness.[29]

A review of literature pertaining to psychosocial factors and childhood obesity noted the possibility of a bidirectional relationship with depression and anxiety, suggesting that it is possible that depression is both a cause and a consequence of obesity; a linear relationship between BMI and low body self-esteem in girls, in contrast to a U-shaped relationship in boys; unhealthy weight control behaviors (eg, unhealthy diets); and eating disorder symptoms, including binge eating episodes, a drive for thinness, and impulse regulation.[44] Weight-based stigmatization and teasing, and weight and shape concerns, were 2 important mediating factors. Specifically, obesity is considered to be a particularly stigmatizing and socially unacceptable condition of childhood, with long-lasting effects related to lower levels of education and family income, higher poverty, and lower marriage rates in later young adulthood.[44]

INTERVENTIONS IN SELECTED HIGH-RISK POPULATIONS

The importance of cultural influences is key for many high-risk populations. Caprio and colleagues[45] summarized investigations pertaining to various cultures as part of a consensus statement for Shaping America's Health and the Obesity Society. Regarding body size, they noted that Latinas tend to favor a thin figure for themselves and a plumper figure for their children, whereas African American women and men were more likely to prefer a large body size for women. Feeding practices also have cultural determinants based in part on, "Affordability, availability of foods and ingredients, palatability, familiarity, and perceived healthfulness prompt immigrant families to retain or discard certain traditional foods and to adopt novel foods associated with the mainstream culture."[45] Children from immigrant Mexican households, for example, may resist parental efforts to promote lower-calorie traditional foods prepared at home in favor of higher calorie foods and favor the higher-calorie foods, beverages, and snacks from the mainstream culture.[45] Cultural patterns may also determine the types of foods considered to be healthy or unhealthy. Among Hmong immigrants in California, frozen or canned foods, as well as school meals, are considered unhealthy, in part, because they are not considered to be fresh.[45] The scientific literature pertaining to these topics is vast and growing. A current National Library of Medicine Pub Med search for "obesity and culture" (May 2016) revealed more than 10,000 citations. The following examples provide a snapshot of interventions in selected high-risk groups.

Black and African American Communities

Researchers have noted the importance of community context in setting the agenda for African American obesity interventions.[46,47] Employment, safety, academic advancement, substance use disorders, incarceration, dysfunctional social networks, and violence may not only be of more immediate concern than calorie intake or physical activity, they may also play important roles in mediating unhealthy eating.[46,47] Additional mediating environmental factors include availability and access to high quality foods, and physical activity resources.[47]

Biologic factors that may contribute to difficulties in weight management among African Americans include lower energy expenditures when sleeping, exercising, or resting; increased propensity for fat storage; higher steady-state ghrelin levels, leading to increased hunger; lower peptide tyrosine production after meals, leading to lower satiety; and decreased energy cost of activity after diet-induced weight loss.[46] Inclusion of a formal maintenance program was associated with lower percentage of regained weight for African American (as well as white) women and there is some evidence that including cultural adaptations may improve outcomes among African American women.[46] The exact composition of effective cultural adaptations, however, seems to be poorly differentiated in the literature.[46] Multidimensional approaches are recommended for future efforts.[46]

United States Immigrant Populations

A recent review identified only 20 of 684 potentially relevant articles that met selection criteria for evaluation.[48] Selection criteria were as follows: (1) the intervention targeted an immigrant population in the US, (2) the intervention objective was the prevention or control of obesity, (3) the study examined measured (vs self-reported) outcomes related to obesity, (4) the findings were published in a peer-reviewed journal, and (5) the article was written in English.[48] Most of the interventions targeted Latinos, predominantly of Mexican origin, and their emphasis was on multiple activities, including diet, physical activity, sleep, and screen time. Successful interventions were characterized by community engagement and/or participation that included placement within community structures and settings, and leveraging community resources to achieve a cultural focus, without which the interventions generally did not work.[48] Child interventions that incorporated parenting practices and promoted a healthy home environment were also effective.[48] A key problem has been that the possible moderating role of acculturation on obesity-related outcomes is rarely considered, even though immigrant weight gain has been overwhelmingly linked to their level of acculturation.[48] The investigators concluded that, notwithstanding the paucity of data on effective interventions, novel obesity prevention strategies to reduce migration-related obesity inequalities are warranted to help inform health policies and programs.[48]

American Indian Communities

"Healthy Children, Strong Families" provides an example of obesity interventions targeted specifically for American Indians.[49] As part of community engagement efforts, it was noted that recognition of obesity was low despite evidence of a high prevalence of both being overweight and obesity. It was also noted that the views of holistic health in the American Indian community might make interventions focused on defining a particular disease ineffective. Investigators were pleasantly surprised at the effectiveness of mailed lessons; however, home visits by mentors, although appreciated, did not seem to make a difference in outcomes. For the future, investigators emphasized the importance of intergenerational inclusion; the availability of fun, easy, interactive learning materials; inclusion of health-related children's books; and a focus on reducing family and environmental barriers to change. Although work specific to American Indian groups is in its infancy, efforts such as this emphasize the common themes, which speak to the importance of community engagement and attention to contextual influences on the family.

Native Hawaiian and Pacific Islander Communities

The PILI 'Ohana project presents an example of obesity prevention efforts among native Hawaiian and Pacific Islander communities.[50] Once again, community context was identified as a key factor. Elements unique to Native Hawaiians and Pacific Islanders included a preference for ethnocultural activities as a form of exercise, such as hula for native Hawaiians and ballroom dancing for Filipinos. Socially derived eating expectations were important to Pacific Islanders, including social pressures from within their own culture to eat and/or prepare large servings of calorie-dense food such as dishes with Spam, canned corned beef, and side dishes with high-fat mayonnaise. Through 8 years of community-based work, researchers were able to mobilize communities to improve food sovereignty and organic and traditional Hawaiian farming.[50]

Rural Appalachia

The Behavioral Risk Factor Surveillance Survey has identified Rural Appalachia as being at the epicenter of the national obesity epidemic.[51] Because unhealthy behaviors such as smoking, failure to meet recommendations for fruit and vegetable consumption, and low levels of physical activity are entrenched in the region,[51] innovative methods are needed so that families can acquire new knowledge. Adolescents, particularly disadvantaged and minority students, are targeted as primary family change agents, with the program building on an existing network of 76 science clubs organized in collaboration between communities in West Virginia and West Virginia University's Health Science and Technology Academy.[51] Club members are encouraged to enroll in and graduate from college. They are taught the science that underlies health care, including new knowledge about the importance and implications of lifestyle choices. Cognitive learning is emphasized as a prerequisite for changing behavior. Teachers and students are trained in the conduct of community-based participatory research.[51] Formal research projects are developed, sent through an approved Institutional Review Board, and implemented. From September 2011 to May 2012 there were 744 students in the program and 400 projects in place, 224 of which were related to obesity.[51] As of this writing, this is still a work in progress, so ultimate effectiveness remains to be determined. However, its unique design offers insights into new ideas for community collaboration in an environment in which changing behaviors for health has been an elusive goal.[51]

INTERNATIONAL PERSPECTIVES

According to the WHO, a rising global epidemic of overweight and obesity, so-called globesity, is spreading across the world. Once considered a problem only for industrialized and high-income countries, worldwide obesity has more than doubled since 1980 and is now also prevalent in low- and middle-income countries.[16,17] Despite that infectious diseases and undernutrition remain a challenge, low- and middle-income countries are experiencing a rapid rise in noncommunicable disease risk factors such as obesity and overweight, especially among urban communities.[18] In fact, 65% of the world's population lives in a country where overweight and obesity-related mortality is much higher than underweight-related mortality.

Globalization forces, including free trade, economic growth, and urbanization, seem also to be driving the global obesity epidemic, especially in low- and middle-income countries. These macrolevel mechanisms can promote nutrition transition, a term for the obesity-inducing shift from traditional to Western diets that accompanies modernization and wealth, by changing food and built environments and spreading new technologies.[52]

There is some evidence that the global public health community is taking the rise in obesity seriously (eg, increasing surveillance).[53] However, the obesity epidemic is not only increasing but no country has also reported decreased rates in the last 3 decades.[46–52] Although obesity may be a global issue, the challenges all begin at local levels considering that dietary, economic, cultural, and lifestyle factors are so widely varied across countries. The WHO's action plan to fight the global obesity epidemic recommends a population-based multisector, multidisciplinary, and culturally relevant approach. Changes must be multilateral to meet the complexity of cultural traditions and dietary norms of the world's many ethnic groups. It is important to continue surveillance and monitoring obesity trends and tailor public-health intervention toward specific population groups. By working with local communities, stakeholders can better develop strategies that address both nutrition and physical activity to reduce obesity prevalence.[53]

POLICY RECOMMENDATIONS AND PRIMARY CARE

Several scientific organizations have published recommendations and guidelines for primary care providers to address obesity prevention and treatment. The Institute of Medicine (IOM) in its most recent report, "Accelerating Progress in Obesity Prevention,"[54] recommends 4 strategies to expand the role of health care providers and to encourage them to support and advocate publicly for several policy changes:

1. Provide standardized care and advocate for healthy community environments. Disseminate healthy lifestyle recommendations and materials as part of primary prevention efforts in the primary care setting. Physician counseling is effective in promoting healthy behavior. Data show that adults with high BMI who report that their doctors have told them they are overweight are more likely to have accurate perceptions of their own weight.[48–55] They are also more likely to be interested in losing weight and to have tried losing weight. Yet a third of obese patients say their doctors did not tell them they were overweight.[48–55]
2. Ensure coverage of, access to, and incentives for routine obesity prevention, screening, diagnosis, and treatment. The US Preventive Services Task Force recommends screening all adults for obesity and that clinicians offer or refer patients with a BMI greater than 30 kg/m^2 to intensive, multicomponent behavioral interventions. Implementation of capacity building within the primary care setting, such as improvements to organizational systems or care models used by providers, are key for effective practices.
3. Encourage active living and healthy eating at work. The IOM suggests that providers use a multifaceted approach to patient education, recognizing that patients may have different learning styles, needs, and preferences.
4. Encourage healthy weight gain during pregnancy and breastfeeding and promote breastfeeding-friendly environments.

FUTURE DIRECTIONS IN PRIMARY CARE

Primary care providers commonly evaluate and treat obesity and health-related conditions. Nonetheless, there is a recognized need to expand their role to include advocacy, modeling healthy lifestyle behaviors in the community, and counseling individuals and families about obesity prevention.[54]

Research

There is a significant need to identify safe and effective methods of providing weight management to patients with unhealthy weight encountered in primary care practices.[56] Obesity is a chronic condition on which the social determinants of health have considerable impact. Sharing responsibility and resources for the management of obesity has considerable promise. However, additional research and tools to facilitate primary care providers and their practices to locate community resources to partner with are warranted to improve obesity rates in their communities.[56]

Practice

Patients with complex health conditions, particularly among underserved communities, are not easily addressed in a typical physician-directed office visit of 15- or 20-minute duration. Nonetheless, the high prevalence of overweight and obesity in the US suggests that a patient's weight status should always be addressed and placed at the center of their overall health care. Providers can also actively promote the prevention and treatment of obesity through efforts in community settings. Moreover, practice recommendations, such as weight status assessment and monitoring, healthy lifestyle promotion through motivational interviewing, treatment, clinician skill development, clinic infrastructure development, community program referrals, community health education, multisector community initiatives, and policy advocacy, are among the necessary steps for effective interventions. Unfortunately, data show that only 12% of physician office visits of all child or adult patients included counseling about nutrition or diet.[54] Lack of time to obtain relevant information from individual and family contexts may be a major impediment to addressing healthy weight. Additional barriers include provider's lack of awareness of the issue, lack of comfort or skill counseling families on the issue, need for organizational prompts, and lack of familiarity with available community resources for lifestyle counseling or obesity prevention programs.[57]

SUMMARY

Identifying successful models that integrate primary care, public health, and community-based efforts is important to obesity prevention, particularly among underserved populations. Primary care providers play an important role in obesity interventions, consistent with current recommendations from scientific and professional organizations.

Outside of their clinical role, primary care providers can also serve as role models, educators, and promoters of healthy lifestyle practices, and serve as leaders in community-based obesity prevention initiatives.

REFERENCES

1. US Centers for Disease Control and Prevention. Defining adult overweight and obesity. Available at: http://www.cdc.gov/obesity/adult/defining.html. Accessed February 25, 2016.
2. US Centers for Disease Control and Prevention. Division of Nutrition, Physical Activity and Obesity. Available at: http://www.cdc.gov/obesity/childhood/defining.html. Accessed February 25, 2016.
3. Ogden CL, Carroll MD, Kit BK, et al. Prevalence of childhood and adult obesity in the United States, 2011-2012. JAMA 2014;311(8):806–14.
4. National Institute of Diabetes and Digestive and Kidney Diseases. Overweight and Obesity Statistics. 2012. NIH Publication No. 04-4158. Available at: http://www.niddk.nih.gov/health-information/health-statistics/Pages/overweight-obesity-statistics.aspx. Accessed January 11, 2016.
5. Gallup and Healthways. State of American well-being: 2014 obesity rankings. 2015. Available at: http://info.healthways.com/hubfs/Well-Being_Index/2014_Data/Gallup-Healthways_State_of_American_Well-Being_2014_Obesity_Rankings.pdf?t=1452282314786. Accessed January 11, 2016.
6. America's Health Rankings. Obesity. 2016. Available at: http://www.americashealthrankings.org/ALL/Obesity. Accessed January 11, 2016.
7. Wang Y, Beydoun MA. The obesity epidemic in the United States–gender, age, socioeconomic, racial/ethnic, and geographic characteristics: a systematic review and meta-regression analysis. Epidemiol Rev 2007;29:6–28.
8. United States Centers for Disease Control and Prevention. Adult Obesity Facts. 2015. Available at: http://www.cdc.gov/obesity/data/adult.html. Accessed January 13, 2016.

9. Anon. Food Research and Action Center (FRAC). Why low-income and food insecure people are vulnerable to obesity. Available at: http://frac.org/initiatives/hunger-and-obesity/why-are-low-income-and-food-insecure-people-vulnerable-to-obesity/. Accessed January 10, 2016.

10. Pampel FC, Denney JT, Krueger PM. Obesity, SES, and economic development: a test of the reversal hypothesis. Soc Sci Med 2012;74(7):1073–81.

11. Nau C, Schwartz BS, Bandeen-Roche K, et al. Community socioeconomic deprivation and obesity trajectories in children using electronic health records. Obesity (Silver Spring) 2015;23(1):207–12.

12. Leddy MA, Schulkin J, Power ML. Consequences of high incarceration rate and high obesity prevalence on the prison system. J Correct Health Care 2009;15(4):318–27.

13. Clarke JG, Waring ME. Overweight, obesity, and weight change among incarcerated women. J Correct Health Care 2012;18(4):285–92.

14. Tsai J, Rosenheck RA. Obesity among chronically homeless adults: is it a problem? Public Health Rep 2013;128(1):29–36.

15. Christeson W, Taggart AD, Messner-Zidell S. Too fat to fight: retired military leaders want junk foods out of America's schools. New York: Mission Readiness; 2010.

16. Levine RS, Kilbourne BJ, Kihlberg CH, et al. Military and civilian approaches to the U.S. obesity epidemic. Chapter 9. In: Brennan VM, Kumanyika SK, Zambrana RE, editors. Obesity interventions in underserved communities. Baltimore (MD): Johns Hopkins University Press; 2014. p. 176–92.

17. World Health Organization Global Health Observatory (GHO) data. Obesity. Available at: http://www.who.int/gho/ncd/risk_factors/obesity_text/en/. Accessed January 10, 2016.

18. World Health Organization Media Centre. Obesity and Overweight. Fact sheet No311. 2015. Available at: http://www.who.int/mediacentre/factsheets/fs311/en/. Accessed January 10, 2016.

19. USDA. U.S. Department of Agriculture. Creating Access to Healthy, Affordable Food. Food Deserts. 2016. Available at: https://apps.ams.usda.gov/fooddeserts/fooddeserts.aspx. Accessed January 12, 2016.

20. Institute of Medicine. Hunger and obesity: understanding a food insecurity paradigm: workshop summary. Washington, DC: The National Academies Press; 2011. Provides a comprehensive discussion by experts from many disciplines of issues related to the coexistence of food insecurity and obesity.

21. Larson NI, Story MT. Food insecurity and weight status among U.S. children and families: a review of the literature. Am J Prev Med 2011;40(2):166–73.

22. Frongillo EA, Bernal J. Understanding the coexistence of food insecurity and obesity. Curr Pediatr Rep 2014;2(4):284–90.

23. Hartline-Grafton H. Understanding the connections: food insecurity and obesity. 2015. Available at: http://frac.org/pdf/frac_brief_understanding_the_connections.pdf. Accessed February 10, 2016.

24. Larson NI, Story MT, Nelson MC. Neighborhood environments: disparities in access to healthy foods in the U.S. Am J Prev Med 2009;36(1):74–81.

25. McDermott AJ, Stephens MB. Cost of eating: whole foods versus convenience foods in a low-income model. Fam Med 2010 Apr;42(4):280–4.

26. Economic Research Service, UD Department of Agriculture. Access to Affordable and Nutritious Food. Measuring and understanding food deserts and their consequences: report to congress. Washington, DC: USDA Administrative Publication No. (AP-036), June 2009. p. 160.

27. Williams JD, Crockett D, Harrison RL, et al. The role of food culture and marketing activity in health disparities. Prev Med 2012;55(5):382–6.
28. Grier SA, Kumanyika SK. The context for choice: health implications of targeted food and beverage marketing to African Americans. Am J Public Health 2008; 98(9):1616–29.
29. National Institute of Heart, Lung, and Blood Disease. What Are the Health Risks of Overweight and Obesity? 2012. Available at: http://www.nhlbi.nih.gov/health/health-topics/topics/obe/risks. Accessed January 14, 2016.
30. McGinnis JM, Gootman JA, Kraak VI. Food marketing to children and youth: threat or opportunity? Washington, DC: National Academies Press; 2006.
31. The State of Obesity. A project of the Trust for America's Health and the Robert Wood Johnson Foundation Special Report: Racial and ethnic disparities in Obesity. Policy Recommendations. 2016. Available at: http://stateofobesity.org/disparities/. Accessed January 12, 2016.
32. National Recreation and Park Association. Parks and recreation in underserved areas: a public health perspective. Ashburn (VA): National Recreation and Parks Association. Available at: http://www.nrpa.org/uploadedFiles/nrpa.org/Publications_and_Research/Research/Papers/Parks-Rec-Underserved-Areas.pdf. Accessed January 15, 2016.
33. Gordon-Larsen P, Nelson MC, Page P, et al. Inequality in the built environment underlies key health disparities in physical activity and obesity. Pediatrics 2006; 117(2):417–24.
34. Barrett MA, Miller D, Frumkin H. Parks and health: aligning incentives to create innovations in chronic disease prevention. Prev Chronic Dis 2014;11:E63.
35. Khan LK, Sobush K, Keener D, et al. Recommended community strategies and measurements to prevent obesity in the United States. MMWR Recomm Rep 2009;58(RR-7):1–26.
36. Leung CW, Epel ES, Willett WC, et al. Household food insecurity is positively associated with depression among low-income supplemental nutrition assistance program participants and income-eligible nonparticipants. J Nutr 2015;145(3): 622–7.
37. Liu Y, Njai RS, Greenlund KJ, et al. Relationships between housing and food insecurity, frequent mental distress, and insufficient sleep among adults in 12 US States, 2009. Prev Chronic Dis 2014;11:E37.
38. Paredes S, Ribeiro L. Cortisol: the villain in metabolic syndrome. Rev Assoc Med Bras 2014;60(1):84–92.
39. Miller WL, Auchus RJ. The molecular biology, biochemistry, and physiology of human steroidogenesis and its disorders. Endocr Rev 2011;32(1):81–151.
40. McAllister EJ, Dhurandhar NV, Keith SW, et al. Ten putative contributors to the obesity epidemic. Crit Rev Food Sci Nutr 2009;49(10):868–913.
41. Block JP, He Y, Zaslavsky AM, et al. Psychosocial stress and change in weight among US adults. Am J Epidemiol 2009;170(2):181–92.
42. Calle EE, Thun MJ. Obesity and cancer. Oncogene 2004;23(38):6365–78.
43. Brennan VM, Kumanyika SK, Zambrana RE. Introduction: advancing a new conversation about obesity in the underserved. Obesity interventions in underserved communities: evidence and directions. Baltimore (MD): Johns Hopkins University Press; 2014. p. 1–21.
44. Russell-Mayhew S, McVey G, Bardick A, et al. Mental health, wellness, and childhood overweight/obesity. J Obes 2012;2012:281801.
45. Caprio S, Daniels SR, Drewnowski A, et al. Influence of race, ethnicity, and culture on childhood obesity: implications for prevention and treatment: a consensus

statement of Shaping America's Health and the Obesity Society. Diabetes Care 2008;31(11):2211–21.

46. Kumanyika SK, Prewitt TE, Banks J, et al. In the way or on the way?. In: Brennan VM, Kumanyika SK, Zambrana RE, editors. Obesity interventions in underserved communities: evidence and directions. Baltimore (MD): Johns Hopkins University Press; 2014. p. 151–61.

47. Tussing-Humphreys LM, Fitzgibbon ML, Kong A, et al. Weight loss maintenance in African American women: a systematic review of the behavioral lifestyle intervention literature. J Obes 2013;2013:437369.

48. Tovar A, Renzaho AM, Guerrero AD, et al. A systematic review of obesity prevention intervention studies among immigrant populations in the US. Curr Obes Rep 2014;3:206–22.

49. Adams A, Cronin KA, Group. HCR. Healthy children, strong families: obesity prevention for preschool American Indian children and their families. In: Brennan VM, Kumanyika SK, Zambrana RE, editors. Obesity Interventions in underserved communities: evidence and directions. Baltimore (MD): Johns Hopkins University Press; 2014. p. 344–52.

50. Kaholokula JK, Kekauoha P, Dillard A, et al. The PILI 'Ohana Project: a community-academic partnership to achieve metabolic health equity in Hawai'i. Hawaii J Med Public Health 2014;73(12 Suppl 3):29–33.

51. Branch RA, Chester AL, Hanks S, et al. Obesity management organized by adolescents in rural Appalachia. In: Brennan VM, Kumanyika SK, Zambrana RE, editors. Obesity interventions in underserved communities: evidence and directions. Baltimore (MD): Johns Hopkins University Press; 2014. p. 205–13.

52. Popkin BM. The world is fat. Sci Am 2007;297(3):88–95.

53. Ng M, Fleming T, Robinson M, et al. Global, regional, and national prevalence of overweight and obesity in children and adults during 1980-2013: a systematic analysis for the Global Burden of Disease Study 2013. Lancet 2014;384(9945): 766–81.

54. Committee on Accelerating Progress in Obesity Prevention and Institute of Medicine. Accelerating progress in obesity prevention: solving the weight of the nation. Baltimore (MD): National Academies Press; 2012.

55. Post RE, Mainous AG 3rd, Gregorie SH, et al. The influence of physician acknowledgment of patients' weight status on patient perceptions of overweight and obesity in the United States. Arch Intern Med 2011;171(4):316–21.

56. Wadden TA, Volger S, Tsai AG, et al. Managing obesity in primary care practice: an overview with perspective from the POWER-UP study. Int J Obes 2013; 37(Suppl 1):S3–11.

57. Vine M, Hargreaves MB, Briefel RR, et al. Expanding the role of primary care in the prevention and treatment of childhood obesity: a review of clinic- and community-based recommendations and interventions. J Obes 2013;2013: 172035.

Exercise and Sports Medicine Issues in Underserved Populations

Vincent Morelli, MD[a],*, Daniel L. Bedney, MD[b],
Arie (Eric) Dadush, MD[b]

KEYWORDS

- Exercise • Underserved • Sports medicine • Socioeconomic status

KEY POINTS

- Primary care providers can make a strong argument for exercise promotion in underserved communities.
- The benefits are vitally important in adolescent physical, cognitive, and psychological development as well as in adult disease prevention and treatment.
- In counseling such patients, we should take into account a patient's readiness for change and the barriers to exercise.

EXERCISE IN UNDERSERVED COMMUNITIES

As discussed in other articles in this issue, the untoward health effects brought on by lower socioeconomic status (SES) and higher allostatic load (AL) can be significant. In this article the authors briefly recap the effects of low SES on adolescent development (both physical and psychological) and on adult burden of disease. The authors then examine how exercise might help to ameliorate these untoward health effects in underserved populations.

DEMOGRAPHICS

The World Health Organization and the American College of Sports Medicine recommend 150 minutes per week of moderate to vigorous physical activity (MVPA) in adults and 60 - minutes per day in children and adolescents.[1,2] (MVPA is any activity whereby one is breathing harder than usual but can still carry on a conversation.) In the United States,

Disclosure: The authors of this work report no direct financial interest in the subject matter or any material discussed in this article.
[a] Sports Medicine Fellowship, Department of Family and Community Medicine, Meharry Medical College, 1005 Dr D. B. Todd Boulevard, Nashville, TN 37208, USA; [b] Department of Family and Community Medicine, Meharry Medical College, 1005 Dr D. B. Todd Boulevard, Nashville, TN 37208, USA
* Corresponding author.
E-mail address: vmorelli@mmc.edu

Prim Care Clin Office Pract 44 (2017) 141–154
http://dx.doi.org/10.1016/j.pop.2016.09.015
0095-4543/17/© 2016 Elsevier Inc. All rights reserved.

only 42% of children and 8% of adolescents meet these modest recommendations,[3,4] with underserved children (black and Hispanics) exhibiting the lowest levels of physical activity. The lowest levels of physical activity are seen in children with poorly educated mothers, those living in high-crime neighborhoods, those from low-income families, those with few adult role models, those in schools lacking sufficient physical education (PE) classes, and those living in communities with low community-based physical activity opportunities.[5,6] In addition, as children age from 9 to 15 years, the time spent in MVPA drops significantly, again with the greatest declines seen in children of low-income families (and girls).[7] Contributing to the problem is the fact that in 2014 only 3.6% of elementary schools, 3.4% of middle schools, and 4.0% of high schools nationwide required daily PE for all students (US DHHS, Centers for Disease Control and Prevention. Results from the School Health Policy and Practices Study 2014. Available at: www.cdc.gov/healthyyouth/data/shpps/pdf/shpps-508-final_101315.pdf. Accessed November 8, 2016.), thus, disregarding the recommendations of the nation's Healthy People 2020 goals.[8]

Among adults, less than 50% of US adults meet current exercise recommendations (less than 15% in some studies); those of low SES have even lower levels of compliance.[9] African American women have the lowest exercise rates (only 34% exercise) of any race/sex demographic group.[10–12]

PHYSICAL DEVELOPMENT IN UNDERSERVED POPULATIONS
Normal Adolescent Physical Development, the Effects of Low Socioeconomic Status and the Role of Exercise

Adolescence, the developmental stage leading to physical, sexual, and psychosocial maturation, is mediated by hormonal, genetic, and environmental factors. Whether or not socioeconomic factors affect physical development and maturation is the topic of this section of inquiry.

The normal child to adolescent transition is mediated by neuroendocrine changes. Gonadotropin-releasing hormone (GnRH), essentially dormant since birth, is activated (by largely unknown triggers) leading to an increased secretion of gonadotrophs: follicle-stimulating hormone and luteinizing hormone from the pituitary. Increased secretion, in turn, promotes the production of androgens and estrogens from the ovaries and testes. Concomitantly, the same triggers that stimulate GnRH secretion also incite corticotrophin-releasing hormone secretion from the hypothalamus, which then stimulates the anterior pituitary to secrete adrenocorticotropic hormone, acting on the adrenal glands to increase the secretion of the *adrenal* androgens dehydroepiandrosterone and androstenedione. The elevated levels of estrogens and gonadal and adrenal androgens begin to initiate sexual development and simultaneously stimulate an increase in the release of growth hormone from the pituitary. Together these well-orchestrated changes lead to an increase in physical stature, the development of secondary sexual characteristics, and the ultimate transition into adulthood.[13–16]

The questions before us are as follows: (1) Are there any untoward effects if this normal developmental cascade is altered? (2) Can SES or AL affect this cascade and contribute to these untoward effects? (3) If so, can exercise favorably influence or mitigate such alterations? In answer to the first question, if normal development is altered, there *are* possible untoward effects. Early menarche has been associated with an increased risk of breast cancer,[17] heart disease,[18–20] asthma,[21,22] insulin resistance,[23] metabolic syndrome,[23] coping strategies,[24] and all-cause mortality.[25] No similar data regarding future health risks in boys could be found.

The second question, positing if SES can increase the likelihood of early menarche and its untoward effects, can be answered by reviewing epidemiologic data.

Generally, the age of the onset of puberty in the United States has been decreasing since the 1950s (menarche 12.9 years in 1948 and 12.4 years in 1994); although African American girls reach menarche 8 months earlier than Caucasian girls,[26] most studies attribute this to race *not* SES.[27] In fact, some studies specifically examining the role of SES on menarche found earlier menarche in girls of *high* SES.[28] Overall, however, although there is fear of low SES facilitating early menarche, as of 2015 the literature has not definitively documented this.[29] Except in cases of significant malnutrition, the authors found no studies unequivocally demonstrating any adverse effects of AL or low SES on age of menarche (with its increased burden of disease), the development of secondary sexual characteristics, or physical development in adolescence.[30]

In light of the answers to the first two questions, the answer to the third question seems moot. However, let us make a few points with respect to exercise, physical development, and disease prevention in this population. It is well established that adolescent and adult health issues occur disproportionately in underserved communities (eg, heart disease, diabetes, adolescent and adult obesity, asthma, cancers) and that AL is a known contributor to this burden of disease. It is also established that physical activity can decrease AL and ameliorate many of these adult health issues. Therefore, because those with lower SES have lower levels of physical activity,[31] and because childhood habits are proven to carry strongly forward into adulthood,[32–34] instilling a habit of exercise during adolescence is perhaps the primary care provider's best way of enhancing mental health and school performance in adolescents and fostering long-term economic success and health in adults who have carried forward a habit of activity from childhood.[35,36]

BRAIN DEVELOPMENT IN UNDERSERVED POPULATIONS

In order to look at brain development in underserved populations, normal brain development must be briefly reviewed first. The cognitive and structural deficits that occur in underserved or impoverished populations can then be discussed. Finally, it is then possible to examine the effects that exercise has on brain structure and function and to examine how these effects may ameliorate some of the deficits caused by stressful or underserved conditions.

Normal Adolescent Brain Development

As a child grows from adolescence to adulthood, the amount of gray matter (neurons) decreases as selective elimination of redundant pathways (pruning) takes place. Conversely, the amount of cortical white matter (myelin coated axons) increases as more and more cell-to-cell connections are formalized.[37] These connections continue to form through early adulthood and are important in learning, imagination, memory, and physical memory. Any arrest in white matter growth during this time could lead to potential interconnectivity deficits and impaired learning.

One specific area of importance when looking at white matter development is the prefrontal cortex. The white matter connections formed in this area (the seat of impulse control, decision making, delayed gratification, goal-directed behavior) are not complete until a person reaches their mid 20s.[38–40] In addition to this delayed white matter development, the adolescent brain has also been found to have a relative lack of mood modulating and behavioral control neurotransmitters (eg, serotonin) and an excess excitatory neurotransmitters (eg, glutamate, dopamine). It is important for parents, teachers, and policy makers to keep in mind that the end result of all this is that the normal adolescent brain is relatively more excitable and is lacking in impulse control and executive function. Any factors that further delay or impede maturation in these areas could be expected to compound these deficits and lead to further learning and behavioral problems and risky behaviors.[41]

THE EFFECT OF BEING UNDERSERVED ON ADOLESCENT BRAIN DEVELOPMENT

It has been shown that children in socioeconomically stressed conditions (eg, less than 150% of US federal poverty levels) have lower brain electrical activity, altered verbal centers,[42,43] up to 10% less gray matter, and smaller brain volumes in areas critical to learning, such as memory (eg, hippocampus), executive functioning, and impulse control (eg, frontal lobes).[44–48]

In addition, these children form fewer network connections between emotional and control centers (eg, the prefrontal cortex)[49] and have slower overall brain growth. These structural difference have been associated with lower test scores,[48,50] shorter attention spans,[51,52] lower reading comprehension, more disruptive behavior, rule breaking, aggression, and hyperactive behavior. Not only do these structural deficits affect the developing child but these disparities in brain structure have also been proven to persist into adulthood with resultant heightened threat response activity, lower responses to positive social stimuli, lower college enrollment and graduation rates,[53] lower wages and income, and more physical and psychological maladies.[54]

One interesting study examining the cognitive effects of socioeconomic stress followed more than 5000 adopted children and showed that those adopted into low-income homes scored 13 IQ points lower than their counterparts adopted into higher-income families,[55] effects postulated to be due to higher levels of stress, lack of parenteral interaction, limited mental stimulation, and poor nutrition.[56,57]

The Effects of Physical Activity and the Developing Brain

The question we face is as follows: Can exercise ameliorate any of the earlier noted stress-induced metabolic, structural, and behavioral changes?

The authors could find no prospective studies examining the effects of exercise on the *structure* of the "low socioeconomic brain," but several prospective studies looked at the effects of exercise on *academic and cognitive performance* in low-income adolescents. One study examining attention span and reading comprehension in low-income adolescents[52] found that aerobic exercise improved both attention span and reading comprehension to a greater degree in low-income students than their higher-income counterparts. The study recommended that "schools serving low-income adolescents should consider implementing brief sessions of aerobic exercise during the school day."[52]

Another study[58] examining fitness and cognitive performance in 83,000 children in the New York City Public School found that, although all children improved academic performance with increased fitness, the effect was most pronounced in impoverished youths, especially boys.

As mentioned earlier, although the authors could find no prospective studies evaluating exercise's effect on allostatic load or brain structure, relevant observations can be made from existing studies examining the differences between fit and unfit *nonimpoverished* children.

Structurally, regular physical activity has been shown to enhance neurogenesis via increased levels of brain-derived neurotropic factor[59,60] and serotonin.[61] This enhanced neurogenesis may account for the structural advantages seen in the brains of fit children. In other words, physically fit children have been shown to have larger hippocampal volumes (memory storage and association area)[62] and larger basal ganglia volumes (areas important in task completion).

Cognitively, again in nonimpoverished children, exercise has been shown to improve attention span[63] and mental processing speed.[64] It has been shown to enhance learning, especially with challenging subjects,[65] and to strengthen multi-tasking ability[66] resulting in higher test scores.[67–69] Fit children also have superior relational or associative memory (able to associate dissimilar bits of information), an area important in learning and imagination. In summary, physically fit children have an increased ability to focus, learn, process, and shut out distractions and conflicting impulses,[70,71] all qualities that would be especially desirable in impoverished populations.

THE IMPORTANCE OF EXERCISE IN UNDERSERVED POPULATIONS

Although, as mentioned earlier, the authors could find no prospective trials specifically evaluating the impact of exercise on AL in *underserved communities*, the literature does make a strong case for promoting exercise in these communities for disease prevention and neurologic, academic, and psychological development.

Various reviews note that our stress response has evolved as a means to enhance survival in the face of physical threat, readying ourselves for action (ie, fight or flight) that could save us. Today, however, when physical threat is less imminent and stress is more often caused by prolonged exposure to emotional or social factors, an action outlet is often unavailable to dissipate our pent-up hormonal readiness. It is thought that the energy meant to be mobilized for *fight or flight* is today, instead, stored in visceral fat. It is thought that the prolonged hormonal changes that occur during chronic stress can lead to central obesity, hypertension, dyslipidemia, metabolic syndrome, cardiovascular maladaptation, and neurologic changes resulting in cognitive and mood disturbances.[72] Physical inactivity likely fuels this fire, whereas exercise has been shown to mitigate the effects of such chronic stress and individual markers of AL.[73–76] It is, therefore, vital in our underserved communities, where chronic psychosocial stress is prevalent, that primary care providers educate patients about the heightened risks of inactivity and energetically promote AL-reducing exercise.

In summation, lack of exercise in underserved communities most certainly contributes to developmental delay, increased behavioral problems, and poor academic performance in our children. This finding is vitally important for policy makers to keep in mind because often PE classes are the first to be eliminated when school budgets come under scrutiny. Such curriculum shrinkage will disproportionately affect our underserved populations because 51% of US public school children come from low-income families (2013 data)[48] and because alternative recreation sites/access to safe playgrounds may be limited. It is the authors' opinion that the ameliorating effects of exercise are a critical unguent in our underserved communities and that thoughtful policy must focus on exercise promotion, the elimination of AL, and the abolition of poverty. This point is critical if a nation's children, and, thus, a nation, are to reach their full intellectual potential.

THE MAJOR HEALTH PROBLEMS IN UNDERSERVED *ADULT* POPULATIONS

Most of the significant health issues faced in underserved communities have been addressed in detail in other articles in this issue. The authors' intent here is not to rehash these issues but instead to briefly mention them, then to discuss the role that exercise might play in treatment and prevention. Hypertension, diabetes, asthma, hyperlipidemia, and depression are 5 of the most common medical problems disproportionately encountered in underserved communities.[77] In addition, as explained in Oluwadamilola O. Olaku and Emmanuel A. Taylor's article, "Cancer in the Medically Underserved Population," in this issue, colorectal and breast cancer are the two most common presenting cancers, with increased mortality in these communities.[78,79]

EXERCISE *AS TREATMENT* IN ADULT UNDERSERVED POPULATIONS

Although exercise has been documented to have beneficial effects in a multitude of medical conditions, including the 5 common maladies mentioned earlier,[80] the authors could find no studies documenting the benefits of exercise *selectively* in these conditions in medically underserved populations (MUPs). Therefore, the benefits of exercise discussed later are discussed in reference to normal or nonunderserved communities, which may or may not accurately project onto underserved populations.

Hypertension

Hypertension is the most common medical problem at underserved clinics[77]; studies have shown that aerobic exercise, strength training, and isometric exercise will all reduce blood pressure.[80] The decrease in pressure brought on by exercise (15 mm Hg systolic and 4 mm Hg diastolic) has been shown to persist for 4 to 10 hours and up to 22 hours after exercise.[81] This exercise-induced reduction is of eye-opening importance because a reduction in systolic blood pressure of only 2 mm Hg has been shown to reduce risk of cardiovascular mortality by 7%.[82] The potential impact of exercise is significant.

Diabetes Type II

Physical activity along with diet and medication are the mainstays for the treatment of type II diabetes.[83–85] Exercise results in increased insulin sensitivity and enhanced uptake of glucose by muscle.[80] It has been shown to reduce glycosylated hemoglobin (HbA1c) by 0.4% to 0.6%, a reduction comparable with metformin,[80] and to reduce fasting glucose. Combining aerobic and resistance training produces the greatest reduction of HbA1c.[86] Recent data also suggest that postprandial glucose (rather than fasting glucose or HbA1c) may better correlate with diabetes mortality. Unlike most medications, physical activity has been shown to significantly reduce this postprandial parameter as well.[87,88] Again, whether the effects of exercise seen here can be extrapolated equally to underserved communities is unknown.

Asthma

Physical training has been shown to improve asthmatic symptoms and asthmatic quality of life.[89] Asthmatic patients can enjoy 6 to 9 more symptom-free days per month with aerobic training than those who do not participate in aerobic training.[90–92] Exercise, of course, can trigger bronchoconstriction[93] in patients with exercise-induced asthma; but despite this, exercise has been proven to be safe and beneficial, even in high-intensity workouts if symptoms are controlled.[94] As discussed earlier, studies are needed to specifically address the effects of exercise on asthmatic patients in underserved communities.

Hyperlipidemia

Elevations of cholesterol and triglycerides are known risk factors for atherosclerosis and heart disease. Physical activity[95,96] has been shown to improve these lipid profiles[97,98] by selectively improving skeletal muscles utilization of lipids.[99] Both low-density lipoprotein and triglycerides are lowered with intense exercise,[100] whereas cardioprotective high-density lipoprotein (HDL) is increased with prolonged aerobic exercise (a minimum of 120 minutes weekly). Every HDL increase of 0.025 mmol/L decreases cardiovascular risk by 2% in men and 3% in women.[101,102] Although specific studies addressing physical activity's benefit in cardiovascular disease selectively in underserved communities are lacking, potential benefits are significant.

Depression

Common in underserved communities, one of the main symptoms of major depressive disorder is fatigue.[103] It has been theorized that inactivity can exacerbate this problem[80] and that, conversely, physical activity can help reduce these symptoms and enhance feelings of well-being.[104] There is evidence that aerobic exercise is as effective as pharmacotherapy in the short-term and that patients who exercise (with or without pharmacotherapy) have less depressive symptoms over the long-term as well.[105,106] These benefits of exercise are thought to be due to multiple factors, including hormonal changes,[107] distraction from sad thoughts,[80] and actually inducing neurologic structural changes (eg, increasing hippocampal volume: there is a noted decrease in hippocampal volume in depression).[108,109]

EXERCISE AS *DISEASE PREVENTION* IN ADULT UNDERSERVED POPULATIONS

Primary care physicians not only treat acute and chronic disease but also endeavor to screen and prevent such disease. The topic of screening inadequacies in underserved communities is beyond the scope of this article; however, they are well addressed in the literature.[77] For the authors' purposes in this article, it is important to recognize the preventative effects of exercise on 2 cancers that are commonly screened for: the two most common cancers presenting in underserved conditions.

Colorectal Cancer

In the United States, a higher incidence of colorectal cancer (CRC) is found in underserved communities. (In Europe such an association is not found.)[79,110–112] This finding is due both to inadequate screening and greater exposure to risk factors (see Oluwadamilola O. Olaku and Emmanuel A. Taylor's article, "Cancer in the Medically Underserved Population," in this issue). One of these risk factors, inactivity, is notably more prevalent in underserved communities and can clearly be addressed by exercise promotion. In the general population, physical activity has been demonstrated to prevent CRC in men and women,[113] with moderate or vigorous exercise shown to reduce colon cancer risk by 40%.[114] In addition, exercise *after* diagnosis has been shown to decrease total CRC-specific mortality (by 39%) in patients who increase in their physical activity to as little 5 hours of normal-pace walking per week.[115]

Breast Cancer

Although the incidence of breast cancer is greater in white women and women of high SES,[116] most studies have found that black women and those of lower SES have higher mortality.[117] This finding is likely linked to late stage of presentation, obesity, lower levels of physical activity, lower levels of education,[118,119] and differing treatment regimes.[120]

Physical activity offers a dose-dependent risk reduction in breast cancer.[121] The average risk reduction with moderate to vigorous physical activity is 25% to 30%, although the exact frequency and duration of exercise to achieve this benefit is unclear.[122] With higher cancer mortality among underserved women, one would assume that studies examining the effects of exercise on this mortality would have been done. However, once again, the authors could find no literature specifically addressing the effects of exercise on breast cancer incidence or mortality *specifically* on women of low SES.[121]

BARRIERS TO EXERCISE IN UNDERSERVED POPULATIONS

With all the known benefits of exercise, why do not more underserved patients exercise? The top reasons for not exercising in MUPs are as follows: not having access to exercise equipment, not having time to exercise, excessive cost, general health concerns (not healthy enough to exercise), lack of exercise companionship, feeling uncomfortable or embarrassed exercising, child care responsibilities, lack of motivation, concerns of safety in neighborhood, and low personal functioning.[72,123–125]

SUMMARY

In conclusion, primary care providers can make a strong argument for exercise promotion in underserved communities. The benefits are vitally important in adolescent physical, cognitive, and psychological development as well as in adult disease prevention and treatment. In counseling such patients, we should take into account a patient's readiness for change and the barriers to exercise as discussed earlier.

REFERENCES

1. Fact Sheet Physical Activity. Global recommendations on physical activity for health. Available at: http://www.euro.who.int/__data/assets/pdf_file/0005/288041/WHO-Fact-Sheet-PA-2015.pdf. Accessed February 29, 2016.
2. ACSM, AHA Support federal physical activity guidelines. Available at: https://www.acsm.org/about-acsm/media-room/acsm-in-the-news/2011/08/01/acsm-aha-support-federal-physical-activity-guidelines. Accessed February 29, 2016.
3. Whitt-Glover MC, Taylor WC, Floyd MF, et al. Disparities in physical activity and sedentary behaviors among US children and adolescents: prevalence, correlates, and intervention implications. J Public Health Policy 2009;30:S309–34.
4. Troiano RP, Berrigan D, Dodd KW, et al. Physical activity in the United States measured by accelerometer. Med Sci Sports Exerc 2008;40:181.
5. Gordon-Larsen P, McMurray RG, Popkin BM. Adolescent physical activity and inactivity vary by ethnicity: the National Longitudinal Study of Adolescent Health. J Pediatr 1999;135:301–6.
6. Gordon-Larsen P, McMurray RG, Popkin BM. Determinants of adolescent physical activity and inactivity patterns. Pediatrics 2000;105:e83.
7. Nader PR, Bradley RH, Houts RM, et al. Moderate-to-vigorous physical activity from ages 9 to 15 years. JAMA 2008;300(3):295–305.
8. Centers for Disease Control and Prevention. Healthy People 2020. Available at: http://www.cdc.gov/nchs/healthy_people/hp2020.htm. Accessed February 29, 2016.
9. Taylor WC, Baranowski T, Young DR. Physical activity interventions in low-income, ethnic minority, and populations with disability. Am J Prev Med 1998;15:334–43.
10. Schrop SL, Pendleton BF, McCord G, et al. The medically underserved: who is likely to exercise and why? J Health Care Poor Underserved 2006;17:276–89.
11. Parks SE, Housemann RA, Brownson RC. Differential correlates of physical activity in urban and rural adults of various socioeconomic backgrounds in the United States. J Epidemiol Community Health 2003;57:29–35.

12. Healthy People 2020. Physical activity. Available at: http://www.healthypeople. gov/2020/topics-objectives/topic/physical-activity. Accessed February 29, 2016.
13. Chulani VL, Gordon LP. Adolescent growth and development. Prim Care 2014; 41:465–87.
14. Colvin CW, Abdullatif H. Anatomy of female puberty: the clinical relevance of developmental changes in the reproductive system. Clin Anat 2013;26:115–29.
15. Tena-Sempere M. Ghrelin, the gonadal axis and the onset of puberty. Endocr Dev 2013;25:69–82.
16. Lee Y, Styne D. Influences on the onset and tempo of puberty in human beings and implications for adolescent psychological development. Horm Behav 2013; 64:250–61.
17. Kotsopoulos J, Lubinski J, Lynch HT. Age at menarche and the risk of breast cancer in BRCA1 and BRCA2 mutation carriers. Cancer Causes Control 2005; 16(6):667–74.
18. Ong KK, Ahmed ML, Dunger DB. Lessons from large population studies on timing and tempo of puberty (secular trends and relation to body size): the European trend. Mol Cell Endocrinol 2006;254-255:8–12.
19. Allison CM, Hyde JS. Early menarche: confluence of biological and contextual factors. Sex Roles 2013;68:55–64.
20. Canoy D, Beral V, Balkwill A, et al, Million Women Study Collaborators*. Age at menarche and risks of coronary heart and other vascular diseases in a large UK cohort. Circulation 2015;131(3):237–44.
21. Castro-Rodriguez JA. A new childhood asthma phenotype: obese with early menarche. Paediatr Respir Rev 2016;18:85–9.
22. Lieberoth S, Gade E. Early menarche is associated with increased risk of asthma: prospective population-based study of twins. Respir Med 2015;109:565–71.
23. Lim SW, Ahn JH, Lee JA, et al. Early menarche is associated with metabolic syndrome and insulin resistance in premenopausal Korean women. Eur J Pediatr 2016;175:97–104.
24. Alcalá-Herrera V, Marván ML. Early menarche, depressive symptoms, and coping strategies. J Adolesc 2014;37:905–13.
25. Tamakoshi K, Yatsuya H, Tamakoshi A, et al. Early age at menarche associated with increased all-cause mortality. Eur J Epidemiol 2011;26:771–8.
26. Ramnitz MS, Lodish MB. Racial disparities in pubertal development. Semin Reprod Med 2013;31:333–9.
27. Wu T, Mendola P, Buck GM. Ethnic differences in the presence of secondary sex characteristics and menarche among US girls: the Third National Health and Nutrition Examination Survey, 1988-1994. Pediatrics 2002;110:752–7.
28. Krzyżanowska M, Mascie-Taylor CG, Thalabard JC. Biosocial correlates of age at menarche in a British cohort. Ann Hum Biol 2015;31:1–6.
29. Krieger N, Kiang MV, Kosheleva A. Age at menarche: 50-year socioeconomic trends among US-born black and white women. Am J Public Health 2015; 105:388–97.
30. McIntyre MH. Adult stature, body proportions and age at menarche in the United States National Health and Nutrition Survey (NHANES) III. Ann Hum Biol 2011;38:716–20.
31. Sallis JF, Zakarian JM, Hovell MF, et al. Ethnic, socioeconomic, and sex differences in physical activity among adolescents. J Clin Epidemiol 1996;49:125–34.
32. Tripodi A, Severi S, Midili S, et al. "Community projects" in Modena (Italy): promote regular physical activity and healthy nutrition habits since childhood. Int J Pediatr Obes 2011;6(Suppl 2):54–6.

33. te Velde SJ, Twisk JW, Brug J. Tracking of fruit and vegetable consumption from adolescence into adulthood and its longitudinal association with overweight. Br J Nutr 2007;98:431–8.

34. Cleland V, Dwyer T, Venn A. Which domains of childhood physical activity predict physical activity in adulthood? A 20-year prospective tracking study. Br J Sports Med 2012;46:595–602.

35. Koivusilta LK, Nupponen H, Rimpelä AH. Adolescent physical activity predicts high education and socio-economic position in adulthood. Eur J Public Health 2012;22:203–9.

36. Aarnio M, Winter T, Kujala U, et al. Associations of health related behaviour, social relationships, and health status with persistent physical activity and inactivity: a study of Finnish adolescent twins. Br J Sports Med 2002;36:360–4.

37. Gogtay N, Giedd JN, Lusk L, et al. Dynamic mapping of human cortical development during childhood through early adulthood. Proc Natl Acad Sci U S A 2004;101:8174–9.

38. Casey BJ, Thomas KM, Welsh TF, et al. Dissociation of response conflict, attentional selection, and expectancy with functional magnetic resonance imaging. Proc Natl Acad Sci 2000;97:8728–33.

39. Casey BJ, Tottenham N, Fossella J. Clinical, imaging, lesion and genetic approaches toward a model of cognitive control. Dev Psychobiol 2002;40:237–54.

40. Casey BJ, Tottenham N, Liston C, et al. Imaging the developing brain: what have we learned about cognitive development? Trends Cogn Sci 2005;9:104–10.

41. Hare TA, Tottenham N, Galvan A, et al. Biological substrates of emotional reactivity and regulation in adolescence during an emotional go-nogo task. Biol Psychiatry 2008;63:927–34.

42. Hackman DA, Farah MJ, Meaney MJ. Socioeconomic status and the brain: mechanistic insights from human and animal research. Nat Rev Neurosci 2010;11:651–9.

43. Noble KG, Wolmetz ME, Ochs LG, et al. Brain-behavior relationships in reading acquisition are modulated by socioeconomic factors. Dev Sci 2006;9:642–54.

44. Kishiyama MM, Boyce WT, Jimenez AM, et al. Socioeconomic disparities affect prefrontal function in children. J Cogn Neurosci 2009;21:1106–15.

45. Noble KG, Engelhardt LE, Brito NH, et al. Socioeconomic disparities in neurocognitive development in the first two years of life. Dev Psychobiol 2015;57: 535–51.

46. Noble KG, Houston SM, Brito NH, et al. Family income, parental education and brain structure in children and adolescents. Nat Neurosci 2015;18:773–8.

47. Hanson JL, Hair N, Shen DG, et al. Family poverty affects the rate of human infant brain growth. PLoS One 2013;8:e80954.

48. Hair NL, Hanson JL, Wolfe BL, et al. Association of child poverty, brain development, and academic achievement. JAMA Pediatr 2015;169:822–9.

49. Javanbakht A, King AP, Evans GW, et al. Childhood poverty predicts adult amygdala and frontal activity and connectivity in response to emotional faces. Front Behav Neurosci 2015;9:154.

50. Haveman R, Wolfe B. The determinants of children's attainments: a review of methods and findings. J Econ Lit 1995;33:1829–78.

51. Mezzacappa E. Alerting, orienting, and executive attention: developmental properties and socio demographic correlates epidemiological sample of young, urban children. Child Dev 2004;75:1373–86.

52. Tine M. Acute aerobic exercise: an intervention for the selective visual attention and reading comprehension of low-income adolescents. Front Psychol 2014;5:575.

53. Institute of Education Sciences. National Center for Education Statistics. Assessment of educational progress. Nations Report Card. 2015. Available at: http://nces.ed.gov/nationsreportcard/. Accessed February 29, 2016.

54. Restuccia D, Urrutia C. Intergenerational persistence of earnings: the role of early and college education. Am Econ Rev 2004;94:1354–78.

55. Duyme M, Dumaret AC, Tomkiewicz S. How can we boost IQs of "dull children"? A late adoption study. Proc Natl Acad Sci U S A 1999;96:8790–4.

56. Luby JL, Barch DM, Belden A, et al. Maternal support in early childhood predicts larger hippocampal volumes at school age. Proc Natl Acad Sci U S A 2012;109:2854–9.

57. Luby JL, Belden A, Botteron K, et al. The effects of poverty on childhood brain development: the mediating effect of caregiving and stressful life events. JAMA Pediatr 2013;167:1135–42.

58. Bezold CP, Konty KJ, Day SE, et al. The effects of changes in physical fitness on academic performance among New York City youth. J Adolesc Health 2014;55: 774–81.

59. Cotman CW, Berchtold NC, Christie L. Exercise builds brain health: key roles of growth factor cascades and inflammation. Trends Neurosci 2007;30:464–72.

60. Phillips C, Baktir MA, Srivatsan M, et al. Neuroprotective effects of physical activity on the brain: a closer look at trophic factor signaling. Front Cell Neurosci 2014;20(8):170.

61. Klempin F, Beis D, Mosienko V, et al. Serotonin is required for exercise-induced adult hippocampal neurogenesis. J Neurosci 2013;33:8270–5.

62. Erickson KI, Prakash RS, Voss MW, et al. Aerobic fitness is associated with hippocampal volume in elderly humans. Hippocampus 2009;19:1030–9.

63. Hillman CH, Buck SM, Themanson JR, et al. Aerobic fitness and cognitive development: event-related brain potential and task performance indices of executive control in preadolescent children. Dev Psychol 2009;45:114–29.

64. Hillman CH, Castelli DM, Buck SM. Aerobic fitness and neurocognitive function in healthy preadolescent children. Med Sci Sports Exerc 2005;37:1967–74.

65. Raine LB, Lee HK, Saliba BJ, et al. The influence of childhood aerobic fitness on learning and memory. PLoS One 2013;8:e72666.

66. Chaddock L, Neider MB, Lutz A, et al. Role of childhood aerobic fitness in successful street crossing. Med Sci Sports Exerc 2012;44:749–53.

67. Castelli DM, Hillman CH, Buck SM, et al. Physical fitness and academic achievement in third-and fifth-grade students. J Sport Exerc Psychol 2007;29: 239–52.

68. Donnelly JE, Greene JL, Gibson CA, et al. Physical Activity Across the Curriculum (PAAC): a randomized controlled trial to promote physical activity and diminish overweight and obesity in elementary school children. Prev Med 2009;49:336–41.

69. Etnier JL, Nowell PM, Landers DM, et al. A meta-regression to examine the relationship between aerobic fitness and cognitive performance. Brain Res Rev 2006;52:119–30.

70. Chaddock L, Erickson KI, Prakash RS, et al. Basal ganglia volume is associated with aerobic fitness in preadolescent children. Dev Neurosci 2010;32:249–56.

71. Chaddock L, Erickson KI, Prakash RS, et al. A functional MRI investigation of the association between childhood aerobic fitness and neurocognitive control. Biol Psychol 2012;89:260–8.

72. Tsasoulis A, Fountoulakis S. The protective role of exercise on stress system dysregulation and comorbidities. Ann N Y Acad Sci 2006;1083:196–213.

73. Salmon P. Effects of physical exercise on anxiety, depression, and sensitivity to stress: a unifying theory. Clin Psychol Rev 2001;21:33–61.
74. Crews DJ, Landers DM. A meta-analytic review of aerobic fitness and reactively to psychosocial stressors. Med Sci Sports Exerc 1987;19:S114–20.
75. Traustadóttir T, Bosch PR, Matt KS. The HPA axis response to stress in women: effects of aging and fitness. Psychoneuroendocrinology 2005;30:399–402.
76. Blumenthal JA, Fredrickson M, Kuhn CM, et al. Aerobic exercise reduces levels of cardiovascular and sympathoadrenal response to mental stress in subjects without prior evidence of myocardial ischemia. Am J Cardiol 1990;65:93–8.
77. HRSA Health Center Program. National data. Available at: http://bphc.hrsa.gov/uds/datacenter.aspx?q=tall&year=2014&state. Accessed March 1, 2016.
78. Siegel R, Naishadham D, Jemal A. Cancer statistics, 2012. CA Cancer J Clin 2012;62:10–29.
79. Doubeni CA, Laiyemo AO, Major JM, et al. Socioeconomic status and the risk of colorectal cancer: an analysis of more than a half million adults in the National Institutes of Health-AARP Diet and Health Study. Cancer 2012;118:3636–44.
80. Pedersen BK, Saltin B. Exercise as medicine—evidence for prescribing exercise as therapy in 26 different chronic diseases. Scand J Med Sci Sports 2015;25:1–72.
81. Pescatello LS, Franklin BA, Fagard R, et al. American College of Sports Medicine position stand. Exercise and hypertension. Med Sci Sports Exerc 2004; 36:533–53.
82. Lewington S, Clarke R, Qizilbash N, et al. Age-specific relevance of usual blood pressure to vascular mortality: a meta-analysis of individual data for one million adults in 61 prospective studies. Lancet 2002;360:1903–13.
83. Joslin EP, Root EF, White P. The treatment of diabetes mellitus. Philadelphia: Lea & Febiger; 1959.
84. Albright A, Franz M, Hornsby G, et al. American College of Sports Medicine position stand. Exercise and type 2 diabetes. Med Sci Sports Exerc 2000;32: 1345–60.
85. American Diabetes Association. Clinical practice recommendations. Diabetes Care 2013;36(Suppl 1):S3.
86. Church TS, Blair SN, Cocreham S, et al. Effects of aerobic and resistance training on hemoglobin A1c levels in patients with type 2 diabetes: a randomized controlled trial. JAMA 2010;304:2253.
87. MacLeod SF, Terada T, Chahal BS, et al. Exercise lowers postprandial glucose but not fasting glucose in type 2 diabetes: a meta-analysis of studies using continuous glucose monitoring. Diabetes Metab Res Rev 2013;29:593–603.
88. Kearney ML, Thyfault JP. Exercise and postprandial glycemic control in type 2 diabetes. Curr Diabetes Rev 2016;12(3):199–210.
89. Carson KV, Chandratilleke MG, Picot J, et al. Physical training for asthma. Cochrane Database Syst Rev 2013;(9):CD001116.
90. Mendes FA, Gonçalves RC, Nunes MP, et al. Effects of aerobic training on psychosocial morbidity and symptoms in patients with asthma: a randomized clinical trial. Chest 2010;138:331–7.
91. Mendes FA, Almeida FM, Cukier A, et al. Effects of aerobic training on airway inflammation in asthmatic patients. Med Sci Sports Exerc 2011;43:197–203.
92. Gonçalves RC, Nunes MPT, Cukier A, et al. Efeito de um programa de condicionamento físico aeróbio nos aspectos psicossociais, na qualidade de vida, nos sintomas e no óxido nítrico exalado de portadores de asma persistente moderada ou grave. [Effects of an aerobic physical training program on psychosocial

characteristics, quality of life, symptoms and exhaled nitric oxide in individuals with moderate or severe persistent asthma]. Rev Bras Fisioter 2008;12:127–35 [in Portuguese].

93. Carlsen KH, Carlsen KC. Exercise induced asthma. Paediatr Respir Rev 2002;3: 154.

94. Emtner M, Herala M, Stalenheim G. High-intensity physical training in adults with asthma. A 10-week rehabilitation program. Chest 1996;109:323–30.

95. Thelle DS, Foorde OH, Try K, et al. The Tromsøo heart study. Methods and main results of the cross-sectional study. Acta Med Scand 1976;200:107–18.

96. Forde OH, Thelle DS, Arnesen E, et al. Distribution of high density lipoprotein cholesterol according to relative body weight, cigarette smoking and leisure time physical activity. The Cardiovascular Disease Study in Finnmark 1977. Acta Med Scand 1986;219:167–71.

97. Prong NP. Short term effects of exercise on plasma lipids and lipoproteins in humans. Sports Med 1993;16:431–48.

98. National Institutes of Health Consensus Development Panel. Triglyceride, DLD, and CHD. JAMA 1993;269:505–20.

99. Earnest CP, Artero EG, Sui X, et al. Maximal estimated cardio-respiratory fitness, cardiometabolic risk factors, and metabolic syndrome in the Aerobics Center Longitudinal Study. Mayo Clin Proc 2013;88:259–70.

100. Mann S, Beedie C, Jimenez A. Differential effects of aerobic exercise, resistance training and combined exercise modalities on cholesterol and the lipid profile: review, synthesis and recommendations. Sports Med 2014;44:211–21.

101. Pasternak RC, Grundy SM, Levy D, et al. Spectrum of risk factors for CHD. J Am Coll Cardiol 1990;27:964–1047.

102. Nicklas BJ, Katzel LI, Busby-Whitehead J, et al. Increases in high-density lipoprotein cholesterol with endurance exercise training are blunted in obese compared with lean men. Metabolism 1997;46:556–61.

103. American Psychiatric Association. Diagnostic and statistical manual of mental disorders. 5th edition. Washington, DC: American Psychiatric Association; 2013.

104. Cooney GM, Dwan K, Greig CA, et al. Exercise for depression. Cochrane Database Syst Rev 2013;(9):CD004366.

105. Blumenthal JA, Babyak MA, Moore KA, et al. Effects of exercise training on older patients with major depression. Arch Intern Med 1999;159:2349–56.

106. Babyak M, Blumenthal JA, Herman S, et al. Exercise treatment for major depression: maintenance of therapeutic benefit at 10 months. Psychosom Med 2000; 62:633–8.

107. Mynors-Wallis LM, Gath DH, Day A, et al. Randomised controlled trial of problem solving treatment, antidepressant medication, and combined treatment for major depression in primary care. BMJ 2000;320:26–30.

108. Pajonk FG, Wobrock T, Gruber O, et al. Hippocampal plasticity in response to exercise in schizophrenia. Arch Gen Psychiatry 2010;67:133–43.

109. Manji HK, Moore GJ, Chen G. Clinical and preclinical evidence for the neurotrophic effects of mood stabilizers: implications for the pathophysiology and treatment of manic-depressive illness. Biol Psychiatry 2000;48:740–54.

110. Aarts MJ, Lemmens VE, Louwman MW, et al. Socioeconomic status and changing inequalities in colorectal cancer? A review of the associations with risk, treatment and outcome. Eur J Cancer 2010;46:2681–95.

111. Leufkens AM, Van Duijnhoven FJ, Boshuizen HC, et al. Educational level and risk of colorectal cancer in EPIC with specific reference to tumor location. Int J Cancer 2012;130:622–30.

112. Brooke HL, Talbäck M, Martling A. Socioeconomic position and incidence of colorectal cancer in the Swedish population. Cancer Epidemiol 2016;40:188–95.

113. Samad AK, Taylor RS, Marshall T, et al. A meta-analysis of the association of physical activity with reduced risk of colorectal cancer. Colorectal Dis 2005;7: 204–13.

114. Thune I, Furberg AS. Physical activity and cancer risk: dose-response and cancer, all sites and site-specific. Med Sci Sports Exerc 2001;33(6 Suppl):S530–50.

115. Van Blarigan EL, Meyerhardt JA. Role of physical activity and diet after colorectal cancer diagnosis. J Clin Oncol 2015;33:1825–34.

116. Goldberg M, Calderon-Margalit R. Socioeconomic disparities in breast cancer incidence and survival among parous women: findings from a population-based cohort, 1964-2008. BMC Cancer 2015;15:921.

117. Thomson CS, Hole DJ, Twelves CJ, et al. Prognostic factors in women with breast cancer: distribution by socioeconomic status and effect on differences in survival. J Epidemiol Community Health 2001;55:308–15.

118. Centers for Disease Control and Prevention. Vital signs: racial disparities in breast cancer severity—United States, 2005-2009. MMWR Morb Mortal Wkly Rep 2012;61:922.

119. Parise CA, Caggiano V. Disparities in race/ethnicity and socioeconomic status: risk of mortality of breast cancer patients in the California Cancer Registry, 2000–2010. BMC Cancer 2013;13:449.

120. Bradley CJ, Given CW, Roberts C. Race, socioeconomic status and breast cancer treatment and survival. J Natl Cancer Inst 2002;94:490.

121. Brown JC, Winters-Stone K, Lee A, et al. Cancer, physical activity, and exercise. Compr Physiol 2012;2:2775–809.

122. Friedenreich CM, Cust AE. Physical activity and breast cancer risk: impact of timing, type and dose of activity and population sub-group effects. Br J Sports Med 2008;42:636–47.

123. Brownson RC, Baker EA, Housemann RA, et al. Environmental and policy determinants of physical activity in the United States. Am J Public Health 2001;91: 1995–2003.

124. Burton NW, Turrell G, Oldenburg B. Participation in recreational physical activity; why do socioeconomic groups differ? Health Educ Behav 2003;30:225–44.

125. Seefeldt V, Malina RM, Clark MA. Factors affecting levels of physical activity in adults. Sports Med 2002;32:143–68.

Environmental Justice and Underserved Communities

Vincent Morelli, MD[a],*, Carol Ziegler, DNP, APRN, NP-C, RD[b], Omotayo Fawibe, MD[c]

KEYWORDS

- Environmental justice • Toxins • Air pollution • Ingested pollutants

KEY POINTS

- Environmental justice has wide social, economic, and educational implications.
- Air pollution has the highest environmental risk with dangers from gases, organic compounds, and toxic materials.
- Carbon monoxide, nitric oxide, or nitrogen dioxide, sulfur dioxide, and ozone pose higher dangers for the poor.
- Exposure to metals in air pollution (eg, mercury, lead, cadmium, and manganese) can cause cognitive disorders, nervous system diseases, cancers, and mental illness.
- There is currently some controversy about the possible carcinogenic dangers of ingesting pollutants from water, soil, and food (eg, bisphenol A, arsenic).

ENVIRONMENTAL JUSTICE

The idea of environmental justice (EJ) arose in the 1980s, bringing to light the concept that the burdens of environmental exposure should be fairly distributed without undue costs being placed on those with low socioeconomic status (SES). The concept was formally written into US policy by executive order in 1994, with policy creation, implementation, and enforcement tasked to the Interagency Working Group on Environmental Justice under the US Department of Agriculture.

When EJ issues are studied, the location of waste disposal sites, manufacturing facilities, energy plants, highways, airports, and toxic waste sites, are mapped against SES or minority groupings. Most North American, Asian, and African studies have documented higher concentrations of pollutants in underserved or low SES communities.[1] Such disparities have important health implications. For example, the

Disclosure Statement: The authors of this work report no direct financial interest in the subject matter or any material discussed in this article.

[a] Sports Medicine Fellowship, Department of Family and Community Medicine, Meharry Medical College, 1005 Dr D. B. Todd Boulevard, Nashville, TN 37208, USA; [b] Vanderbilt University School of Nursing, 461 21st Avenue, South, Nashville, TN 37240, USA; [c] Department of Family and Community Medicine, Meharry Medical College, Nashville, TN 37208, USA
* Corresponding author.
E-mail address: vmorelli@mmc.edu

prevalence of asthma in some underserved communities in the United States is twice that of the national average (9% of US children have asthma vs 22% in some underserved communities).[2]

EJ issues also have wider social implications due to the interrelatedness of crime, education, poverty, and pollution. For example, a recent air toxin per youth crime mapping study found an association between airborne manganese, mercury, and particulate matter (PM) with higher rates of youth involvement with the juvenile justice system.[3] Although the study methodology could not definitively link exposure to EJ concerns, the implications demand further study. Other studies have noted that mononitrogen oxide (NO_x), ozone, heavy metals, and other pollutants are associated with neurologic deficits, behavioral problems, aggressive behavior, slowed learning, and other cognitive deficits, all important from health, human potential, and social policy perspectives.

ENVIRONMENTAL TOXINS

The Centers for Disease Control and Prevention (CDC) Fourth National Report on Human Exposure to Environmental Chemicals (2009, updated in 2015) includes data on 265 toxins. Exposures may be the result of inhalation (eg, motor vehicle emission, industrial air pollution), ingestion (eg, from tainted foods, ground water), or percutaneous absorption. Compounds, such as pesticides, heavy metals, phenols, fungicides, herbicides, parabens, phthalates, polyaromatic hydrocarbons, volatile organic compounds (VOCs), and tobacco smoke, are included in the analysis. For each chemical in the report, the CDC provides mean blood and urine levels, as well as the 75th, 90th, and 95th percentile levels, so that individuals or groups can be compared with population standards. The best method of detection (blood or urine) for each of the chemicals is also noted and 93 of the compounds have more in-depth biomonitoring data.[4]

The report, however, does not establish what levels may be harmful to an individual's health. These must be obtained from other sources. For example, the CDC provides population comparison levels for arsenic; the Environmental Protection Agency (EPA) monitors and sets the safe levels for air, drinking water, and soil; the Food and Drug Administration (FDA) sets safe food and bottled water levels; and the Occupational Safety and Health Administration (OSHA) is tasked with formulating and monitoring harmful workplace levels. (The EPA, FDA, and OSHA are also tasked with enforcement, so that companies found in violation of guidelines may be fined as set out in their respective policies.)

There are many mechanisms by which toxins may cause injury. Exposures may induce an inhalant allergic response, direct toxic effects on cellular mechanics (eg, lead, arsenic, mercury), endocrine disrupting effects (bisphenol A [BPA], phthalates),[5] direct DNA damage, or may create epigenetic changes (see later discussion). In most cases, free radical formation, oxidative stress, and inflammation[6] are thought to contribute to the injury. Other factors, such as whether the particles are solid, liquid, or gas; electrostatic charge; particle size; site of deposition; and lung response must also be taken into consideration.[7]

The concept of epigenetic change is a relatively recent construct that primary care providers (PCPs) working with underserved populations would do well to keep in mind. This is a growing area of research in which changes in gene expression without alterations in DNA sequence have been shown to contribute to untoward health effects.[8] Briefly, the concept is that environmental, social, physical, nutritional, or chemical stressors can lead to modifications (eg, methylation, acetylation) of the proteins surrounding DNA.[9,10] These modifications can lead to changes in gene expression, which can then be passed on to future generations. Environmentally induced epigenetic mechanisms have been proposed for diabetes and obesity,[11] asthma and food allergies,[12,13] autoimmune disease,[14] psychiatric diseases,[15] cardiovascular disease,[16] cancer,[17,18] and others.

In light of the vast number of potentially noxious compounds, the various mechanisms of injury and the complexities involved in monitoring, a detailed discussion of individual toxins is beyond the scope of this article. However, it will serve the PCP working in underserved communities, in which EJ issues are of concern, to have a general understanding of environmental toxins and their health effects. Armed with an appropriate perspective and a heightened index of suspicion, the PCP should then be able to locate helpful resources, to undertake proper methods of screening and detection, and to educate patients in methods of avoidance or amelioration. This article is meant to help guide the PCP in this pursuit.

AIR POLLUTION

In 2013, 87% of the world's population lived in areas that exceeded World Health Organization (WHO) Air Quality Guidelines. WHO data published in 2014 estimate that 7 million deaths per year are attributable to air pollution, making air pollution the world's largest single environmental health risk.[19] As previously stated, many studies have shown that this burden is borne disproportionately by underserved populations, with both outdoor and indoor air pollution contributing to the disparity.[20]

The chemical makeup of air pollution consists of:

1. Gases (carbon monoxide [CO], sulfur oxides, nitrogen oxides, ground-level or bad ozone, and VOCs)
2. Organic compounds (polycyclic aromatic hydrocarbons, VOCs)
3. Toxic metals (chromium, copper, manganese, lead, vanadium, antimony).

It is a complex, cross-reacting, ever-changing mixture, depending on weather patterns and industrial release. Ninety-eight percent of the urban air pollution consists of gases or vapor-phase compounds: CO, nitrogen dioxide (NO_2), nitric oxide (NO), ozone, sulfur dioxide (SO_2), or volatile hydrocarbons. Each of these components can act independently to produce adverse health effects, or they can chemically interact to form combined or secondary pollutants. The effects of these combined pollutants are less studied (with the exception of ozone) and largely unknown.

Besides grouping air pollution by chemical makeup, pollutants can also be grouped according to particle size. This is relevant because only small particles (<10 microns) are able to enter the lower airways and cause the most significant damage. Particles with a diameter of 2.5 to 10 μm (PM10) are called coarse particles. Those less than 2.5 μm (PM2.5), the most harmful category, are designated as fine particles. Those less than 1 μm are called ultrafine or nanoparticles.

This article briefly reviews the categories of gases, organic compounds, metals, and PM, so that the PCP may have a fundamental knowledge of terminology, properties, health effects, and approach to monitoring and mitigation.

THE GASES

Ninety-eight percent of urban air pollution consists of gases (CO, NO_2, NO, ozone, SO_2), which vary depending on regional differences in traffic, industry, wind, weather patterns, and so forth. It is a ubiquitous, itinerant, ever-changing, noxious ether, which bleeds across borders and cycles into the earth's very respirations.

Carbon Monoxide

CO, colloquially known as the silent killer, arises from the incomplete combustion of gas, coal or wood, traffic exhaust, furnaces, heaters, and wood or propane stoves. CO is a colorless, odorless gas that binds tightly to hemoglobin, creating carboxyhemoglobin, essentially displacing oxygen and rendering an affected person hypoxic. Because symptoms can be nonspecific (headache, nausea, vomiting, dizziness, depression, memory loss, irritability, fatigue, subjective weakness) and because carboxyhemoglobin's bright red hue may mask tissue hypoxia (making patients appear a healthy pink while being hypoxic at the cellular level), PCPs must maintain a high level of suspicion in effected areas.

Normal carboxyhemoglobin to hemoglobin ratio is less than 5%, while smokers or auto mechanics may have up to 9%. Symptoms usually occur in the 10% to 30% range.[21]

In addition to its direct toxic effects, CO is also a short-lived greenhouse gas. It has an additional indirect greenhouse effect by slowing the breakdown of methane and ozone, both more potent greenhouse gases. Greenhouse gases contribute to increased ozone formation (see later discussion) and all of the climate change effects noted in this article.

Mononitrogen Oxides, Nitric Oxide, and Nitrogen Dioxide

Any combustion in the presence of nitrogen found in coal or oil in power plants, vehicular exhaust (especially biodiesel), or natural sources will create NOx. NOx adds the brownish hue to urban smog and can contribute to acid rain formation (see later discussion).

NOx can react to form nitric acid, which can penetrate lung tissue and cause cardiorespiratory effects, including bronchitis, chronic obstructive pulmonary disease (COPD), and heart disease. It can also react with sunlight to create ozone, which further contributes to cardiorespiratory disease and neurotoxic effects, including impaired executive function and lower learning abilities (see later discussion). The implications of these neurotoxic effects are particularity worrisome in underserved communities where EJ concerns have been documented.[1,22]

Ozone

Good ozone in the upper atmosphere (stratosphere) is protective because it serves to absorb harmful UVB light, which, if unchecked, can cause significant human skin problems and can damage plant and animal DNA. Depletion of this ozone layer is concerning.

Bad ozone in the lower atmosphere (troposphere) is formed when sunlight reacts with partially combusted fossil fuels (NOx and organic compounds) from autos or industrial plants. This ozone has been proven to interfere with plant photosynthesis, stunt plant growth, and decrease crop yields.[23] In humans, it has been linked to increased inflammation, oxidative stress, asthma, bronchitis, overall respiratory morbidity and mortality, heart attacks and cardiovascular mortality,[24,25] and possibly diabetes.[26] The EPA has stated that both short-term and long-term ozone exposure can "harm the respiratory system causing significant symptoms and imposing significant costs on American families." It goes on to say that there is "likely a causal relationship"[27] between ozone and cardiovascular disease.

Finally, and especially important in underserved communities with higher pollution levels, ozone has been linked to neurotoxic effects, including decreased attention and short-term memory.[28]

Allowable air pollution levels of 70 parts per billion (ppb) have been set by the EPA and recent studies[29,30] have validated that these levels are safe, documenting no harmful cardiopulmonary effects from either short or prolonged ozone exposure at levels near or below EPA standards.

It should be noted that besides ozone's direct health effects on plants and animals, bad or low-level ozone is also a harmful greenhouse gas, trapping heat radiating from the earth and contributing to climate change. An increase in ozone would then result in a disastrous cycle, with increased ozone as a greenhouse gas contributing to global warming. Global warming leads to warmer, stagnant air, which, in turn, creates conditions for the formation of more ozone, further contributing to global warming. It is projected that if pollution remains at its current levels, climate change could nearly double the number of unhealthy AQI (air quality index) days (days when ozone levels are hazardous for everyone) by 2050.[31]

Currently, ozone mapping is the only reasonable way to track ozone because there are no clinically useful biomarkers for individual patient ozone detection.[32] In its 2015 updated ozone regulations, the EPA increased ground monitoring in 33 at-risk states.

Because ozone is largely formed by the conversion of traffic toxins by sunlight, it makes sense that ozone should peak in the late morning to early afternoon, after sunlight has had a chance to play its generative role on the fresh inflow of morning vehicle exhaust.[33]

PCPs caring for underserved patients in high ozone areas should advise them to stay indoors during these times and on high pollution days. They may also advise patients to use indoor air filters if possible, limit physical exertion near roads or industrial sources, and to mitigate parenteral and psychosocial stressors (see later discussion).[34]

Sulfur Dioxide

Sources for SO2 include coal burning power plants, other industries, and volcanoes. It is also used as a preservative in wine, dried fruit, and other foods. SO2 exposure can result in respiratory symptoms and asthma exacerbations.[2,35] Exposure has also been linked to preterm birth, which this is especially important in underserved communities where higher rates of exposure and health care access disparities exist. No neurologic or cardiovascular effects have been documented with SO2. SO2 can also react to form sulfuric acid, which contributes to the formation of acid rain, with its well-known detrimental effects on biodiversity, plant, and animal species. The EPA 1-hour exposure limit is 75 ppb.

Organic Compounds in Air Pollution

These compounds arise from vehicle and industrial fuels, soil erosion, or secondary formation (eg, benzene, toluene, xylene, VOCs). VOCs can cause direct harmful effects (suspected carcinogens linked to leukemia) or can be oxidized to join the ranks of particulate air pollution (see later discussion). They can also contribute to the formation of ozone-causing effects as previously noted. VOCs are grouped as either methane or nonmethane VOCs (NMVOCs). Methane is a greenhouse gas contributing to global warming, whereas NMVOCs, as alluded to, may be a direct carcinogen.

METALS IN AIR POLLUTION

Metals, such as chromium, zinc, copper, nickel, manganese, lead, vanadium, antimony, and barium, are known toxins and are monitored by the EPA. Fifty metals have been identified in coal, 35 in crude oil, and 18 in gasoline.[36,37] Because of combustion, these metals enter the atmosphere, usually as constituents of PM (see later discussion).

Although a complete review of air-metal pollutants is beyond the scope of this article, a few of the more common offenders are discussed so that PCPs working in underserved and overburdened communities may get a general idea and become more aware of potential health impacts.

Mercury

Most harmful mercury exposure in the United States comes from methyl mercury after consumption of fish. However, other inorganic sources of mercury are important in underserved communities and include noncompliant coal burning power plants and other industrial sources.

Prenatal exposure to mercury has been associated with lower IQ, delayed cognitive development, and decreased memory, attention, language, and spatial cognition.[38–40] It has been associated with spontaneous abortions, stillbirths, and congenital malformations (eg, cerebral palsy and mental retardation),[39,41] as well as leukemia.[42] Mercury can cause clinical symptoms, including loss of appetite, weight loss, sleeping disorders, personality changes, memory deficits, depression, headache, tremor, and dermatitis. It has also been linked to antisocial behavior and youth involvement with the juvenile justice system.[3] In the United States, it is estimated that industrial mercury emissions could contribute to lower IQ in 300,000 to 600,000 children,[43] and that the cost of lost productivity and lower intelligence caused by mercury is $8.7 billion annually.[44] All of this is especially important in underserved communities with potentially higher exposure and potentially decreased awareness, monitoring, and access to health care.

Lead

Lead exposure may come from house paint used before 1978 when lead-based paint was banned, plumbing installed before 1987 when lead pipe soldering was banned, soil contaminated with lead from urban sources (eg, leaded gasoline, decaying lead-based paint), and industrial facilities making lead-based products.

Lead toxicity is a well-known entity. Toxic levels can cause cardiovascular, renal, skeletal, and neurologic complications. Nonspecific symptoms, such as nausea, vomiting, abdominal pain, irritability, lethargy, headache, and difficulty concentrating and learning, usually develop early and slowly progress as lead builds up in the body. Lead's effects are especially toxic to the developing nervous system and can cause permanent learning deficits and behavior problems in children. It is known to reduce the prefrontal cortical gray matter area, an area involved in impulse control and executive function, and as such has been strongly associated with aggressive and antisocial behavior, delinquency, and violent crimes.[45,46] Again, all of this is of great interest in underserved communities where both lead toxicity and behavioral problems are more likely to exist.

A toxic level for children, as set by the CDC, is above 5 μg/dL of blood. However no safe level of lead has been established.

Cadmium

Exposure to cadmium comes from cigarette smoke, fossil fuel combustion, mining, manufacturing of nickel-cadmium batteries, pigments, and the creation of plastic stabilizers. Cadmium exposure has been associated COPD; renal failure; osteopenia; and prostate, lung, and testicular cancer.[47] Again, this is important in underserved communities where both combustion byproducts and second-hand smoke (SHS) are more prevalent.

Manganese

Toxic manganese exposure is usually related to steel or aluminum production plants and, although it is among the least toxic elements, high manganese exposure can lead to neurologic effects by altering serotonin and dopamine levels, leading to depression, mood swings, compulsive behaviors, psychosis, and Parkinson-like symptoms. It has also been documented to have neurobehavioral effects, including anxiety, aggression, impulsivity, emotional instability, poor planning, and fatigue.[3]

AIR POLLUTION GROUPING BY PARTICLE SIZE

Common sources of PM10 are ground dust, tire wear emissions, soot from wood combustion, construction works, and mining operations. PM2.5, the most injurious category of PM and thus the most studied, commonly originates from diesel exhaust (contributing to more than 40 toxic pollutants), car exhaust, oil refineries, metal processing facilities, power plants (especially coal burning plants in China, India, and unfiltered plants in the United States), ground dust (eg, sands arising from the Arabian and Saharan deserts), and wild fires. Ultrafine particles may originate from automobile exhaust, jet exhaust, printer toner, photocopiers, and natural sources.[48]

Particulate Matter 2.5

Particles are perhaps the most studied air pollutants and are particularly pathogenic because they are able to evade the body's defenses and penetrate deep into the lungs where, in the case of smaller particles, they may enter the bloodstream. The American Heart Association estimates that in the United States, PM2.5 air pollution contributes to 60,000 deaths per year in the United States with global estimates at 3.3 million premature deaths per year.[49]

Although PM2.5 levels have decreased in most developed countries, industrial practices in Southeast Asia and China have contributed to the recent 20% global increase.[50] The makeup of PM2.5 varies depending on local conditions. In Mexico City in 2006, for example, 55% of PM2.5 was made up of from fossil fuel carbons, 16% from mineral dust, 10% from sulfates, 7% from nitrates, 3% from ammonium, and 9% from various other sources. Bundled into these various other sources are the heavy metals produced by traffic and industrial sources as previously discussed.

PM2.5 has been associated with increased morbidity and mortality from cardiovascular disease (eg, hypertension, coronary artery disease, atherosclerosis and carotid artery intimal thickening, congestive heart failure, myocardial infarction),[51–53] pulmonary disease (eg, asthma, bronchitis,[54] respiratory infections including tuberculosis,[55] pulmonary embolism,[56] and lung cancer).[57,58] It has also been shown to decrease lung function (eg, forced vital capacity, forced expiratory volume in 1 second, respiratory flow rate).[59]

Of special note is that the harmful cardiovascular and pulmonary effects are seen even at low levels of long-term PM2.5 exposure (ie, 5–35 µg/m3). As a reference, the US EPA standard is 12 µg/m3 annual average, whereas Beijing's average from 2010 to 2012 was 100 µg/m3.[60] It is estimated that a 10 µg/m3 increase in average 24-hour PM2.5 exposure increases the relative risk for cardiovascular mortality up to 1.0% and will contribute to 1 premature death per day in a region of 5 million people, potentially leading to the early mortality of tens of thousands of individuals per year in the United States alone.[61,62]

In addition to cardiopulmonary disease, long-term exposure to air pollution has also been linked to neurologic and cognitive function deficits. Pollutants can enter the central nervous system (CNS) via the lung-circulation-CNS pathway or can directly access the CNS through the olfactory mucosa. In either case, the pollutants cause either direct toxicity or may induce damage by activating inflammatory cascades and eliciting free radical formation. These changes will eventually lead to impaired neurogenesis, clinical manifestations, and cognitive-behavioral changes (see later discussion).[63–65]

In utero, PM2.5 exposure in specific windows may have different neurologic sequela. PM2.5 exposure at 31 to 38 weeks has been associated with lower IQ, at 32 to 36 weeks with slower reaction times, at 20 to 26 weeks with decreased attention, and at 12 to 20 weeks with decreased general memory in girls.[66] Overall, PM2.5 exposure in utero has been linked to poorer memory, attention, executive function,[66] psychomotor development,[67] learning, and IQ.[68] It has also been associated with increased autism[69,70] and attention deficit hyperactivity disorder (ADHD). The long-lasting learning impairment, self-esteem issues, and behavioral problems of these latter 2 maladies can be devastating to the individual and costly to society.[71] As could be expected, PM2.5 and PM10 exposure has been associated with increased criminality.[3] All of this is especially evident and worrisome in underserved children living less than 500 m from a freeway or major road.[54]

In adults, the strongest neurologic links to air pollution have been noted with stroke, Parkinson disease, and multiple sclerosis. It has also been linked to Alzheimer disease in genetically susceptible individuals. Cognitively, PM2.5 particles have been associated with poor verbal learning, spatial learning, and memory.[72]

Peak carbon and PM2.5 concentrations occur in the mornings with rush hour traffic.[73] Therefore, PCPs should caution patients to avoid strenuous exercise during these times. For interested PCPs, global satellite maps of PM2.5 have been created and are available online.[74] It should be remembered that when considering the effects of air pollutants, both indoor (SHS or indoor fires for cooking) and outdoor air quality must be considered.

A note on second-hand cigarette smoke particulate matter 2.5

Although the composition of cigarette PM2.5 differs from that of air pollution PM2.5, it has been noted to have similar harmful effects.[60] To underscore the highly toxic effect of SHS, it is noted that living for a year in a polluted city such as Beijing, with an average PM2.5 concentration of 100μg/m3, is the equivalent of smoking just 1.2 cigarettes per week; thus one can only imagine the noxious effect of smoking a pack per day or living in a household where SHS exposure is constant. PCPs working in underserved areas with vastly higher rates of smoking and SHS (11 × greater risk of child SHS exposure in low SES households)[75] need to be aware of these dangers so that avoidance and behavior modification can be emphasized.

GENERAL AIR POLLUTION COUNSELING

As previously stated, when counseling patients regarding air pollution in general, PCPs caring for underserved patients in high pollution areas should advise them to stay indoors on high pollution days, clean indoor air with filters if possible, and limit physical exertion near roads or industrial sources, especially in the late morning or early afternoons when pollutant concentrations and ozone conversion may be highest.

INGESTED POLLUTANTS: WATER, SOIL, AND FOOD CONTAMINATION

Ingested water, soil, and food pollutants can all have adverse effects. As with air pollutants, these toxins vary widely in composition (eg, infectious agents, organic contaminants, inorganic heavy metals) and can come from a variety of sources, including industrial contamination, agricultural runoff, and food storage methods (plastic lining of canned goods). BPA and arsenic (see later discussion) are meant to serve as examples of potential harmful ingestible compounds. These 2 examples are meant only to heighten PCP awareness, not to imply that these examples are more prevalent or more toxic than other ingestible pollutants. The EPA monitors 87 microorganisms, disinfectants, organic compounds, inorganic chemicals, and radionuclides in rivers and public water supplies, each of which is potentially offensive. The FDA tests food and food packaging materials for more than 60 infectious agents, 484 pesticide residues, and many other heavy metals and other chemical contaminants.

Bisphenol A

BPA is used in making polycarbonates, which are found in products such as plastic dinnerware, eyeglass lenses, compact discs, toys, epoxy-based paints, water bottles, and home flooring. One of the most ubiquitous uses of BPA are in the protective linings of canned foods and beverages from which it has been found to leach into canned foods, especially acidic foods such as canned tomato products. In a recent study, 75 participants were split into 2 groups. The first group consumed 5 days of canned soup followed by 5 days without canned consumption. The second group did the reverse. Those consuming canned soup were found to have urinary BPA levels 1000% greater than those consuming only fresh foods.[76] BPA's weak estrogenic properties have been the intense focus of studies since the early 2000s when the concept of endocrine-disrupting compounds came to the forefront. BPA has been detected in 41% of US streams surveyed in 30 states[77] and has been found in the urine of 92% of people older than 6 years of age.[78]

Although the FDA and European Food and Safety Authority currently conclude that, "exposure to BPA at current levels is safe,"[79,80] the Chapel Hill Consensus Statement on BPA disagrees, stating that "BPA concentrations found in the human body are similar to those found in laboratory animals that have been associated with organizational changes of prostate, breast, testis, mammary glands, immune systems and brain."[81] A recent 2015 review concluded, "BPA may increase susceptibility to mammary and prostate cancer."[82] In addition links to hypertension, thyroid function obesity, asthma, and other cardiovascular diseases have been noted.[83–85]

The greatest concern of BPA exposure, however, is the potential risk for pregnant women, infants, and children. Several studies have stated that BPA's neurodevelopmental and behavioral effects are of the greatest concern,[83] and have shown early BPA exposure to be associated with aggressive behavior, ADHD, depression, and anxiety, indicating disruption of brain development during critical, formative windows.[86] It has also been classified as a reproductive toxicant and a recent 2014 review highlights the evidence for decreased uterine receptivity, increased implantation failure, adverse birth outcomes, sexual dysfunction, and testicular toxicant effects.[87] Such effects also may be passed on to future generations through genetic and epigenetic mechanisms (see later discussion).[88,89]

Although BPA has been shown to be biodegradable and is thought not to bioaccumulate,[90] it is still possible that untoward human effects might occur. This is because BPA is so prevalent and exposure is ongoing and prolonged. All of this, especially the prolonged exposure and neurobehavioral effects, is important when assessing BPAs effects in underserved communities. All of the recent studies the authors could find explicitly addressing BPA in underserved communities[91,92] found that those with low SES had significantly higher BPA levels.

The EPA reference dose of 50 μg/kg/d is the recommended safe level of exposure to BPA; however, animal studies have shown effects at much lower doses.

Arsenic

Arsenic is used in many industrial processes (ie, making metal alloys) and in the production of pressure-treated woods (scheduled to be phased out beginning in 2003 but still prevalent in many older houses). Once in the soil, it can be absorbed and concentrated in plants, most notably in leafy vegetables and rice. The main source of arsenic exposure, however, is from the natural diffusion of inorganic arsenic into groundwater. Groundwater in the US Southwest, Nevada, New England, Michigan, Wisconsin, Minnesota, and the Dakotas is known to have higher levels. In a Nevada town, for example, naturally elevated groundwater levels accounted for an average urinary arsenic level 4 times that of the average US population level.[93] It is significantly higher in other countries (ie, Bangladesh, Mongolia, Vietnam, Cambodia). In Bangladesh, levels have been noted to be 50 times higher than US standards and for Inner Mongolia the average level may be up to 70 times higher.[94]

Arsenic has been linked to skin and bladder cancer,[95,96] as well as dermal keratosis, vasospasm, and peripheral neuropathy. These effects have been associated with urinary levels as low as 50 to 100 μg/L in chronically exposed populations, a level found in roughly 5% to 10% of the US population in 2009 to 2010. WHO and EPA standards for arsenic safety is 10 ppb for both food and water consumption. China has a food standard of 150 ppb.

Overall, the authors could find relatively few studies assessing public drinking water or soil contamination in underserved communities[97–102] but those found validated EJ concerns and found excessive toxin levels in underserved communities. Much of this discrepancy was found in rural communities with small or underfunded municipal water systems.

SUMMARY

Because underserved communities are likely to have higher pollution levels, PCPs working in these areas should be prepared to investigate potential occurrences, educate patients, and mitigate effects while waiting for or advocating for larger scale policy changes. Again, PCPs should understand that no standard approach to air, water, or food toxin exposure is possible. Instead, because different communities experience different exposure, depending on industrial contributions; agricultural runoff; traffic patterns; and the prevalence of other infectious, organic, or inorganic toxins, a more individualized and site-specific approach in necessary. It is important for the PCP to be aware of her of his particular community and the environmental factors at play.

REFERENCES

1. Hajat A, Hsia C, O'Neill MS. Socioeconomic disparities and air pollution exposure: a global review. Curr Environ Health Rep 2015;2:440–50.
2. Bai Y, Hillemeier MM, Lengerich EJ. Racial/ethnic disparities in symptom severity among children hospitalized with asthma. J Health Care Poor Underserved 2007;18:54–61.
3. Haynes EN, Chen A, Ryan P, et al. Exposure to airborne metals and particulate matter and risk for youth adjudicated for criminal activity. Environ Res 2011;111: 1243–8.

4. Centers for Disease Control and Prevention. National Biomonitoring Program. Biomonitoring Summaries. Available at: http://www.cdc.gov/biomonitoring/biomonitoring_summaries.html. Accessed May 28, 2016.
5. Rosenfeld CS. Bisphenol A and phthalate endocrine disruption of parental and social behaviors. Front Neurosci 2015;9:57.
6. Bengalli R, Molteni E, Longhin E, et al. Release of IL-1 β triggered by Milan summer PM10: molecular pathways involved in the cytokine release. Biomed Res Int 2013;2013:158093.
7. Suhaimi NF, Jalaludin J. Biomarker as a research tool in linking exposure to air particles and respiratory health. Biomed Res Int 2015;2015:962853.
8. Olden K, Lin YS, Gruber D, et al. Epigenome: biosensor of cumulative exposure to chemical and nonchemical stressors related to environmental justice. Am J Public Health 2014;104:1816–21.
9. Feil R. Environmental and nutritional effects on the epigenetic regulation of genes. Mutat Res 2006;600:46–57.
10. Vandegehuchte MB, Janssen CR. Epigenetics and its implications for ecotoxicology. Ecotoxicology 2011;20:607–24.
11. Slomko H, Heo HJ, Einstein FH. Minireview: epigenetics of obesity and diabetes in humans. Endocrinology 2012;153(3):1025–30.
12. Bégin P, Nadeau KC. Epigenetic regulation of asthma and allergic disease. Allergy Asthma Clin Immunol 2014;10:27.
13. Hong X, Wang X. Early life precursors, epigenetics, and the development of food allergy. Semin Immunopathol 2012;34:655–69.
14. Javierre BM, Hernando H, Ballestar E. Environmental triggers and epigenetic deregulation in autoimmune disease. Discov Med 2011;12:535–45.
15. Klengel T, Pape J, Binder EB, et al. The role of DNA methylation in stress-related psychiatric disorders. Neuropharmacology 2014;80:115–32.
16. Saban KL, Mathews HL. Epigenetics and social context: implications for disparity in cardiovascular disease. Aging Dis 2014;5:346–55.
17. Herceg Z, Vaissière T. Epigenetic mechanisms and cancer: an interface between the environment and the genome. Epigenetics 2011;6:804–19.
18. Kanwal R, Gupta K, Gupta S. Cancer epigenetics: an introduction. Methods Mol Biol 2015;1238:3–25.
19. World Health Organization. Media Centre. 7 million premature deaths annually linked to air pollution. Available at: http://www.who.int/mediacentre/news/releases/2014/air-pollution/en/. Accessed March 7, 2016.
20. Calderón-Garcidueñas L, Kulesza RJ. Megacities air pollution problems: Mexico City metropolitan area critical issues on the central nervous system pediatric impact. Environ Res 2015;137:157–69.
21. Hampson NB, Piantadosi CA, Thom SR, et al. Practice recommendations in the diagnosis, management, and prevention of carbon monoxide poisoning. Am J Respir Crit Care Med 2012;186:1095–101.
22. Gatto NM, Henderson VW, Hodis HN, et al. Components of air pollution and cognitive function in middle aged and older adults in Los Angeles. Neurotoxicology 2014;40:1–7.
23. Iglesias DJ, Calatayud A, Barreno E, et al. Responses of citrus plants to ozone: leaf biochemistry, antioxidant mechanisms and lipid peroxidation. Plant Physiol Biochem 2006;44:125–31.
24. Jerrett M, Burnett RT, Pope CA, et al. Long-Term ozone exposure and mortality. N Engl J Med 2009;360:1085–95.

25. Weinhold B. Ozone nation: EPA standard panned by the people. Environ Health Perspect 2008;116:A302–5.

26. Kodavanti UP. Air pollution and insulin resistance: do all roads lead to Rome? Diabetes 2015;64:712–4.

27. United States Environmental Protection Agency. The National Ambient Air Quality Standards for Ozone. Ozone and Health. Available at: https://www.epa.gov/sites/production/files/2016-04/documents/20151001healthfs.pdf. Accessed October 26, 2016.

28. Chen JC, Schwartz J. Neurobehavioral effects of ambient air pollution on cognitive performance in US adults. Neurotoxicology 2009;30:231–9.

29. Goodman JE, Prueitt RL, Sax SN. Weight-of-evidence evaluation of short-term ozone exposure and cardiovascular effects. Crit Rev Toxicol 2014;44:725–90.

30. Prueitt RL, Lynch HN. Weight-of-evidence evaluation of long-term ozone exposure and cardiovascular effects. Crit Rev Toxicol 2014;44:791–822.

31. Lei H, Wuebbles DJ, Liang XZ. Projected risk of high ozone episodes in 2050. Atmospheric Environment 2012;59:567–77.

32. Goodman JE, Prueitt RL. Ozone exposure and systemic biomarkers: evaluation of evidence for adverse cardiovascular health impacts. Crit Rev Toxicol 2015;45:412–52.

33. Molina LT, Kolb CE, deFoy B, et al. Air quality in North America's most populous city – Overview of the MCMA 2003 campaign. Atmos Chem Phys 2007;7:2447–73.

34. Shankardass K, McConnell R, Jerrett M, et al. Parental stress increases the effect of traffic-related air pollution on childhood asthma incidence. Proc Natl Acad Sci U S A 2009;106:12406–11.

35. American Lung Association. Trends in asthma morbidity and mortality. Chicago (IL): Epidemiology and Statistical Unit, Research and Health Education Division; 2012. Available at: http://www.lung.org/assets/documents/research/asthma-trend-report.pdf. Accessed on January 30, 2016.

36. Jungers RH, Lee RE, von Lehmden DJ. The EPA national fuel surveillance network. Trace constituents in gasoline and commercial gasoline fuel additives. Environ Health Perspect 1975;10:143–50.

37. Cheung KL, Ntziachristos L, Tzamkiozis T, et al. Emissions of particulate trace elements, metals and organic species from gasoline, diesel, and biodiesel passenger vehicles and their relation to oxidative potential. Aerosol Sci Technol 2010;44:500–13.

38. Grandjean P, Weihe P, White RF, et al. Cognitive deficit in 7-year-old children with prenatal exposure to methylmercury. Neurotoxicol Teratol 1997;19:417–28.

39. Harada M. Minamata disease: Methylmercury poisoning in Japan caused by environmental pollution. Crit Rev Toxicol 1995;25:1–24.

40. Davidson PW, Myers GJ, Cox C, et al. Effects of prenatal and postnatal methylmercury exposure from fish consumption on neurodevelopment: outcomes at 66 months of age in the Seychelles Child Development Study. JAMA 1998;280:701–7.

41. Sikorski R, Juszkiewicz T, Paszkowski T, et al. Women in dental surgeries: reproductive hazards in occupational exposure to metallic mercury. Int Arch Occup Environ Health 1987;59:551–7.

42. Yorifuji T, Tsuda T, Kawakami N. Age standardized cancer mortality ratios in areas heavily exposed to methyl mercury. Int Arch Occup Environ Health 2007;80:679–88.

43. Trasande L, Schechter C, Haynes KA, et al. Applying cost analyses to drive policy that protects children: Mercury as a case study. Ann N Y Acad Sci 2006; 1076:911–23.

44. Trasande L, Landrigan PJ, Schechter C. Public health and economic consequences of methyl mercury toxicity to the developing brain. Environ Health Perspect 2005;113:590–6.

45. Brower MC, Price BH. Neuropsychiatry of frontal lobe dysfunction in violent and criminal behaviour: a critical review. J Neurol Neurosurg Psychiatry 2001;71: 720–6.

46. Braun JM, Froehlich TE, Daniels JL, et al. Association of environmental toxicants and conduct disorder in U.S. children: NHANES 2001–2004. Environ Health Perspect 2008;116:956–62.

47. Bertin G, Averbeck D. Cadmium: cellular effects, modifications of biomolecules, modulation of DNA repair and genotoxic consequences (a review). Biochimie 2006;88:1549–59.

48. United States Environmental Protection Agency, 2002. Health Assessment Document for Diesel Engine Exhaust. Washington, DC: National Center for Environmental Assessment, USEPA; 2002. p. 669.

49. Lelieveld J, Evans JS. The contribution of outdoor air pollution sources to premature mortality on a global scale. Nature 2015;525:367–71.

50. Brauer M, Freedman G, Frostad J, et al. Ambient air pollution exposure estimation for the global burden of disease 2013. Environ Sci Technol 2016;50:79–88.

51. McGuinn LA, Ward-Caviness CK, Neas LM, et al. Association between satellite-based estimates of long-term PM2.5 exposure and coronary artery disease. Environ Res 2016;145:9–17.

52. Giorgini P, Di Giosia P, Grassi D, et al. Air Pollution Exposure and Blood Pressure: An Updated Review of the Literature. Curr Pharm Des 2015;22:28–51.

53. Kunzli N, Jerrett M, Mack WJ, et al. Ambient air pollution and atherosclerosis in Los Angeles. Environ Health Perspect 2005;113:201–6.

54. Chen Z, Salam MT, Eckel SP, et al. Chronic effects of air pollution on respiratory health in Southern California children: findings from the Southern California Children's Health Study. J Thorac Dis 2015;7:46–58.

55. Ghio AJ. Particle exposures and infections. Infection 2014;42:459–67.

56. Spiezia L, Campello E, Bon M, et al. Short-term exposure to high levels of air pollution as a risk factor for acute isolated pulmonary embolism. Thromb Res 2014;134:259–63.

57. Zhou F, Li S, Jia W, et al. Effects of diesel exhaust particles on microRNA-21 in human bronchial epithelial cells and potential carcinogenic mechanisms. Mol Med Rep 2015;12:2329–35.

58. Brunekreef B, Beelen R, Hoek G, et al. Effects of long-term exposure to traffic-related air pollution on respiratory and cardiovascular mortality in the Netherlands: the NLCS-AIR study. Res Rep Health Eff Inst 2009;139:5–71.

59. Wu S, Deng F, Hao Y, et al. Chemical constituents of fine particulate air pollution and pulmonary function in healthy adults: the Healthy Volunteer Natural Relocation study. J Hazard Mater 2013;260:183–91.

60. Pope CA 3rd, Burnett RT, Turner MC, et al. Lung cancer and cardiovascular disease mortality associated with ambient air pollution and cigarette smoke: shape of the exposure–response relationships. Environ Health Perspect 2011;119: 1616–21.

61. Pope CA 3rd, Dockery DW. Health effects of fine particulate air pollution: lines that connect. J Air Waste Manag Assoc 2006;56:709–42.

62. Brook RD, Franklin B, Cascio W, et al, Expert panel on population and prevention science of the American Heart Association. Air pollution and cardiovascular disease: a statement for healthcare professionals from the expert panel on population and prevention science. Circulation 2004;109:2655–71.

63. Genc S, Zadeoglulari Z, Fuss SH, et al. The adverse effects of air pollution on the nervous system. J Toxicol 2012;2012:782462.

64. Costa LG, Cole TB, Coburn J, et al. Neurotoxicity of traffic-related air pollution. Neurotoxicology 2015 [pii: S0161-813(15) 30024–30033].

65. Gerlofs-Nijland ME, van Berlo D, Cassee FR, et al. Effect of prolonged exposure to diesel engine exhaust on proinflammatory markers in different regions of the rat brain. Part Fibre Toxicol 2010;7:12.

66. Chiu YM, Hsu HL, Coull BA, et al. Prenatal particulate air pollution and neurodevelopment in urban children: examining sensitive windows and sex-specific associations. Environ Int 2015;87:56–65.

67. Guxens M, Garcia-Esteban R, Giorgis-Allemand L, et al. Air pollution during pregnancy and childhood cognitive and psychomotor development. Epidemiology 2014;25:636–47.

68. Edwards SC, Jedrychowski W, Butscher M, et al. Prenatal exposure to airborne polycyclic aromatic hydrocarbons and children's intelligence at 5 years of age in a prospective cohort study in Poland. Environ. Health Perspect 2010;118: 1326–31.

69. Volk HE, Lurmann F, Penfold B, et al. Traffic related air pollution, particulate matter, and autism. JAMA Psychiatry 2013;70:71–7.

70. Suades-González E, Gascon M, Guxens M, et al. Air pollution and neuropsychological development: a review of the latest evidence. Endocrinology 2015;156: 3473–82.

71. Siddique S, Banerfee J, Ray MR, et al. Attention deficit hyperactivity disorder in children chronically exposed to high level of vehicular pollution. Eur J Pediatr 2011;170:923–9.

72. Win-Shwe TT, Yamamoto S, Fujitani Y, et al. Spatial learning and memory function-related gene expression in the hippocampus of mouse exposed to nanoparticle-rich diesel exhaust. Neurotoxicology 2008;29:940–7.

73. Eiguren-Fernandez A, Miguel AH, Froines JR, et al. Seasonal and spatial variation of poly cyclic aromatic hydrocarbons in vapor-phase and PM2.5 in southern California and rural communities. Aerosol Sci Technol 2004;38:447–55.

74. van Donkelaar A, Martin RV, Brauer M, et al. Global estimates of ambient fine particulate matter concentrations from satellite-based aerosol optical depth: development and application. Environ Health Perspect 2010;118:847–55.

75. Pisinger C, Hammer-Helmich L, Andreasen AH, et al. Social disparities in children's exposure to second hand smoke at home: a repeated cross-sectional survey. Environ Health 2012;11:65.

76. Carwile JL, Ye X, Zhou X, et al. Canned soup consumption and urinary bisphenol A: a randomized crossover trial. JAMA 2011;306:2218–20.

77. Kolpin DW, Furlong ET, Meyer MT, et al. Pharmaceuticals, hormones, and other organic wastewater contaminants in U.S. streams, 1999-2000: a national reconnaissance. Environ Sci Technol 2002;36:1202–11.

78. Trasande L, Attina TM, Blustein J. Association between urinary bisphenol A concentration and obesity prevalence in children and adolescents. JAMA 2012;308: 1113–21.

79. US Food & Drug Administration.Bisphenol A (BPA): Use in Food Contact Application. Available at: http://www.fda.gov/NewsEvents/PublicHealthFocus/ucm064437.htm. Accessed October 26, 2016.

80. EFSA. Bisphenol A. Available at: http://www.efsa.europa.eu/en/topics/topic/bisphenol. Accessed March 9, 2016.

81. vom Saal FS, Akingbemi BT, Belcher SM, et al. Chapel Hill bisphenol A expert panel consensus statement: integration of mechanisms, effects in animals and potential to impact human health at current levels of exposure. Reprod Toxicol 2007;24:131–8.

82. Seachrist DD, Bonk KW, Ho SM, et al. A review of the carcinogenic potential of bisphenol A. Reprod Toxicol 2016;59:167–82.

83. Rochester JR. Bisphenol A and human health: a review of the literature. Reprod Toxicol 2013;42:132–55.

84. Lang IA, Galloway TS, Scarlett A, et al. Association of urinary bisphenol A concentration with medical disorders and laboratory abnormalities in adults. JAMA 2008;300:1303–10.

85. vom Saal FS, Myers JP. Bisphenol A and risk of metabolic disorders. JAMA 2008;300:1353–5.

86. Mustieles V, Pérez-Lobato R, Olea N, et al. Human exposure and neurobehavior. Neurotoxicology 2015;49:174–84.

87. Peretz J, Vrooman L, Ricke WA, et al. Bisphenol A and reproductive health: update of experimental and human evidence, 2007-2013. Environ Health Perspect 2014;122:775–86.

88. Bernal AJ, Jirtle RL. Epigenomic disruption: the effects of early developmental exposures. Birth Defects Res A Clin Mol Teratol 2010;88:938–44.

89. Ryan KK, Haller AM, Sorrell JE, et al. Perinatal exposure to bisphenol-A and the development of metabolic syndrome in CD-1 mice. Endocrinology 2010;151:2603–12.

90. Negri-Cesi P. Bisphenol A interaction with brain development and functions. Dose Response 2015;13. 1559325815590394.

91. Nelson JW, Scammell MK, Hatch EE, et al. Social disparities in exposures to bisphenol A and polyfluoroalkyl chemicals: a cross-sectional study within NHANES 2003-2006. Environ Health 2012;11:10.

92. Tyrrell J, Melzer D, Henley W, et al. Associations between socioeconomic status and environmental toxicant concentrations in adults in the USA: NHANES 2001-2010. Environ Int 2013;59:328–35.

93. Caldwell KL, Jones RL, Verdon CP, et al. Levels of urinary total and speciated arsenic in the U.S. Population: National Health and Nutrition Examination Survey 2003-2004. J Expo Sci Environ Epidemiol 2009;19:59–68.

94. Sun G, Xu Y, Li X, et al. Urinary arsenic metabolites in children and adults exposed to arsenic in drinking water in Inner Mongolia, China. Environ Health Perspect 2007;115:648–52.

95. Ioch LM, Zierold K, Anderson HA. Association of arsenic-contaminated drinking-water with prevalence of skin cancer in Wisconsin's Fox River Valley. J Health Popul Nutr 2006;24:206–13.

96. Chu HD, Crawford-Brown DJ. Inorganic arsenic in drinking water and bladder cancer: a meta-analysis for dose-response assessment. Int J Environ Res Public Health 2006;3:316–22.

97. Heaney C, Wilson S, Wilson O, et al. Use of community-owned and -managed research to assess the vulnerability of water and sewer services in marginalized

and underserved environmental justice communities. J Environ Health 2011;74: 8–17.

98. Delpla I, Benmarhnia T. Investigating social inequalities in exposure to drinking water contaminants in rural areas. Environ Pollut 2015;207:88–96.

99. Cushing L, Morello-Frosch R, Wander M, et al. The haves, the have-nots, and the health of everyone: the relationship between social inequality and environmental quality. Annu Rev Public Health 2015;36:193–209.

100. Balazs CL, Ray I. The drinking water disparities framework: on the origins and persistence of inequities in exposure. Am J Public Health 2014;104:603–11.

101. Balazs CL, Morello-Frosch R, Hubbard AE, et al. Environmental justice implications of arsenic contamination in California's San Joaquin Valley: a cross-sectional, cluster-design examining exposure and compliance in community drinking water systems. Environ Health 2012;11:84.

102. Diawara MM, Litt JS, Unis D, et al. Arsenic, cadmium, lead, and mercury in surface soils, Pueblo, Colorado: implications for population health risk. Environ Geochem Health 2006;28:297–315.

Climate Change and Underserved Communities

Carol Ziegler, DNP, APRN, NP-C, RD[a,b], Vincent Morelli, MD[c,*], Omotayo Fawibe, MD[b]

KEYWORDS

- Climate change ● Global warming ● Greenhouse gases ● Greenhouse gas emissions
- Patient education

KEY POINTS

- Climate change is a threat to the basic necessities of life, especially for the most vulnerable. These necessities include health, shelter, food, and water.
- Climate change will have direct health impact on populations seen in primary care.
- The effects of climate change must be dampened with adaptation and mitigation strategies.

A GLOBAL PERSPECTIVE ON CLIMATE CHANGE

The Intergovernmental Panel on Climate Change defines climate change as a change in the state of the climate that persists for an extended period, typically decades, and can be identified by the variability of its properties. It is also any change in climate over time, whether due to natural variability or as a result of human activity.[1] Climate change is not currently widely accepted as a health hazard by health care professionals in the United States; yet it is the single greatest global health threat of the twenty-first century.[2] The effects of climate change on global health are so enormous that in the next few decades billions of lives will be affected.[2] The concept of climate change, despite skepticism and political opposition, is valid. Available science concludes with 90% certainty that the earth's climate has warmed over the past few decades as a result of greenhouse gas emissions from human activities.[1,3] Moreover, no credible body of climate scientists have found an alternate explanation for the rising global temperature.

Disclosure Statement: The authors of this work report no direct financial interest in the subject matter or any material discussed in this article.
[a] Vanderbilt University School of Nursing, Nashville, 461 21st Ave South, Nashville, TN 37240, USA; [b] Department of Family & Community Medicine, Meharry Medical College, 1005 Dr D. B. Todd Boulevard, Nashville, TN 37208, USA; [c] Sports Medicine Fellowship, Department of Family and Community Medicine, Meharry Medical College, 1005 Dr D. B. Todd Boulevard, Nashville, TN 37208, USA
* Corresponding author.
E-mail address: vmorelli@mmc.edu

Prim Care Clin Office Pract 44 (2017) 171–184
http://dx.doi.org/10.1016/j.pop.2016.09.017
0095-4543/17/© 2016 Elsevier Inc. All rights reserved.

Climate change occurs due to an imbalance between incoming and outgoing radiation in the atmosphere.[4] When solar radiation from sunlight enters the atmosphere, some of the radiation is absorbed by the earth's surface and emitted as infrared radiation. Greenhouse gases, such as carbon dioxide (CO_2), methane (CH_4) and nitrous oxide (N_2O), absorb the infrared radiation, heating up the lower atmosphere.[5,6] These greenhouse gases can occur naturally or from human activities. Fluctuations in the temperature of the lower atmosphere have occurred in the past due to variations in concentrations of naturally occurring greenhouse gases. The significant rise in global temperatures now experienced, however, is due to a rise in the concentration of global greenhouse gases in the atmosphere due to various human activities. CO_2 accounts for 76% of greenhouse gas emissions and is a product of petroleum product combustion, natural gas, and coal. CH_4 is a product of landfills, coal mines, and oil and gas operations and accounts for 16% of emissions, whereas N_2O accounts for 5% of emissions and is a product of nitrogen fertilizers, burning biomass, and waste management processes. Finally, fluorinated gases account for 2% of emissions and are a product of industrial processes like refrigeration (**Fig. 1**).[7]

Since the industrial revolution, atmospheric concentration of CO_2 has increased from 280 parts per million to approximately 395 parts per million today.[3,5] This has led to record-high global temperatures. The planet's average temperature has increased by 0.8°C since 1880 and if the current trend of CO_2 emission levels remains stable, it is predicted that the planet's average temperature will increase by an additional 1.8°C to 5.8°C by the end of the twenty-first century.[5] This is expected to have an impact on basic human needs like food, water, shelter, and health. Increased global temperature will disrupt the water cycle because warmer air retains more moisture, causing flooding in some areas and drought in others; this will affect crop yield from farming and even livestock productivity. Increased temperature can also lead to heat waves increasing the incidence of heat-related illnesses. Heat waves can also increase the ambient level of some air pollutants, which can increase morbidity and mortality related to cardiorespiratory conditions. Also, flooding or drought can affect the geographic distribution of vector-borne diseases, such as malaria and dengue fever. Increased global temperature will also increase ocean

■ Carbon dioxide (from fossil fuel burning, forestry, industrial processes)

■ Methane (from landfills, coal mines, oil & gas operations)

■ Nitrous oxide (from nitrogen fertilizers, burning biomass & waste management processes)

■ Fluorinated gases (from industrial processes like refrigeration)

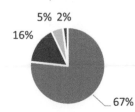

Fig. 1. Global greenhouse gas emissions.

temperatures, potentially disrupting the aquatic ecosystem and affecting industries like fishing. The increased global temperature will also cause sea levels to rise as a result of melting sea ice, forcing migration of coastal dwellers and leading to a host of other challenges (**Fig. 2**).[3,5,7]

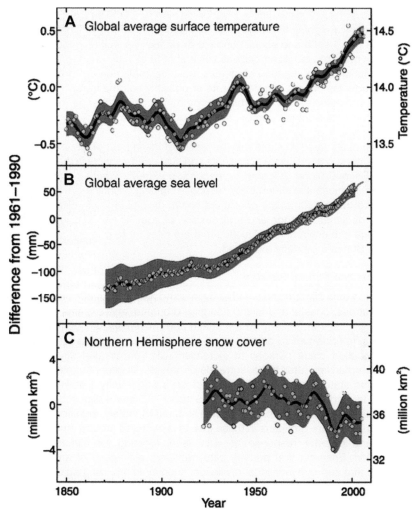

Fig. 2. Changes in temperature, sea level, and Northern Hemisphere snow cover.[1] Observed changes in (a) global average surface temperature, (b) global average sea level from tide gauge (*blue*) and satellite (*red*) data, and (c) Northern Hemisphere snow cover for March–April. All differences are relative to corresponding averages for the period 1961 to 1990. Smoothed curves represent decadal averaged values whereas circles show yearly values. The shaded areas are the uncertainty intervals estimated (a and b) from a comprehensive analysis of known uncertainties and (c) from the time series. (*From* IPCC. Climate change 2007: Synthesis report. Contribution of working groups I, II and III to the fourth assessment report of the intergovernmental panel on climate change. 2007. Available at: http://www.ipcc.ch/publications_and_data/ar4/syr/en/contents.html. Accessed March 6, 2016; with permission.)

CLIMATE CHANGE IN THE PRIMARY CARE SETTING

Climate change is a phenomenon that is real but is still approached with skepticism. It is the duty of health care practitioners to learn about the various impacts of climate change and serve as an informant for their patients as well as serving as sentinels for the public health sector when health crises erupt due to climate change. Although the impact of climate change will be seen across the globe, low-income and middle-income countries (LMICs) with minimal resources along with the susceptible groups in wealthy countries are going to be the most negatively impacted by climate change. In the United States, health and socioeconomic disparities as well as geographic location leave the most marginalized citizens vulnerable to climate change. Policies promoting adaptation and mitigation strategies must be implemented to both dampen some of the adverse effects and decelerate or possibly halt the trend of the change. Primary care providers play a vital role in promoting climate change mitigation and activism through their unique perspective and ability to make it personally relevant to health.

Although primary care providers may be aware of the impact of climate change on global health, most are not aware of its acute and sustained impacts in their local practice setting. Beyond being prepared to respond to extreme weather events through disaster preparedness and emergency response training, frontline providers should be attentive to the local impacts on patient health associated with climate change. The process of climate change and a discussion of specific health issues related to climate change and environmental justice that are relevant to primary care providers in the United States are briefly explained.

Climate Events and Natural Disasters

Increases in extreme climate and weather events and natural disasters, including hurricanes, tornadoes, coastal and inland flooding, droughts, and extreme temperature fluctuations, will have an impact on the health and movement of populations in the United States. In underserved communities, lack of adequate resources for evacuation and relocation place persons at increased risk from natural disasters. Case studies of communities after the occurrence of natural disasters suggest that lower socioeconomic status has a negative impact on a community's ability to prepare for, respond to, and recover from natural disasters.[8–11] Natural disasters often result in mass casualties with a spectrum of injuries and, unfortunately, significant mortality. The role of primary care providers in these events is centered around emergency preparedness and disaster response as well as advocating for climate mitigation and adaptation. Ensuring that primary care providers are aware of and promoting interventions that improve individual resilience, such as immunizing against vaccine-preventable illnesses, such as pneumonia, influenza, and tetanus; maintaining infection control in health care settings; and educating patients about nutrition and exercise as well as optimally managing chronic illnesses, is imperative to maximizing patient resilience.[12] Mitigation and adaptation are discussed later; however, emergency preparedness and disaster response are outside of the scope of this article. Primary care providers should avail themselves of training and information related to specific disaster risk and response relevant to their respective regions. Mental health impacts associated with such events are discussed later.

Extreme Temperatures

The American Meteorological Society declared 2014 the hottest year on record.[13] Extreme fluctuations in temperature, both increases in intensity of heat and duration of heat waves, rapid shifts in hot and cold temperatures, and altered patterns of extreme cold are occurring globally and across the United States. Several studies have demonstrated that cold (for normal) and hot (for normal) ambient temperatures are associated with increased risk of mortality in regions across the globe.[14] Although both hot and cold temperatures seem associated with increased risk of mortality across regions, the impact associated with heat, termed *thermal injury*, is observed more rapidly and is typically shorter in duration (the isolated impact of heat on mortality), whereas cold temperatures seem to have a more delayed but longer-lasting impacts.[14]

In addition to impacts from hyperthermia and hypothermia, both of which are emergent conditions not managed in primary care, temperature extremes increase morbidity and mortality with respect to respiratory and cardiovascular systems. Extreme or unseasonably cold temperatures place persons at increased risk of death from cardiovascular disease and respiratory illnesses. Persons with chronic respiratory illnesses, such as asthma and chronic obstructive pulmonary disease (COPD), as well as cardiovascular and cerebrovascular diseases are observed to experience increased mortality in colder temperatures.[15–18] Extreme temperature fluctuations have been observed to increase cardiovascular mortality and morbidity and these impacts disproportionately affect the elderly, small children, people with low socioeconomic status, and those with comorbidities, such as diabetes, hypertension, and kidney disease.[19]

Outside of the direct impact of heat and cold stress on the body's thermoregulatory system, heat waves have been associated with increased exacerbations in cardiovascular disease, asthma, and COPD, and these increases seem related to the temperature itself as well as outdoor and indoor air pollution and humidity.[20] Primary care providers should be aware of the potential impacts of extreme temperature on patients with cardiovascular and respiratory illnesses so that they are able to rapidly optimize management strategies and assist patients in adapting to temperature changes. Educating patients about safety in extreme temperatures, air quality information, and warnings and how to react to them and communicating with local agencies to assist patients in obtaining housing or climate control devices are critical aspects of providing care for those at risk to climate and temperature-related stress.

Vector-Borne Illnesses

Changes in temperature, humidity, and seasonal weather and flooding patterns have broadened the geographic range and seasonal survivability of many vectors of disease. This increase in seasonal and geographic range of common vectors, combined with increased human population density in urban centers and increased human mobility, will broaden the distribution and increase the prevalence of vector-borne and waterborne illnesses. Human mobility and migration patterns due to extreme and insidious changes in climate, as well as conflict, will likely exacerbate this problem.

Warmer winters and changes in seasonal weather patterns will likely broaden the geographic range and encourage expansion of common vectors (in the United States, notably, rodents, ticks, and mosquitoes) to wider latitudes. Globally, malaria, dengue fever, diarrheal diseases, and cholera are on the rise and this increase is directly attributable to climate change.[5] Barriers to vaccinations and other primary care services as well as increased exposures due to inadequate housing and poor vector control in impoverished communities leave persons living in distressed regions of poverty in the United States, such as in communities of color in the Mississippi Delta, impoverished communities in Appalachia, and the urban poor, at increased risk from infections known as neglected infections of poverty.[21]

In the United States, primary care providers must be aware of the signs, symptoms, and most up-to-date transmission patterns and treatment guidelines for illnesses like leptospirosis, Lyme disease, mosquito-borne encephalitis, and hantavirus as the transmission patterns of these illnesses have been noted to increase with respect to the changing climate.[22] Data on the direct impact of climate change on tick and mosquito-related illness in the United States are limited, but modeling suggests that climate change may shift the onset of tick-related illnesses in the United States, expanding the season for tick-borne infections.[23] It is also expected that emerging and re-emerging infections, such as Zika virus, avian flu, malaria, West Nile virus, and others, will likely increase in prevalence and range, appearing in areas where primary care providers may not be familiar with presenting symptoms. In addition, primary care providers must respond rapidly to apparent changes in seasonal patterns of vector-borne illnesses and new cases of vector-borne illnesses by communicating with their local health departments as well as providing patients with education about prevention of these illnesses and the most up-to-date and evidence-based care and management of the illness once a patient is sick. Ensuring that patients are up to date with regular vaccination schedules will prevent the resurgence of vaccine-preventable illnesses.

Impacts on Mental Health

The impact of climate change on mental health is more difficult to assess and more insidious than the direct impact on physical health. The devastating effects of drought, flooding, and other natural disasters coupled with increased migration from conflicts and food shortages will likely have disturbing impacts on populations. Posttraumatic stress disorder, depression, and acculturation stress may result from the devastating impacts that climate change will have on individuals, families, communities, and even entire countries in cases of conflict, drought, or famine.[24] Survivors of floods and hurricanes have increased rates of stress-associated psychiatric disorders.[25–27] In the United states, unusually warm temperatures are associated with increases in mental health disorders, and exacerbations, such as mood and anxiety-related disorders, as well as dementia are increased in heat waves.[28] Heat waves are also associated with higher levels of community violence in low-income neighborhoods.[29] There is a strong association between climate change and collective violence. Increases in social instability and political unrest are associated with elevated temperatures and extreme precipitation.[30,31] It is highly likely that armed conflict will continue to increase with the destabilization of the global climate system.[32]

In addition to effects directly related to extreme weather events and heat, the economic and social consequences of climate change to individuals and entire industries (like agriculture) as well as the impact of increased social conflict have the potential for deleterious effects on the mental health of individuals and populations.[33–35] Climate change will likely have long-term impacts on seasonality, temperatures, and rainfall, thus having an impact on food security and the health of the agricultural industry.[36] The downstream impact of destabilization of broad-based food security systems globally will disproportionately have an impact on the poor and likely lead to malnutrition as well as increases in metabolic diseases from diminished nutrient density of food and food quality.[37] Additionally, economic distress diminishes patient access to primary care services, limiting their ability to manage chronic illnesses and placing them at increased risk for poor health outcomes. Primary care providers practicing in regions experiencing extreme heat and weather events, conflict, and/or community violence or practicing in regions where industries, such as agriculture, are significant sources of employment and income must be cognizant of the pressures felt by the populations they serve. Conducting mental health evaluations and providing trauma-informed counseling for patients experiencing stress from climate-related events and assessing families for food security are critical roles for the primary care provider practicing in the age of climate change.

ADDRESSING HEALTH DISPARITIES RELATED TO CLIMATE CHANGE

The health effects of climate change will not be uniform across the globe. LMICs that already lack the basic infrastructure to meet the essential health care needs of its citizens, are likely to suffer to a greater extent from the impact of climate change than developed countries. These LMICs have little capacity to prevent and/or treat illnesses due to climate change. Ironically, LMICs are the least responsible for climate change, producing less than 10% of global greenhouse gas emissions.[38]

Certain groups in both LMICs and wealthier countries are more susceptible to adverse health effects from climate change. These susceptible groups include the poor, elderly, children, and patients with underlying chronic diseases. The poor have limited access to quality health care, are more likely to be malnourished, and are more likely to live in residences with poor indoor air quality, all factors that contribute to the greater burden of disease experienced by the poor in relation to climate change. The elderly are also at a greater risk of disease from climate change due to frail health and limited mobility, making them less likely to be able to evacuate in the case of a storm or any extreme weather event related to climate change.[39] Children often have developing immune, respiratory, and neurologic systems, making them more sensitive to the adverse health effects of climate change like extreme weather events, heat, and vector-borne diseases.[40,41] In addition to physiologic immaturity, which makes children living in poor countries vulnerable to the health-related consequences of climate change, their poor living conditions often compound health risks.[42] Children accounted for 88% of yearly deaths attributed to climate change in the early 2000s[43] and 99% of the children lived in LMICs.[44,45] In addition, climate change is thought to worsen the top causes of under–5-year-old child mortality, such as acute respiratory infection, diarrhea, malaria, malnutrition, and neonatal deaths.[38] Patients with underlying chronic diseases, such as COPD or asthma, often have impaired lung function that becomes even further impaired by the effects of climate change.[3] It is known that patients with asthma are particularly sensitive to changes in weather, with hot humid days increasing airway resistance of asthmatics.[3] Rapid rises in temperature and humidity have been associated with increased emergency department visits for asthma.[46] Also, exposure to ground-level ozone, production of which is catalyzed by warmer temperatures, has been found associated with increased emergency department visits and hospitalization due to asthma,[47–49] worse asthma control,[50] and reduced lung function.[51,52] Patients with COPD have been found to have more exacerbations, hospitalizations, and even increased all-cause mortality with exposure to heat.[53,54]

Additional Vulnerable Populations in the United States

Vulnerability to climate change may be increased by marginalized mental and/or physical health status, geographic location, or access to adaptation resources (resources that decrease vulnerability to the impacts of climate change). Although climate change will likely have an impact on persons living in low-resource settings globally, in the United States, several populations have been identified who are at increased risk for morbidity and mortality due to climate change and associated stress (in addition to those described previously): older adults (over age 65), children under age 5, pregnant women, persons living with chronic physical and mental illness and/or addiction, the homeless, and people employed in industries requiring exposure to the outdoors. Additionally, specific geographic regions are at increased risk based on proximity to shorelines, coastal and inland waterways, weather patterns, and availability of natural resources, such as water.[55,56] Specific climate-associated risks related to these vulnerable groups are discussed later.

Regional risk depends on availability of resources, proximity to waterways and flood zones, and regional weather patterns. Climate change will have a disproportionate impact on vulnerable populations, but what traits make a community more vulnerable in the United States? Communities of color, indigenous peoples, those who are isolated geographically, and the poor are least able to respond and adapt to climate change. Currently in the Unites States, the southeastern region is at greatest risk from collective impacts of climate change.[57] The southeastern United States is susceptible to climate-related events, such as hurricanes and extreme weather, tornadoes, and also sea level rise along the coastal states. Heat waves and drought also disproportionately have an impact on the southeastern United States[58]; southern cities, such as Atlanta, Miami, New Orleans, and Tampa, reported increased deaths from extreme heat from 1975 to 2004 relative to an increase in days with temperatures at 95°F or greater.[59] Climate change in the southeastern region will have long-term impacts on water availability and associated stresses from water shortages.[60] Additionally, the southern United States has more people living in rural areas and more people working outdoors in agriculture, both at increased risk for health problems from climate change.[61]

Persons employed in industries, such as utilities, transportation, emergency response, health care, environmental remediation, construction or demolition, landscaping and agriculture, forestry and wildlife management, heavy manufacturing, and warehouse work, are at increased risk from extreme weather and temperature events due to the nature of their work and being exposed regularly to the outdoors.[62,63] Workers in these fields may have increased exposure to temperature variations and precipitation, injury due to extreme weather, and exposure to vector-borne illnesses and outdoor pollutants, including from forest fires and industries.

The homeless and the poor will be disproportionately impacted by climate change. Homeless persons typically have increased severity of chronic disease, specifically cardiovascular disease and respiratory illnesses, due to stress, lifestyle factors, and difficulties accessing health care and other resources. Additionally, the homeless disproportionately suffer from substance use and mental health disorders, giving them multiple risk factors for climate change vulnerabilities.[64–67] Homeless persons tend to congregate in urban areas and, due to their lack of shelter, are at increased risk from extreme temperatures and weather events, outdoor air pollution, and vector-borne illnesses, such as West Nile virus.[68]

ADAPTATION STRATEGIES

Considering that LMICs and susceptible groups are more vulnerable to the adverse health effects of climate change, policies promoting adaptation and mitigation strategies should be implemented. Adaptation refers to actions taken by individuals, communities, and governments to lessen or protect against the impacts of climate change. On the other hand, mitigation refers to actions taken by individuals, communities, and governments to reduce or eliminate greenhouse gas emission, thereby limiting the damage from future climate change. Adaptation strategies for adverse health effects of climate change include improving access to quality health care for vulnerable populations, improving disease surveillance, improving weather forecasting, advancing emergency management, ensuring that health facilities are equipped to handle disasters, educating the public about climate change health impacts, development and dissemination of appropriate vaccines, ensuring food and water safety, and having a good vector control program.[38] Mitigation strategies for adverse health effects of climate change include using energy-efficient and renewable energy sources, reducing deforestation, reforestation, and development of greenhouse gas capture and greenhouse gas sequestration technologies.[33,69]

Aside from individual and community adaptation strategies for dealing with the effects of climate change, primary care providers and primary health systems must be prepared to respond to climate-related shifts in both the short term and long term. Great variability exists in the response and adaptation abilities of primary care systems across the globe.[70] Communities in the United States and abroad need functional adaptation assessments prior to climactic events to determine readiness to respond and react to climate change.[70,71] Knowing the significant impact of climate-associated changes on the health of individual patients and the larger impacts on community and population health, frontline care providers have a responsibility to advocate for climate mitigation policies to reduce greenhouse gas emissions and adaptation strategies aimed at preparing for anticipated impacts on the most vulnerable.[72] Several organizations, such as the International Society of Doctors for the Environment (http://www.isde.org/) and the Climate and Health Council (http://www.climateandhealth.org/), are currently engaged in linking primary care providers with climate change policy activism.

Educating Patients About Impact of Climate Change and Ways to Make a Difference

Because patient with underlying chronic diseases like COPD and asthma are more likely to be impacted by climate change, primary care providers have a vital role to

Table 1 Impact of climate change	
Type	**Effect**
Health	1. Increasing burden of disease from malnutrition (as a result of drought and flooding)[41] 2. Increasing burden of disease from diarrheal diseases (as a result of drought and flooding)[41] 3. Increase mortality and morbidity from cardiovascular diseases and respiratory diseases (as a result of heat waves, fluctuations in weather, and air pollution) 4. Increasing burden of disease from vector-borne diseases (as a result of drought, flooding, and increased or decreased precipitation causing change in distribution of some disease vectors)
Shelter	1. Loss of coastal wetlands (as a result of flooding and storms),[41] which means people who live in coastal communities are less protected from adverse events, such as storms 2. Forced migration (as a result of flooding, drought, and hurricanes)
Food	1. Decline in crop yields and livestock productivity (as a result of drought and flooding) 2. Reduction in fish supply (as a result of warming of ocean bodies)
Water	1. Increased water stress, especially in arid and semiarid areas (as a result of drought)[44] 2. Decrease in availability of safe water (as a result of flooding, rise in sea level, and increase in water temperature, which can cause alga blooms and increase bacteria population in water)[44]

play in informing patients about the impact of climate change on their health. **Table 1** lists and discusses the direct health impacts of climate change.

People can make a difference in slowing climate change by adopting environmental-friendly practices. These include improving home energy efficiency by properly insulating homes; using energy-efficient appliances and recycling; using renewable energy sources when feasible, such as photovoltaic solar panels for electricity and compressed natural gas for automobiles; where possible, walking, cycling, using mass transit, or using energy-efficient cars; using a carbon footprint calculator, which is an online tool found on Web sites, such as the Environmental Protection Agency (https://www3.epa.gov/carbon-footprint-calculator/EPA), to estimate household carbon print to identify areas of improvement; and joining an advocacy group, such as Sierra Club, Greenpeace, or Citizens Climate Lobby, to provide opportunity to learn more about the impact of climate change and also be able to advocate for a change.[5,6,38]

SUMMARY

Primary care providers can act as critical advocates for the populations they serve by promoting climate change mitigation and adaptation strategies to optimize the health spans of patients. As frontline providers, primary care providers are critical informants for policymakers, public health researchers, and patients on the emerging health impacts of climate change. In addition to emergency preparedness in the face of increasing climate-related events, primary care providers must be aware of increased risks to marginalized patients related to both extreme weather and vector-borne illnesses and of mental health and environmental impacts on chronic disease management. By educating emerging health care providers as well as patients about this great threat to public health, primary care providers can increase the resilience of the patients they care for in the face of increasing pressure from climate-related changes.

REFERENCES

1. IPCC. Climate change 2007: Synthesis report. Contribution of working groups I, II and III to the fourth assessment report of the intergovernmental panel on climate change. 2007. Available at: http://www.ipcc.ch/publications_and_data/ar4/syr/en/contents.html. Accessed March 6, 2016.
2. Lim V, Stubbs JW, Nahar N, et al. Politicians must heed health effects of climate change. Lancet 2009;374:973.
3. Bernstein AS, Rice MB. Lungs in a warming world climate change and respiratory health. Chest 2013;143:1455–9.
4. Patz JA. Climate change. In: Frumkin H, editor. Environmental health. San Francisco (CA): Josey-Bass; 2005. p. 238–68.
5. Shuman EK. Global climate change and infectious diseases. Int J Occup Environ Med 2011;2:11–20.
6. Holdstock D. Environmental health: threats and their interactions. Environ Health Insights 2008;2:117–22.
7. Environmental Protection Agency. Climate change. 2010. Available at: www.epa.gov/climatechange. Accessed February 9, 2016.
8. Masozera M, Bailey M, Kerchner C. Distribution of impacts of natural disasters across income groups: a case study of New Orleans. Ecol Econ 2007;63:299–306.
9. Bohle HG, Downing TE, Watts MJ. Climate change and social vulnerability: the sociology and geography of food insecurity. Global Environ Change 1994;4:37–48.

10. Fothergill A, Maestas E, Darlington J. Race, ethnicity and disasters in the United States: a review of the literature. Disasters 1999;23:156–73.
11. Fothergill A, Peek L. Poverty and disasters in the United States: a review of the recent sociological findings. Nat Hazards 2004;32:89–110.
12. Keim M. Building human resilience: the role of public health preparedness and response as an adaptation to climate change. Am J Prev Med 2008;35:508–16.
13. NOAA. International report confirms: 2014 was Earth's warmest year on record. Available at: http://www.noaanews.noaa.gov/stories2015/071615-international-report-confirms-2014-was-earths-warmest-year-on-record.html. Accessed March 6, 2016.
14. Guo Y, Gasparrini A, Armstrong B, et al. Global variation in the effects of ambient temperature on mortality: a systematic evaluation. Epidemiology 2014;25:781–9.
15. The Eurowinter Group. Cold exposure and winter mortality from ischemic heart disease, cerebrovascular disease, respiratory disease, and all causes in warm and cold regions of Europe. Lancet 1997;349:1341–6.
16. Lloyd EL. The role of cold in ischaemic heart disease: a review. Public Health 1991;105:205–15.
17. Pozos RS, Danzl DF. Human physiological responses to cold stress and hypothermia. In: Pandolf KB, Burr RE, editors. Medical aspects of harsh environments. Washington, DC: Borden Institute; 2001. p. 351–82.
18. Barnett A, Dobson A, McElduff P, et al. Cold periods and coronary events: an analysis of populations worldwide. J Epidemiol Community Health 2005;59: 551–7.
19. Liu C, Yavar Z, Sun Q. Cardiovascular response to thermoregulatory challenges. Am J Physiol Heart Circ Physiol 2015;309(11):H1793–812.
20. Kravchenko J, Abernethy AP, Fawzy M, et al. Minimization of heatwave morbidity and mortality. Am J Prev Med 2013;44:274–82.
21. Hotez PJ. Neglected diseases and poverty in "The Other America": the greatest health disparity in the United States? PLoS Negl Trop Dis 2007;1:e159.
22. Gubler DJ, Reiter P, Ebi KL, et al. Climate variability and change in the United States: potential impacts on vector- and rodent-borne diseases. Environ Health Perspect 2001;109(Suppl 2):223–33.
23. Monaghan AJ, Moore SM, Sampson KM, et al. Climate change influences on the annual onset of Lyme disease in the United States. Ticks Tick Borne Dis 2015; 6(5):615–22.
24. Padhy SK, Sarkar S, Panigrahi M, et al. Mental health effects of climate change. Indian J Occup Environ Med 2015;19:3–7.
25. DeSalvo KB, Hyre AD, Ompad DC, et al. Symptoms of posttraumatic stress disorder in a New Orleans workforce following Hurricane Katrina. J Urban Health 2007;84:142–52.
26. McMillen C, North C, Mosley M, et al. Untangling the psychiatric comorbidity of posttraumatic stress disorder in a sample of flood survivors. Compr Psychiatry 2002;43:478–85.
27. Norris FH, Murphy AD, Baker CK, et al. Postdisaster PTSD over four waves of a panel study of Mexico's 1999 flood. J Trauma Stress 2004;17:283–92.
28. Berry HL, Bowen K, Kjellstrom T. Climate change and mental health: a causal pathways framework. Int J Public Health 2010;55:123–32.
29. Mares D. Climate change and levels of violence in socially disadvantaged neighborhood groups. J Urban Health 2013;90:768–83.
30. Levy BS, Sidel VW. Collective violence caused by climate change and how it threatens health and human rights. Health Hum Rights 2014;16:32–40.

31. Hsiang SM, Burke M. Climate, conflict, and social stability: what does the evidence say? Climatic Change 2014;123:39–55.
32. Haines A. Redefining security. 1992. Med Confl Surviv 2009;25:282–5.
33. De Silva MJ, McKenzie K, Harpham T, et al. Social capital and mental illness: a systematic review. J Epidemiol Community Health 2005;59:619–27.
34. Whitley R, McKenzie K. Social capital and psychiatry: review of the literature. Harv Rev Psychiatry 2005;13:71–84.
35. Uphoff EP, Pickett KE, Cabieses B, et al. A systematic review of the relationships between social capital and socioeconomic inequalities in health: a contribution to understanding the psychosocial pathway of health inequalities. Int J Equity Health 2013;12:54.
36. Stevenson TJ, Visser ME, Arnold W, et al. Disrupted seasonal biology impacts health, food security and ecosystems. Proc Biol Sci 2015;282:20151453.
37. Bloem MW, Semba RD, Kraemer K. Castel Gandolfo Workshop: an introduction to the impact of climate change, the economic crisis, and the increase in the food prices on malnutrition. J Nutr 2010;140:132.
38. Kiang K, Graham S, Farrant B. Climate change, child health and the role of the paediatric profession in under-resourced settings. Trop Med Int Health 2013; 18:1053–6.
39. Ebi KL, Sussman FG, Wilbanks TJ. In: Gamble JL, editor. CCSP: Effects of Global Change on Human Health, in Analyses of the effects of global change on human health and welfare and human systems. A report by the U.S. climate change science program and the subcommittee on global change research. Washington, DC: US Environmental Protection Agency; 2008. p. 39–87.
40. National Research Council. Advancing the science of climate change. Washington, DC: National Research Council. The National Academies Press; 2010.
41. Wilbanks TJ, Lankao PR, Bao M, et al. Industry, settlement and society. In: Parry ML, Canziani OF, Palutikof JP, et al, editors. Climate Change 2007: impacts, adaptation and vulnerability. contribution of working group II to the fourth assessment report of the intergovernmental panel on climate change. Cambridge (United Kingdom): Cambridge University Press; 2007. p. 357–90.
42. Bunyavanich S, Landrigan CP, McMichael AJ, et al. The impact of climate change on child health. Ambul Pediatr 2003;3:44–52.
43. McMichael AJ, Woodruff RE, Hales S. Climate change and human health: Present and future risks. Lancet 2006;367:859–69.
44. Patz J, Gibbs H, Foley JA, et al. Climate change and global health: Quantifying a growing ethical crisis. EcoHealth 2007;4:397–405.
45. DARA. Climate Vulnerable Forum. Climate vulnerability monitor. A guide to the cold calculus of a hot planet. 2nd edition. Madrid (Spain): Estudis Graficos Europeos, S.A.; 2012.
46. Mireku N, Wang Y, Ager J, et al. Changes in weather and the effects on pediatric asthma exacerbations. Ann Allergy Asthma Immunol 2009;103:220–4.
47. Moore K, Neugebauer R, Lurmann F, et al. Ambient ozone concentrations cause increased hospitalizations for asthma in children: an 18-year study in Southern California. Environ Health Perspect 2008;116:1063–70.
48. Glad JA, Brink LL, Talbott EO, et al. The relationship of ambient ozone and PM(2.5) levels and asthma emergency department visits: Possible influence of gender and ethnicity. Arch Environ Occup Health 2012;67:103–8.
49. Babin S, Burkom H, Holtry R, et al. Medicaid patient asthma-related acute care visits and their associations with ozone and particulates in Washington, DC, from 1994-2005. Int J Environ Health Res 2008;18:209–21.

50. Meng YY, Wilhelm M, Rull RP, et al. Traffic and outdoor air pollution levels near residences and poorly controlled asthma in adults. Ann Allergy Asthma Immunol 2007;98:455–63.

51. Chan CC, Wu TH. Effects of ambient ozone exposure on mail carriers' peak expiratory flow rates. Environ Health Perspect 2005;113:735–8.

52. Chen PC, Lai YM, Chan CC, et al. Short-term effect of ozone on the pulmonary function of children in primary school. Environ Health Perspect 1999;107:921–5.

53. Lin S, Luo M, Walker RJ, et al. Extreme high temperatures and hospital admissions for respiratory and cardiovascular diseases. Epidemiology 2009;20: 738–46.

54. Zanobetti A, O'Neill MS, Gronlund CJ, et al. Summer temperature variability and long-term survival among elderly people with chronic disease. Proc Natl Acad Sci U S A 2012;109:6608–13.

55. Balbus JM, Malina C. Identifying vulnerable subpopulations for climate change health effects in the United States. J Occup Environ Med 2009;51:33–7.

56. Kim KH, Kabir E, Ara Jahan S. A review of the consequences of global climate change on human health. J Environ Sci Health C Environ Carcinog Ecotoxicol Rev 2014;32:299–318.

57. Gutierrez KS, LePrevost CE. Climate justice in rural Southeastern United States: a review of climate change impacts and effects on human health. Int J Environ Res Public Health 2016;13(2):189.

58. Carter LM, Jones JW, Berry L, et al. In: Melillo JM, Richmond TC, Yohe GW, editors. Southeast and the Caribbean. Climate change impacts in the United States: the third national climate assessment. U.S. Global Change Research Program; 2014. p. 396–417. Ch. 17.

59. Sheridan SC, Kalkstein AJ, Kalkstein LS. Trends in heat-related mortality in the United States, 1975–2004. Nat Hazards 2009;50:145–60.

60. Sun G. Impacts of climate change and variability on water resources in the Southeast USA. In: Ingram KT, Dow K, Carter L, et al, editors. Climate of the Southeast United States. Washington, DC: Springer; 2013. p. 210–36.

61. Portier CJ, Tart KT, Carter SR, et al. A human health perspective on climate change; environmental health perspectives and the national institute of environmental health sciences. Washington, DC: Environmental Health Perspectives and the National Institute of Environmental Health Sciences; 2010.

62. Roelofs C, Wegman DH. Workers: the "climate canaries"?. In: Levy BS, Patz JA, editors. Climate change and public health. New York: Oxford University Press; 2015. p. 18–9.

63. Lundgren K, Kuklane K, Gao C, et al. Effects of heat stress on working populations when facing climate change. Ind Health 2013;51:3–15.

64. Hwang SW. Homelessness and health. Can Med Assoc J 2001;164:229–33.

65. Lee TC, Hanlon JG, Ben-David J, et al. Risk factors for cardiovascular disease in homeless adults. Circulation 2005;111:2629–35.

66. Raoult D, Foucault C, Brouqi P. Infections in the homeless. Lancet Infect Dis 2001; 1:77–84.

67. North CS, Eyrich KM, Pollio D, et al. Are rates of psychiatric disorders in the homeless population changing? Am J Public Health 2004;94:103–8.

68. Ramin B, Svoboda T. Health of the homeless and climate change. J Urban Health 2009;86:654–64.

69. Shea KM. Global climate change and children's health. Pediatrics 2007;120: 1359–67.

70. Van Minh H, Tuan Anh T, Rocklöv J, et al. Primary healthcare system capacities for responding to storm and flood-related health problems: a case study from a rural district in central Vietnam. Glob Health Action 2014;7:23007.
71. Ebi KL, Schmier JK. A stitch in time: improving public health early warning systems for extreme weather events. Epidemiol Rev 2005;27:115–21.
72. Patz JA, Grabow ML, Limaye VS. When it rains, it pours: future climate extremes and health. Ann Glob Health 2014;80:332–44.

International Comparisons in Underserved Health

Issues, Policies, Needs and Projections

Paul Hutchinson, PhD[a], Vincent Morelli, MD[b],*

KEYWORDS

- International health care • Global health care statistics • Health care spending
- Universal health care • Health care technology

KEY POINTS

- Primary care physicians/providers worldwide need to be aware of the issues and obstacles faced by the underserved patients they serve.
- Primary care physicians need to be aware of the changing issues involved with providing health care to underserved populations.
- Primary care physicians can participate in solving current and future challenges such as improving access to care, embracing new technologies, improving patient education, and being sensitive to the social/cultural prejudices.

Globally, there have been vast improvements in health over the past several decades, rapidly decreasing—but not eliminating—disparities between high-income and low-income countries. In the latter, the average life expectancy has increased rapidly—by 9 years in just the period from 1990 to 2012 (**Fig. 1**), and the difference in life expectancy between high-income countries and low-income countries has shrunk from 22 years to 17 years (**Fig. 2**). Excluding sub-Saharan Africa, the life expectancy gap is only 9 years.[1] Both infant mortality and mortality among those less than 5 years of age have decreased by nearly one-half, equivalent to a staggering 17,000 fewer child deaths each day.[1] Mothers are now more likely than ever to survive childbirth; the maternal mortality rate in low-income countries has decreased from 900 per 100,000 live births to 450 per 100,000 live births, largely owing to better prenatal care and increases in facility births. Similar proportional decreases have been evidenced in lower middle and upper middle income countries.[2]

[a] Global Community Health Sciences, Tulane University School of Public Health and Tropical Medicine, 1440 Canal Street, Suite 2210, New Orleans, LA 70112, USA; [b] Department of Family and Community Medicine, Meharry Medical College, 1005 Dr D. B. Todd Boulevard, Nashville, TN 37208, USA
* Corresponding author.
E-mail address: morellivincent@yahoo.com

Prim Care Clin Office Pract 44 (2017) 185–202
http://dx.doi.org/10.1016/j.pop.2016.09.021
0095-4543/17/© 2016 Elsevier Inc. All rights reserved.

primarycare.theclinics.com

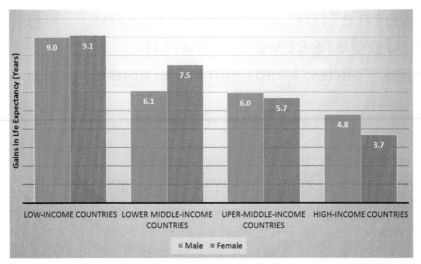

Fig. 1. Years gained in life expectancy 1990 to 2012, by sex and country income group. (*From* World Health Statistics 2014. A wealth of information on global public health. WHO. Available at: http://apps.who.int/iris/bitstream/10665/112739/1/WHO_HIS_HSI_14.1_eng.pdf?ua=1. Accessed June 10, 2016; with permission.)

Households in low-income countries, on average, are enjoying a higher quality of life than ever before. Currently, 90% of the world's population has access to safe drinking water and almost two-thirds have access to adequate sanitation.[1] Measles vaccination rates have reached 80% of children, and nearly three-quarters of births are

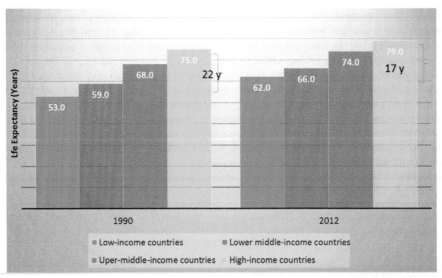

Fig. 2. Life expectancy (years) by level of income. (*From* World Health Statistics 2014. A wealth of information on global public health. WHO. Available at: http://apps.who.int/iris/bitstream/10665/112739/1/WHO_HIS_HSI_14.1_eng.pdf?ua=1. Accessed June 10, 2016; with permission.)

attended by skilled personnel. The percentage of those less than 5 years of age who are underweight decreased by 40%—from 25% in 1990% to 15% in 2009. The education gap between boys and girls has decreased dramatically, and now more than 90% of school-age girls are enrolled in primary school. Better access to family planning has given women more control over their fertility, allowing them to better time and limit births, with resultant decreases in infant and maternal mortality.[3]

In part, these improvements are owing to improved incomes globally. Poverty has decreased dramatically in much of the world. The percentage of people living in extreme poverty has decreased by more than one-half since 1990.[4] In 2015, less than 10% of the world's population was estimated to live on less than $1.90 per day, considered to be the benchmark for poverty. This represents 200 million fewer people living in poverty than in 2012.[5] In recent years, 7 of the 10 fastest growing economies of the past half-decade have been in Africa.[6]

These improvements are also owing to greater international focus, as evidenced by the United Nations Millennium Development Goals, which arose out of the Millennium Summit of the United Nations in 2000 and were intended to improve welfare in developing countries by 2015 through 8 subobjectives (eg, reducing poverty and hunger, improving education, reducing gender inequality, reducing child mortality, improving maternal health, and addressing human immunodeficiency virus (HIV) infection/AIDS, malaria, and other diseases). These objectives, many of which were met well before the 2015 deadline, are now being replaced by the broader and even more ambitious Sustainable Development Goals (available: https://sustainabledevelopment.un.org/post2015/transformingourworld), which also include ensuring prosperity for all and providing better protection for the planet.

In many low-income countries, an epidemiologic transition has begun, largely owing to population shifts, reflected in a change from a preponderance of mortality and morbidity owing to communicable diseases to an increase in the share attributable to noncommunicable diseases of older populations. "Where infectious disease and childhood illnesses related to malnutrition were once the primary causes of death, now children in many parts of the world—outside of sub-Saharan Africa—are more likely to live into an unhealthy adulthood and suffer from eating too much food rather than too little."[7] Over the past few decades, this shift has led to an increase in the importance of diseases such as diabetes, lung cancer, and chronic obstructive pulmonary disease, whereas the shares of other diseases, such as diarrhea, lower respiratory infections, and tuberculosis, have decreased.[7] This is apparent in composite measures of well-being—such as disability-adjusted life years (DALYs)—that combine both morbidity and mortality to give a more accurate picture of the burden of disease. For example, "in 1990, 47% of disability-adjusted life-years (DALYs) worldwide were from communicable, maternal, neonatal, and nutritional disorders, 43% from noncommunicable diseases, and 10% from injuries. By 2010, this had shifted to 35%, 54%, and 11%, respectively."[8]

First-world diseases are increasingly becoming problems globally. Currently, the top 5 causes of years of life lost globally are ischemic heart disease, lower respiratory infections, stroke, diarrheal diseases, and road injuries.[9] Again, although these patterns differ across low-income and high-income countries, convergence is apparent. The top 3 killers in low-income countries (heart disease, lower respiratory infections, stroke) are also in the top 10 in higher income countries. In terms of mortality, cancer now kills more people in low-income and middle-income countries than HIV, malaria, and tuberculosis combined,[10] although the latter diseases represent a larger loss of years of life lost. As a result, many low-income countries face a triple burden of disease: infections, noncommunicable diseases, and injuries. Early childhood conditions (eg, neonatal preterm complications, neonatal encephalitis, diarrheal diseases) and infectious diseases such as malaria and HIV/AIDS continue to afflict developing countries.

Although these gains have been widespread, they have not been shared by all. In sub-Saharan Africa, infectious diseases, childhood illnesses, and maternal causes of death still account for as much as 70% of the burden of disease. In other regions, such as south Asia and Oceania, these conditions account for only one-third of the burden, and less than 20% in all other regions. This discrepancy is readily apparent in mortality statistics. "While the average age of death throughout Latin America, Asia, and north Africa increased by more than 25 years between 1970 and 2010, it rose by less than 10 years in most of sub-Saharan Africa."[7]

DISEASE PATTERNS BY AGE
Under 5 Years of Age

In the past several decades, there have been major shifts in death rates and in the principal causes of death among those younger than 5 years. In 1990, 1 in 10 children died before their fifth birthday. Currently, that number is 1 in 20.[7] In 2000, the 5 major causes of death for those under 5 were acute respiratory infections (17%), diarrheal diseases (13%), prematurity (13%), intrapartum-related complications (11%), and malaria (8%). The top 5 causes of death are currently prematurity (17%), acute respiratory infections (15%), intrapartum-related complications (11%), diarrheal diseases (9%), and malaria (7%), but significant increases have been seen in neonatal sepsis (7%), congenital anomalies (7%), and injuries (6%).[1]

From 2000 to 2012, there were substantial decreases in measles deaths by 80%, HIV/AIDS deaths by 51%, diarrhea by 50%, pneumonia by 40% and malaria by 37% (**Fig. 3**).[1] These reductions have been achieved by multiple means. Countries have vastly improved their immunization rates for killers such as measles and pneumonia. Prevention and treatment for long-standing health issues such as malaria have

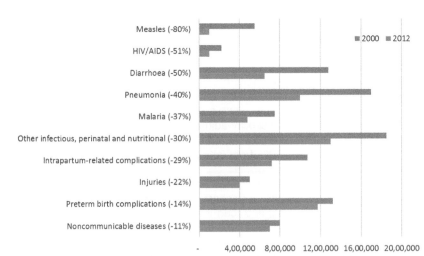

Fig. 3. Changes in major causes of deaths of those under 5 years of age globally, 2000 to 2012. HIV, human immunodeficiency virus. (*From* World Health Statistics 2014. A wealth of information on global public health. WHO. Available at: http://apps.who.int/iris/bitstream/10665/112739/1/WHO_HIS_HSI_14.1_eng.pdf?ua=1. Accessed June 10, 2016; with permission.)

improved, particularly through the development of new therapies and increased use of insecticide-treated nets. Improved sanitation and nutrition, most notably improved breastfeeding rates, have also contributed to improvements in diarrheal diseases.

However, positive trends with many diseases are being countered by negative trends in other areas. Obesity has become a global epidemic, including among children. In 1990, approximately 31 million (5%) children aged less than 5 years were overweight or obese. By 2012, that had increased to around 44 million (6.7%) of children. In Africa alone, the number of overweight children more than doubled, from 4 million to 10 million.[1] Further, "diseases such as diarrhea due to rotavirus and measles continue to kill more than 1 million children under the age of 5 every year, despite effective vaccines against those diseases."[7]

Pediatric/Adolescent

Adolescents, individuals aged 10 to 19 years, constitute 1.2 billion or roughly 17% of the world's population. In general, they are healthy; the vast majority of deaths in this age group are from preventable or treatable causes, such as road traffic injuries, which cause roughly 330 adolescents deaths each day. Although measles deaths are down for this age group, diarrhea, lower respiratory tract infections and meningitis remain among the top 10 causes of death.[11]

Nearly all adolescents become sexually active during this period, and approximately 11% of all births occur to girls aged 15 to 19 years. This marks a decline in recent years, which has translated to lower maternal mortality as well. However, there are more than 2 million adolescents who are HIV positive, and, although deaths have decreased, only 10% to 15% of adolescents in sub-Saharan Africa know their status, placing them at risk for perpetuating transmission and facing declining health themselves. In Sub-Saharan Africa, AIDS remains the number 1 killer among adolescents.[11]

Mental health is also a priority for this age group. Approximately 10% to 20% of children and adolescents worldwide face mental health problems.[12] Globally, "depression is the top cause of illness and disability among adolescents and suicide is the third cause of death."[11] Although approximately one-half of all adult mental health disorders appear by age 14, the majority of these cases are undetected and untreated.[11] Many adolescents face pervasive violence, and approximately 30% of girls aged 15 to 19 years experience intimate partner violence. In the low-income and middle-income countries of Latin America, approximately one-third of deaths among adolescent males are owing to violence.[11]

It is also at this age that many individuals develop harmful health habits. Smoking and its consequences (eg, cancer, heart disease, stroke, lung diseases, diabetes, and chronic obstructive pulmonary disease) is a leading cause of loss of life-years, and it is estimated that 1 in 5 boys aged 13 to 15 and 1 in 10 girls are smokers.[11] Consumption of alcohol can have multiple deleterious effects including increased risky behaviors, unsafe sex, traffic accidents and job related injuries.

Diet and exercise are primary concerns globally among this group, and are often tied to the environments in which adolescents live.[13] Obesity has been increasing in both low-income and high-income countries, and only 25% of adolescents meet the recommended requirements of 60 minutes of moderate activity per day. Lack of iron in diets leading to anemia is the third leading cause of loss of life-years among both girls and boys.[11]

Adults

The world is growing older. As child and other death rates have declined, the average age of the population has increased, leading to a higher proportion of deaths among older populations.[9] Death rates from many diseases have been declining but others have been increasing, including HIV/AIDS, pancreatic cancer, atrial fibrillation and flutter, drug use disorders, diabetes, chronic kidney disease, and sickle cell anaemias.[9] In fact, the number of deaths among adults aged 15 to 49 increased by 44% between 1970 and 2010. Much of this can be attributed to HIV/AIDS, which kills 1.5 million people each year, and increased violence in many parts of the world.[7]

As with adolescents, poor diets and physical inactivity have led to increasing rates of obesity and other lifestyle-related risk factors, including high blood pressure, tobacco smoking, and harmful alcohol use. It is now estimated that fully one-third of adult males globally smoke, including nearly one-half of all males in upper middle income countries. Further, among all adults, dietary risk factors and physical inactivity collectively cause 10% of the disease burden.[7] In 2008, globally 10% of adult males and 14% of adult females were obese.[1] In summary, "we have gone from a world 20 years ago where people weren't getting enough to eat to a world now where too much food and unhealthy food—even in developing countries—is making us sick."[7] Paradoxically, some researchers have noted a double burden of overnutrition and undernutrition within the same households.[14,15] For example, in a 7-country study, Doak and colleagues[14] found that in 6 of the countries, 22% to 66% of households with an underweight person also had an overweight person.

Even with improvements in so many other areas, it is estimated that approximately 1 woman still dies in childbirth every 2 minutes and an additional 20 to 30 experience serious complications.[2] Over time, with increased access to family planning methods, women have gained greater control over their own fertility. In all regions except Sub-Saharan Africa, the total fertility rate is fewer than 3 births per woman. In East Asia and Pacific, Europe and Central Asia and high-income countries, the total fertility rate is less than the replacement level (**Fig. 4**).

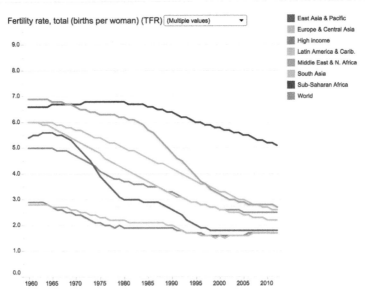

Fig. 4. Global trends in total fertility rates by region, 1960 to 2010. Regional aggregations are for all income levels. (*From* The World Bank. The Data Blog. Between 1960 and 2012, the world average fertility rate halved to 2.5 births per woman. © World Bank. Available at: http://blogs. worldbank.org/opendata/between960-and012-world-average-fertility-rate-halved5-births-woman. Accessed June 10, 2016. Creative Commons Attribution CC BY 3.0 IGO.)

Overall, there was a substantial increase of 37.6% from 1990 to 2010 in the burden of disease attributable to mental health and substance abuse disorders. In 2010, such disorders accounted for 7.4% (183.9 million DALYs) of all DALYs worldwide and were the leading cause of years lived with disability.[16] The problem is particularly acute in Africa, where "pain, anxiety, and depression—which erode quality of life and productivity—are ranked among the highest causes of years lived with disability throughout sub-Saharan Africa." As noted by one researcher, "African nations have not even begun to confront the consequences of exploding cases of mental illness, depression, pain, and the enormous burden of substance abuse that stem from those conditions."[7]

FUNDING

Health spending is a principal determinant of population health but global spending in health is far from equitable, with the preponderance of expenditures occurring in the wealthiest countries. In 2000, the ratio of health care spending per capita in high-income relative to low-income countries was 85 times, $2370 per capita versus $28 per capita. Since then, however, low-income and middle-income countries have renewed their focus on health as a priority area and have more than doubled their expenditures on health, by 129%, 114%, and 162% in low-income, lower middle-income, and upper middle-income countries, respectively. The gap between rich and poor, however, remains wide; in 2011, high-income countries still spent 68 times more per capita on health than low-income countries ($4319 vs $64).[17]

Even with the rapid increase in government spending, the majority of low-income countries fail to spend enough on care. It has been estimated that a minimum basic package of essential health services costs between $34 per capita[18] and $54 per capita.[19] Many low-income countries still currently fail to meet that target.[20]

The impact of spending on health is clear; countries that spend more have greater life expectancy and greater quality of life (**Fig. 5**). Further, "the returns on investing in health are impressive. Reductions in mortality account for about 11% of recent economic growth in low-income and middle-income countries."[21] In short, investing in health leads to a virtuous cycle; better health begets economic growth begets even more improvements in health.

International aid has contributed significantly to a changing global health environment. In 2013, global development assistance for health for low-income and middle-income countries reached an all-time high of $31.3 billion. Much of this increase was owing to increased assistance from the Global Fund to Fight AIDS,

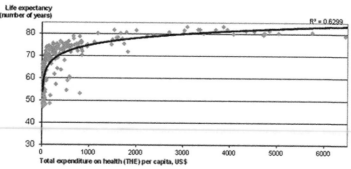

Fig. 5. Life expectancy by total health expenditure per capita. (*From* World Health Organization. Spending on health: a global overview. 2012. Available at: http://www.who.int/mediacentre/factsheets/fs319/en/; with permission.)

Tuberculosis, and Malaria; the GAVI (Global Alliance Vaccine Initiative) Alliance; and bilateral agencies in the United Kingdom. HIV/AIDS (25%) received the largest proportion of health assistance, followed by maternal, newborn, and child health (20%).[8]

Although the effectiveness of international aid has long been a question,[22,23] it is increasingly clear that global health initiatives have substantially improved the health situation in many countries. Since 2000, GAVI has funded vaccinations for 683 million children. Since 1988, the Global Polio Eradication Initiative has helped immunize 2.5 billion children, reducing the number of countries where polio is endemic from 125 to 3. To date, the Global Fund to Fight AIDS, Tuberculosis and Malaria has placed 6.1 million people on antiretroviral therapy, detected and treated 11.2 million cases of tuberculosis, and distributed 360 million insecticide-treated bed nets.[4]

THE WAY FORWARD

So what needs to be done to maintain these positive trends? And what can be done to ameliorate the remaining disparities? In short, what is the way forward? And how can primary care providers contribute?

Improve Access to Health Care

Limited access or complete absence of medical services clearly places many populations at risk for untoward health consequences. In Sub-Saharan Africa, it is estimated that 4 in 10 people do not have access to primary care.[24] Further, even when physical infrastructure is in place, access may be limited owing to scarcity of trained personnel. In low-income countries, for example, there are only 2.4 doctors per 10,000 population on average, far less than the 10 doctors per 10,000 population recommended by the World Health Organization (WHO).[25] The WHO estimates a current worldwide shortage of health workers of 7.2 million with trends indicating a 12.9 million person shortage by 2035.[25] This discrepancy is most evident in Sub-Saharan Africa, which has 25% of the global disease burden but only 3% of the world's health workforce. Within-country differences can be even more dramatic. In South Africa, for example, 43.6% of the population lives in rural areas but only 12% of the country's doctors are stationed in rural health facilities.[26]

Improving access to care can be accomplished even in low resource settings; some low-income and middle-income countries (eg, Sri Lanka, Costa Rica, Cuba) do quite well in ensuring access to care through a number of means, including prioritizing the health sector in public sector funding, establishing tiered referral networks starting at the village level, and innovative delivery systems.

An example of an innovative delivery system can be seen in Bangladesh, a poor country that historically had explosively high fertility rates and underuse of basic health services. Customs and norms in the highly conservative Muslim country restricted female mobility and women's ability to access services for themselves and their children. In 1977, researchers piloted a female-provided "doorstep delivery of care" program in 70 rural villages. After 18 months, contraceptive use had quadrupled and by just 24 months fertility rates had decreased by 25%. In addition, children were healthier, fewer women died of pregnancy-related causes, and child mortality decreased. All of these decreases persisted for more than 2 decades.[27]

Needed policy changes to address such access and shortage issues could include providing financial incentives to health workers to work in rural areas, providing ongoing professional development outside of urban areas, increasing the duration of the residency period during which health workers are given less flexibility with postings, and providing nonfinancial incentives such as free housing, better diagnostic facilities, and access to free or reduced price health care.[28]

Technology can also assist in health care delivery. For example, in many countries of Africa, where cellphone ownership is approaching 90% of adults, technology is already being used with great success. Mobisante, a startup company based in Redmond, Washington, has developed a cellphone-based ultrasound modality. Other companies have piloted mobile eye examinations, electronic medical record keeping, and smartphone microscopes. Still others help patients with medical compliance or assist health care providers with clinical decision making (Health Market Innovations 2016). All told, the WHO has identified 14 ways that cellphones can be used to promote population health.[29]

It is incumbent on the primary care physician working in underserved areas to be aware of these and other technologies to optimize access and health care delivery in their particular local. For example, in the United States, access to specialty care in underserved communities is a significant problem. The 25% of patients from Federally Qualified Health Centers needing specialist consultation often have to wait up to a year for an appointment[30,31] and these long waits have been shown to result in higher rates of chronic disease complications, disability, and death.[32] Such disparities are being addressed by asynchronous electronic consultation between primary care physicians and specialists using a secure Health Insurance Portability and Accountability Act of 1996 (HIPAA)-complaint platform. With specialist assistance, primary care physicians are then able to handle less common/more complex medical conditions. One study[33] showed that 70% of referrals could be handled in this manner, obviating the need for patient specialist appointments and long referral wait times. The average wait time for electronic consultations between physicians in this study was 5 days. Such electronic consultations have proven to be particularly effective in rural and sparsely populated areas.[34] Other studies have noted that telemedicine saves travel time and money for patients, provides better disease management, and increases rapport between specialists and primary care providers, providing education to primary care physicians and enhancing overall collaboration.[35] Technologies such as these will have to be embraced by primary care physicians working in underserved communities if they are to serve their constituents optimally.

Move Toward Universal Health Care Coverage

In many parts of the world, health services are unaffordable to vast numbers of people, and as a consequence individuals may seek care from informal or low-quality providers, forego necessary care, or, perhaps worst of all, suffer impoverishment from debilitating medical expenses, leading to further ill health and a downward cycle deeper into poverty. Carrin and colleagues,[36] looking at household expenditure surveys in 89 countries, found that the costs of accessing health services caused severe financial hardships for 44 million people annually, and an additional 25 million people were thrust into poverty because of such expenditures. Although the global average for household out-of-pocket medical expenditures as a percentage of total expenditures is 19%, in poorer countries it accounts for more than 50% of the total, meaning that poorer households are at greater risk of experiencing catastrophic health expenditures. In short, those least able to afford health care are the ones that must use a higher percentage of their wealth to access that health care.

As a result, the majority of countries have endorsed the idea that health is a fundamental human right, regardless of a person's income,[37] and in recent decades a movement has begun to ensure universal health coverage globally.[38] This means having a health care system that provides health care and financial protection to all citizens.[39] In 2012, the United Nations passed a resolution endorsing universal health coverage as a "pillar of sustainable development and global security." In 2014, a Global Coalition of more than 500 organizations launched a campaign to "Accelerate Access to Universal Health Coverage." According to the coalition, "Each year, 100 million people fall into poverty because they or a family member becomes seriously ill and they have to pay for care out of their own pockets. Around one billion people worldwide can't even access the health care they need, paving the way for disease outbreaks to become catastrophic epidemics."[38]

There is no one way to achieve universal health coverage. "Whether a nation chooses a mixed economy model of coverage, single-payer mode, donor-issued voucher mechanism, or other innovative models of universal financing is not the issue; provision of universal health coverage is the issue facing the entire global health construct."[37] The Lancet Commission on Global Health 2035 proposed 2 pathways toward achieving universal health coverage within the next 20 years: (1) a publicly financed health insurance that covers essential health care interventions or (2) a health insurance program, financed through a range of mechanisms, which covers a broader range of health services from which the poor would be exempt from payment.

Any plan to expand health coverage must tackle a number of fundamental issues. As noted by Marten,[40] the implementation of universal health coverage requires political support for the concept, the government resources to achieve it, and strong oversight to "design, implement, measure and manage complex technical challenges." One of the key challenges involves creating risk pools that promote subsidies from the rich to the poor, from lower risk to higher risk individuals, and from younger, healthier individuals to older ones. Health care providers also need to be incentivized to allocate resources in the most efficient way; health care providers who are expected to take a financial loss from providing care for the poor are apt to reduce the quality of that care or even to stop offering services used by the poor.

A second key challenge is providing coverage to informal workers, who make up 40% to 90% of the population in low-income and middle-income countries. "Most health system stewards employ some mixture of three discrete approaches: (a) using a tax-based system to offer health coverage to all people within a country; (b) enrolling informal workers by "building out" from covering the formal sector through contributory schemes; or (c) employing a combination of tax-based subsidies and contributions to enroll informal workers."[40]

Because of these efforts, approximately 58 countries globally have achieved universal health coverage, including 9 in Africa. Rwanda, for example, uses a mutual insurance scheme paid for by a combination of government and individual contributions of approximately $2 per year. Households that cannot afford to pay the $2 have their copay subsidized by the Global Fund to Fight AIDS, Tuberculosis and Malaria, which funds roughly 1.5 million Rwandans.[37]

Although the role of primary care physicians in policy design and implementation is often limited, it is important for them to be aware of the issues involved and the effects of shortcomings so that they may best advocate for optimal patient care when the opportunity arises.

Reduce Stigma and Prejudice Against Women and Marginalized Populations to Ensure a Safe, Supportive Environment in Which These Underserved Populations Can Fulfill Their Health Care Needs

Stigma—against women, the disabled, the mentally ill, minorities, men who have sex with men, commercial sex workers, injection drug users, among others—can be a huge barrier to care. Certain diseases, such as HIV/AIDS, have long carried devastating stigma—about sexual orientation, about promiscuity, and about divine retribution. Discrimination against people living with HIV and AIDS can prevent infected individuals from getting tested, from seeking treatment, and even from changing risky behaviors.[41] At the extreme, legislation—such as laws against homosexuality—can criminalize behavior, further marginalizing stigmatized populations. Currently, 79 countries have made homosexuality illegal, placing individuals at risk of incarceration if their sexual orientation is revealed through accessing health services.

Power differentials between men and women can determine whether or not women use necessary contraception, become victims of violence, fail to space births appropriately, or even access basic prenatal care or delivery care in a heath facility. A study of 23 low-income countries, for example, found that in none of them did a majority of women have decision making ability alone about their own health care.[42]

The poor also face stigma and discrimination. In the United States, for example, the Affordable Care Act expanded Medicaid coverage to many low-income individuals. However, qualitative interviews have indicated that perceptions of being treated poorly or unfairly because of Medicaid status inhibit many low-income individuals from using the health services to which they are entitled. Allen and colleagues,[43] for example, found

That stigma was most often the result of a provider-patient interaction that felt demeaning, rather than an internalized sense of shame related to receiving public insurance or charity care. An experience of stigma was associated with unmet health needs, poorer perceptions of quality of care, and worse health across several self-reported measures.

The effects of stigma and discrimination on the use of mental health services is perhaps even more pronounced. The WHO estimates that roughly 1 in 4 people will experience a mental or neurologic disorder in their lifetime and that approximately 350 million people worldwide suffer from depression.[44] They further estimate that 76% of people with mental disorders in low-income countries and 85% of people in middle-income countries receive no treatment for their disorder, largely because of stigma and absence of services. High-income countries are not immune either; roughly 35% to 50% of people with mental disorders also do not receive treatment.[44]

Health communication programs can work to reduce stigma against marginalized populations and to shift norms. Ongoing behavior change communication programs still have not reached many populations and are necessary to continue to shift norms and attitudes. In the case of HIV/AIDS, these efforts can include community interactions, such as focus group discussions with people living with HIV, the use of media to educate through entertaining nonstigmatizing "edutainment" messages, engagement with religious and community leaders and celebrities, inclusion of nondiscrimination in institutional and workplace policies, and peer mobilization and support for and by people living with HIV.[41]

To help combat stigma and discrimination, primary care physicians have key responsibilities as role models, advocates of policy change, and protectors of their clients. In Kenya, for example, 15% of HIV-positive individuals reported that a health care worker disclosed their HIV status without their consent.[45] In Lesotho, nearly 23% of people living with HIV stated that it was clear that their HIV records were not kept confidential.[45] Ensuring basic privacy of clients' health and treatment should be a minimal standard for care.

A key responsibility of primary care physicians is to familiarize themselves with human rights and ethics training. This serves 2 purposes. First, it enables primary care physicians to become familiar with their own health rights, including HIV prevention and treatment, universal precautions, and compensation for work-related infection. Second, such training can help to "reduce stigmatizing attitudes in health care settings and to provide health care providers with the skills and tools necessary to ensure patients' rights to informed consent, confidentiality, treatment and non-discrimination."[41]

Improve Surveillance Systems to Detect Threats More Quickly

We live in an increasingly connected world. Airline passengers can move from 1 continent to another in a matter of hours. New and emerging diseases have shown the potential to spread quickly: Ebola, Marburg, Chikungunya, H1N1 influenza, dengue, and most recently Zika. Even places where diseases have been eliminated can experience outbreaks. In 2015, a measles-infected international traveler visiting a theme park in the United States, where measles has been eliminated, is believed to have come into contact with unvaccinated individuals, leading to 147 measles cases across multiple states.

As noted by Bill Gates, the world has been "lucky" with recent outbreaks. The Ebola outbreak in 2014 in western Africa led to approximately 10,000 deaths. The toll, however, could have been far worse if it had not been for the diligent work of dedicated medical professionals, if the disease had been easier to transmit—Ebola is transmitted through bodily fluids—or if the disease had reached a major urban population center. According to Dr Tom Frieden, head of the Centers for Disease Control and Prevention, "With patterns of global travel and trade, disease can spread nearly anywhere within 24 hours. That's why the ability to detect, fight, and prevent these diseases must be developed and strengthened overseas, and not just here in the United States."[46]

Similarly, the influenza outbreak of 2009 also highlighted shortcomings in epidemiologic surveillance and outbreak control. "Shortcomings included the lack of standards for reporting illness, risk factor and mortality data and a mechanism for systematic reporting of epidemiologic data. Such measures would have facilitated direct comparison of data between countries and improved timely understanding of the characteristics and impact of the pandemic."[47]

Currently, only 1 in 5 countries can rapidly detect, respond to, or prevent global health threats caused by emerging infections. Improvements overseas, such as strengthening disease surveillance and laboratory systems for identifying threats, training disease detectives, and building facilities to investigate disease outbreaks make the world—and the United States—more secure.[48]

Achieving better systems to rapidly detect and handle global health threats requires a multifaceted solution. First, health systems need to be strengthened. This goes hand in hand with ensuring universal health coverage, so that disease may be reported quickly without financial concern. Second, there needs to be an abundant supply of health care professionals, most notably a medical reserve corps with training and expertise in epidemics who can respond quickly to threats. Bill Gates advocates pairing such a corps with military forces, who have the logistical capabilities to respond quickly and secure areas. Further, according to Gates, there is a "need to do simulations, germ games, not war games, so that we see where the holes are. The last time a germ game was done in the United States was back in 2001, and it didn't go so well. So far the score is germs: 1, people: 0." Finally, there is an ongoing need for research and development of vaccines and rapid diagnostic tests.[49] Already, research and development seems to have developed a rapid diagnostic test for the Zika virus, which may serve as a model for other new and emerging infectious diseases.[50]

Once again, technology and eHealth can help in dealing with potential outbreaks. For example, *eHealth Africa* developed an Android-based app to help caseworkers trace people who had had contact with Ebola patients. According to Justin Lorenzon, head of software development, "that's a huge deal in controlling an outbreak—making sure that if there's a new case, that it's followed up on and that person is isolated as quickly as possible, so you don't have just a continuation of transmission."[51] The app is an example of how epidemics can lead to innovations that address a current public health crisis. Originally designed to track and prevent polio, eHealth Africa's Ebola contact-tracing app helped to cut reporting times for new Ebola cases by 75%. Lane Goodman of the Center for Health Market Innovations noted that many analysts believe contact tracing was instrumental in helping Nigeria to eradicate the disease.

Primary care physicians are often the front line in detecting outbreaks. A key responsibility in preventing outbreaks is enhanced vigilance to unusual cases and familiarity with the symptoms of emerging diseases. Physicians working in endemic areas have a duty to maintain surveillance systems—reporting all unusual cases as rapidly as possible—so that larger patterns can be detected by surveillance agencies.

Governments Play a Large Role in the Health of Their Populations

Functioning governments are a requisite for good population health. The greatest decrements in health occur in places where governments and nations are failing (eg, Syria, Somalia). Armed conflict can quickly take advanced societies back generations, destroying vital health infrastructure, displacing populations, increasing the risk of disease transmission, and wreaking havoc on morbidity and mortality.[52] Violence can have both direct effects (eg, the loss of life and morbidity from conflict) and indirect effects (eg, the health repercussions of a depleted health care infrastructure).

Governments also play a role in prioritizing health within their public sector budgets. On average, the share of health in aggregate government expenditure is approximately 12%. However, considerable variation exists. Costa Rica spends approximately 28% of the government budget on health; Myanmar spends less than 1%.[20]

Finally, governments, by enforcing contracts, weeding out corruption and abiding by the rule of law, can ensure the maximal effects of public and private spending on health by insisting that limited resources are not leaked from the health system. Transparency International has defined corruption "as the abuse of entrusted power for private gain, which in health care encompasses bribery of regulators and medical professionals, manipulation of information on drug trials, diversion of medicines and supplies, corruption in procurement, and overbilling of insurance companies."[53] In India, unofficial bribes for spots in medical schools can cost up to US$200,000. Kickbacks from clinics and drug companies to physicians for prescribed tests and drugs have led to a climate of distrust between patients and physicians, who are generally not believed to have the well-being of their patients at heart.[54]

Primary care physicians can play an important role by refusing to engage in unethical behaviors, to prioritize patient health over financial gain, and by reporting instances of inappropriate medical conduct. Primary care physicians are encouraged to follow standard ethical of conduct such as the AMA's published code of ethics (available: http://www.ama-assn.org/ama/pub/physician-resources/medical-ethics/code-medical-ethics.page) in their governed areas. Such adherence will foster patient trust and promote "human values" over political expediency or self interest.

Behavioral Economics Is a New Frontier in Changing Healthy Behaviors

One area that has recently emerged for achieving the types of behavior change that can substantially improve health is the field of behavioral economics. Popularized in books such as *Nudge*,[55] *Predictably Irrational*,[56] and *Thinking Fast and Slow*,[57] behavioral economics marries psychology and economics to "nudge" people to change behaviors. This can include gentle nudges—such as reframing choices, getting people to view the future differently, using defaults (eg, automatic refilling of prescriptions or default health insurance plan options) to ensure that people do not succumb to status quo bias, and identity priming (eg, "a lot of people like yourself have started trying medicine *X*, treatment *Y*, or therapy *Z* to deal with problem *Q*") can have huge impacts. To date, these approaches have been small in scale, but promising. Some examples include providing vouchers to keep adolescents in school and avoid early pregnancy/disease, using routine child immunization visits as opportunities to present family planning options to women, making reenrollment in health insurance programs the default, and providing financial incentives to encourage health workers to work with underserved or remote populations.

An ongoing study in Kenya is examining why women fail to adequately plan for delivering in a health facility. This is important because 1 key means of reducing maternal and neonatal mortality is ensuring that women have access to safe, high-quality delivery services at health facilities. During pregnancy, women may express a desire to deliver in a facility but at the time of delivery they may find themselves faced with unexpected barriers that could have been foreseen through better planning. The study is using a key behavioral economics tool—a commitment device—in which women receive cash transfers—both conditional and unrestricted—that encourage them to deliver in a health facility.[58]

Another study examined the issue of early child marriage in Ethiopia, where early marriage is the norm, leading to early childbearing and subsequent increases in maternal and infant mortality. Surveys have found that 19% of girls are married by age 15 and the mean age of marriage is 16 years. Changing the social pressure to marry earlier presented an enormous challenge. The program paired adolescent girls with older female mentors, provided financial incentives for girls to stay in school, enrolled out-of-school girls in livelihood training (eg, basic literacy and numeracy), and engaged communities in problem solving conversations about early marriage. By the endline of the study, girls aged 10 to 14 years were more likely to still be in school and less likely to have gotten married.[59]

As health care technologies and delivery methods continue to evolve, it is vital that primary care physicians express their practical perspective to policy makers so that behavioral economics and other best practices may be used to inform policy creation and revision.

THE ROLE OF THE PRIMARY CARE PHYSICIAN IN ADDRESSING THE CHALLENGES

Primary care physicians in underserved areas are faced with a rapidly changing health environment. As the global epidemiologic transition continues, they will be faced with an increasing diversity of health issues. No longer are noncommunicable diseases the sole purview of first-world countries. Obesity is now a global problem and in many places coexists with undernutrition and more traditional patterns of communicable diseases. Primary care physicians need to be vigilant about addressing this double burden of disease, while also being aware of new and emerging diseases, such as Zika and chikungunya.

Primary care physicians will also have to embrace new technology, which will be essential to both disease surveillance and persistent shortages of health personnel globally. Despite movements toward universal health coverage, both physical and financial access to health care will continue to be a problem. New technology will allow for a greater dependence on telemedicine, which may serve to alleviate the short-term pressure on scarce health services.

As mentioned, primary care physicians working in underserved communities will have to be prepared to enhance access to care, to embrace technology, to be aware of health care policy and WHO universal coverage recommendations, to embrace patient education and the reduction of stigmatization and prejudice, to be aware of and ready to respond to activated disease surveillance systems and to be aware of governmental policy as it relates to health of their populations. To this end, the Centers for Disease Control and Prevention and other agencies have noted the need to enhance training for primary care physicians working in these areas. Education in public and population health,[60] leadership, community engagement, community collaboration and data analysis are all needed.[61,62] Such skills are vital to optimally addressing the chronic medical conditions that account for more than 75% of US health care costs and are disproportionately present in underserved communities. This type of primary care physician training may be even more important in the developing world.

REFERENCES

1. World Health Statistics 2014. A wealth of information on global public health. WHO. Available at: http://apps.who.int/iris/bitstream/10665/112739/1/WHO_HIS_HSI_14.1_eng.pdf?ua=1). Accessed June 10, 2016.
2. UNFPA. United Nations Population Fund. Maternal Health. Available at: http://www.unfpa.org/maternal-health. Accessed March 5, 2016.
3. Cleland J, Bernstein S, Ezeh A, et al. Family planning: the unfinished agenda. Lancet 2006;368:1820–7.
4. Gates B, Gate M. 2015 Gates annual letter: three myths that block progress for the poor. Available at: http://www.gatesfoundation.org/Who-We-Are/Resources-and-Media/Annual-Letters-List/Annual-Letter-2014. Accessed February 29, 2016.
5. World Bank. 2015. Global Monitoring Report: development goals in an era of demographic change. Available at: http://www.worldbank.org/en/publication/global-monitoring-report. Accessed June 10, 2016.
6. The Economist, 2011. Daily chart: Africa's impressive growth. Available at: http://www.economist.com/blogs/dailychart/2011/01/daily_chart. Accessed February 1, 2016.
7. Institute for Health Metrics and Evaluation. 2012. Global burden of disease: massive shifts reshape the health landscape worldwide. Available at: http://www.healthdata.org/news-release/global-burden-disease-massive-shifts-reshape-health-landscape-worldwide. Accessed February 17, 2016.
8. Dieleman JL, Graves CM, Templin T, et al. Global health development assistance remained steady in 2013 but did not align with recipients' disease burden. Health Aff 2013;33:878–86.
9. GBD 2013 Mortality and Causes of Death Collaborators. Global, regional, and national age-sex specific all-cause and cause-specific mortality for 240 causes of death, 1990-2013: a systematic analysis for the Global Burden of Disease Study 2013. Lancet 2015;385:117–71.
10. Allemani C, Weir HK, Carrera H, et al. Global surveillance of cancer survival 1995–2009: analysis of individual data for 25,676,887 patients from 279 population-based registries in 67 countries (CONCORD-2). Lancet 2015;385: 977–1010.
11. World Health Organization. Adolescents: health risks and solutions, WHO Fact Sheet No. 345. Available at: http://www.who.int/mediacentre/factsheets/fs345/en/. Accessed February 18, 2016.

12. Kieling C, Baker-Henningham H, Belfer M, et al. Child and adolescent mental health worldwide: evidence for action. Lancet 2011;378:1515–25.
13. Gordon-Larsen P, McMurray RG, Popkin BM. Determinants of adolescent physical activity and inactivity patterns. Pediatrics 2000;105:E83.
14. Doak CM, Adair LS, Bentley M, et al. The dual burden household and the nutrition transition paradox. Int J Obes (Lond) 2005;29:129–36.
15. Megan J, Brewis A. Paradoxical malnutrition in mother–child pairs: untangling the phenomenon of over- and under-nutrition in underdeveloped economies. Econ Hum Biol 2009;7:28–35.
16. Whiteford HA, Degenhardt L, Rehm J, et al. Global burden of disease attributable to mental and substance use disorders: findings from the Global Burden of Disease Study 2010. Lancet 2013;382:1575–86.
17. The World Bank. Data. Health expenditure per capita. Available at: http://data.worldbank.org/indicator/SH.XPD.PCAP. Accessed on June 10, 2016.
18. World Health Organization. Macroeconomics and Health (CMH). Available at: http://www.who.int/macrohealth/en/. Accessed June 10, 2016.
19. World Health Organization. Constraints to Scaling up the Health Millennium Development Goals: costing and financial analysis gap, The taskforce for innovative international financing for health systems. 2010. Geneva.
20. Tandon A, Fleisher L, Li R, et al. Reprioritizing government spending on health: pushing an elephant up the stairs. Washington, DC: World Bank; 2014. HNP Discussion Paper 85773.
21. Jamison DT, Summers LH, Alleyne G, et al. Global health 2035: a world converging within a generation. Lancet 2013;382:1898–955.
22. Easterly W. The white Man's burden: why the West's efforts to aid the rest have done so much ill and so little good. New York: Penguin Press; 2006.
23. Kaufmann D. Aid effectiveness and governance. World Bank. Available at: https://openknowledge.worldbank.org/handle/10986/4571. Accessed May 14, 2016.
24. Knapp T, Richardson B, Viranna S. Three practical steps to better health for Africans. Available at: http://www.mckinsey.com/industries/healthcare-systems-and-services/our-insights/three-practical-steps-to-better-health-for-africans. Accessed January 13, 2016.
25. World Health Organization. Global Health Observatory (GHO) data. Density of physicians (total number per 1000 population, latest available year). Available at: http://www.who.int/gho/health_workforce/physicians_density/en/. Accessed June 10, 2016.
26. AHP. Africa Health Placements. The Need: No People = No Healthcare. Available at: http://ahp.org.za/the-need/. Accessed June 10, 2016.
27. Joshi S, Schultz TP. Family planning and women's and children's health: long-term consequences of an outreach program in Matlab, Bangladesh. Demography 2015;50:149–80.
28. World Health Organization. Global health workforce alliance. A universal truth: no health without a workforce. Third Global Forum on Human Resources for Health Report. Available at: http://www.who.int/workforcealliance/knowledge/resources/hrhreport2013/en/. Accessed on June 10, 2016.
29. World Health Organization. Health: new horizons for health through mobile technologies, 2011. Available at: http://www.who.int/goe/publications/goe_mhealth_web.pdf. Accessed June 10, 2016.
30. Kim Y, Chen AH, Keith E, et al. Not perfect, but better: primary care providers' experiences with electronic referrals in a safety net health system. J Gen Intern Med 2009;24:614–9.

31. Kim-Hwang JE, Chen AH, Bell DS, et al. Evaluating electronic referrals for specialty care at a public hospital. J Gen Intern Med 2010;25:1123–8.

32. Cook NL, Hicks LS, O'Malley AJ, et al. Access to specialty care and medical services in community health centers. Health Aff (Millwood) 2007;26:1459–68.

33. Olayiwola JN, Anderson D, Jepeal N. Electronic consultations to improve the primary care- specialty care interface for cardiology in the medically underserved: a cluster-randomized controlled trial. Ann Fam Med 2016;14:133–40.

34. O'Gorman LD, Hogenbirk JC, Warry W. Clinical telemedicine utilization in Ontario over the Ontario Telemedicine Network. Telemed J E Health 2016;22:473–9.

35. Meyers L, Gibbs D. Building a telehealth network through collaboration: the story of the Nebraska statewide telehealth network. Crit Care Nurs Q 2012;35:346–52.

36. Carrin G, Mathauer I, Xu K, et al. Universal coverage of health services: tailoring its implementation. Bull World Health Organ 2008;86:857–63.

37. Garrett LA, Chowdhury MR, Pablos-Méndez A. All for universal health coverage. Lancet 2009;374:1294–9.

38. Rockefeller Foundation. Universal health coverage: a commitment to close the gap. 2013. Available at: https://www.rockefellerfoundation.org/report/universal-health-coverage-a-commitment-to-close-the-gap/. Accessed June 10, 2016.

39. World Health Organization. What is universal health coverage? Available at: http://www.who.int/features/qa/universal_health_coverage/en/. Accessed March 19, 2016.

40. The World Bank. Marten R. Investing in health. Ten (Plus One) things to think about when planning and implementing universal health coverage. Available at: http://blogs.worldbank.org/health/ten-plus-one-things-think-about-when-planning-and-implementing-universal-health-coverage. Accessed June 10, 2016.

41. UNAIDS. May 15, 2012. Key programmes to reduce stigma and discrimination and increase access to justice in national HIV responses. Available at: http://www.unaids.org/en/resources/documents/2012/Key_Human_Rights_Programmes. Accessed June 10, 2016.

42. Kishor S, Subaiya L. 2008. 2008. Understanding women's empowerment: a comparative analysis of Demographic and Health Surveys (DHS) data. DHS Comparative Reports No. 20. Calverton, Maryland, USA: Macro International. Available at: http://dhsprogram.com/publications/publication-cr20-comparative-reports.cfm#sthash.NtUHytt2.dpuf. Accessed June 10, 2016.

43. Allen H, Wright BJ, Harding K, et al. The role of stigma in access to health care for the poor. Milbank Q 2014;92:289–318.

44. World Health Organization. Mental disorders. Fact sheet number 396; 2015. Available at: http://www.who.int/mediacentre/factsheets/fs396/en/. Accessed January 15, 2016.

45. The people living with HIV Stigma index: Kenya. 2009. Available at: http://www.stigmaindex.org/sites/default/files/reports/Kenya%20People%20Living%20with%20HIV%20Stigma%20Index%20Report%202009.pdf. Accessed March 3, 2016.

46. Centers for Disease Control and Prevention. 2013. Measles Still Threatens Security. Available at: http://www.cdc.gov/media/releases/2013/p1205-meales-threat.html. Accessed February 14, 2016.

47. Briand S, Mounts A, Chamberland M. Challenges of global surveillance during an influenza pandemic. Public Health 2011;125:247–56.

48. Centers for Disease Control and Prevention. Press Release, December 16, 2013. CDC looks back at 2013 health challenges, ahead to 2014 health worries. Available at: https://www.cdc.gov/media/releases/2013/p1216-eoy2013.html. Accessed June 10, 2016.

49. Gates, B. 2015. Ted Talks: the next outbreak: we're not ready. Available at: https://www.ted.com/talks/bill_gates_the_next_disaster_we_re_not_ready/transcript?language=en. Accessed June 10, 2016.

50. Biocan. 2016. Zika virus rapid test. Available at: http://www.zikatest.com/?page_id=24. Accessed March 3, 2016.

51. Center for Health market innovations, 2016. Available at: http://healthmarket innovations.org/blog/developing-countries-lead-way-mobile-health-technologies. Accessed March 8, 2016.

52. Murray CJ, King G, Lopez AD, et al. Armed conflict as a public health problem. BMJ 2002;324:346–9.

53. Jain A, Nundy S, Abbasi K. Corruption: medicine's dirty open secret. BMJ 2014; 348:g4184.

54. Berger D. Corruption ruins the doctor-patient relationship. BMJ 2014;348:g3169.

55. Thaler RH, Sunstein C. Nudge: improving decisions about health, wealth, and happiness. New Haven (CT): Yale University Press; 2008.

56. Ariely D. Predictably irrational: the hidden forces that shape our decisions. Harper Perennial; 2007.

57. Kahneman D. Thinking, Fast and Slow. New York: Farrar, Straus and Giroux; 2011.

58. Cohen J, McConnell M. Behavioral economics in reproductive health initiative. 2016. Impact of pre-commitment to delivery facilities on the quality of maternal and neonatal care. Available at: http://www.beri-research.org/research/sub-saharan-africa/kenya-quality-delivery-facilities/. Accessed March 5, 2016.

59. Erulkar A, Muthengi E. Evaluation of Berhane Hewan: a program to delay child marriage in rural Ethiopia. Int Perspect Sex Reprod Health 2009;35:6–14.

60. Maeshiro R, Koo D, Keck CW. Integration of public health into medical education: an introduction to the supplement. Am J Prev Med 2011;41:S145–8.

61. Elliott L, McBride TD. Health care system collaboration to address chronic diseases: a nationwide snapshot from state public health practitioners. Prev Chronic Dis 2014;11:E152.

62. Institute of Medicine. Primary care and public health: exploring integration to improve population health. Released March 28, 2012. Available at: http://www.nationalacademies.org/hmd/Reports/2012/Primary-Care-and-Public-Health.aspx. Accessed March 30, 2016.

Moving?

Make sure your subscription moves with you!

To notify us of your new address, find your **Clinics Account Number** (located on your mailing label above your name), and contact customer service at:

Email: journalscustomerservice-usa@elsevier.com

800-654-2452 (subscribers in the U.S. & Canada)
314-447-8871 (subscribers outside of the U.S. & Canada)

Fax number: 314-447-8029

Elsevier Health Sciences Division
Subscription Customer Service
3251 Riverport Lane
Maryland Heights, MO 63043

*To ensure uninterrupted delivery of your subscription, please notify us at least 4 weeks in advance of move.

Printed and bound by CPI Group (UK) Ltd, Croydon, CR0 4YY

07/10/2024

01040505-0001